Substance Abuse Disorders

World Psychiatric Association Evidence and Experience in Psychiatry Series

Series Editor: Helen Herrman, WPA Secretary for Publications, University of Melbourne, Australia

Depressive Disorders, 3e
Edited by Helen Herrman, Mario Maj and Norman Sartorius
ISBN: 9780470987209

Substance Abuse Disorders
Edited by Hamid Ghodse, Helen Herrman, Mario Maj and Norman Sartorius
ISBN: 9780470745106

Trauma and Mental Health: Resilience and Post-Traumatic Stress Disorders
Edited by Dan J Stein, Matthew J Friedman and Carlos Blanco
ISBN: 9780470688977

Schizophrenia 2e
Edited by Mario Maj, Norman Sartorius
ISBN: 9780470849644

Dementia 2e
Edited by Mario Maj, Norman Sartorius
ISBN: 9780470849637

Obsessive-Compulsive Disorders 2e
Edited by Mario Maj, Norman Sartorius, Ahmed Okasha, Joseph Zohar
ISBN: 9780470849668

Bipolar Disorders
Edited by Mario Maj, Hagop S Akiskal, Juan José López-Ibor, Norman Sartorius
ISBN: 9780471560371

Eating Disorders
Edited by Mario Maj, Kathrine Halmi, Juan José López-Ibor, Norman Sartorius
ISBN: 9780470848654

Phobias
Edited by Mario Maj, Hagop S Akiskal, Juan José López-Ibor, Ahmed Okasha
ISBN: 9780470858332

Personality Disorders
Edited by Mario Maj, Hagop S Akiskal, Juan E Mezzich
ISBN: 9780470090367

Somatoform Disorders
Edited by Mario Maj, Hagop S Akiskal, Juan E Mezzich, Ahmed Okasha
ISBN: 9780470016121

Current Science and Clinical Practice Series

Series Editor: Helen Herrman, WPA Secretary for Publications, University of Melbourne, Australia

Schizophrenia
Edited by Wolfgang Gaebell
ISBN: 9780470710548

Obsessive Compulsive Disorder
Edited by Joseph Zohar
ISBN: 9780470711255

Other World Psychiatric Association titles

Series Editor (2005–): Helen Herrman, WPA Secretary for Publications, University of Melbourne, Australia

Special Populations

The Mental Health of Children and Adolescents: an area of global neglect
Edited by Helmut Remschmidt, Barry Nurcombe, Myron L. Belfer, Norman Sartorius and Ahmed Okasha
ISBN: 9780470512456

Contemporary Topics in Women's Mental Health: global perspectives in a changing society
Edited by Prabha S. Chandra, Helen Herrman, Marianne Kastrup, Marta Rondon, Unaiza Niaz, Ahmed Okasha, Jane Fisher
ISBN: 9780470754115

Families and Mental Disorders
Edited by Norman Sartorius, Julian Leff, Juan José López-Ibor, Mario Maj, Ahmed Okasha
ISBN: 9780470023822

Disasters and Mental Health
Edited by Juan José López-Ibor, George Christodoulou, Mario Maj, Norman Sartorius, Ahmed Okasha
ISBN: 9780470021231

Parenthood and Mental Health: A bridge between infant and adult psychiatry
Edited by Sam Tyano, Miri Keren, Helen Herrman and John Cox
ISBN: 9780470747223

Approaches to Practice and Research

Religion and Psychiatry: beyond boundaries
Edited by Peter J Verhagen, Herman M van Praag, Juan José López-Ibor, John Cox, Driss Moussaoui
ISBN: 9780470694718

Psychiatric Diagnosis: challenges and prospects
Edited by Ihsan M. Salloum and Juan E. Mezzich
ISBN: 9780470725696

Recovery in Mental Health: reshaping scientific and clinical responsibilities
By Michaela Amering and Margit Schmolke
ISBN: 9780470997963

Handbook of Service User Involvement in Mental Health Research
Edited by Jan Wallcraft, Beate Schrank and Michaela Amering
ISBN: 9780470997956

Psychiatrists and Traditional Healers: unwitting partners in global mental health
Edited by Mario Incayawar, Ronald Wintrob and Lise Bouchard,
ISBN: 9780470516836

Psychiatric Diagnosis and Classification
Edited by Mario Maj, Wolfgang Gaebel, Juan José López-Ibor, Norman Sartorius
ISBN: 9780471496816

Psychiatry in Society
Edited by Norman Sartorius, Wolfgang Gaebel, Juan José López-Ibor, Mario Maj
ISBN: 9780471496823

Psychiatry as a Neuroscience
Edited by Juan José López-Ibor, Wolfgang Gaebel, Mario Maj, Norman Sartorius
ISBN: 9780471496564

Early Detection and Management of Mental Disorders
Edited by Mario Maj, Juan José López-Ibor, Norman Sartorius, Mitsumoto Sato, Ahmed Okasha
ISBN: 9780470010839

World Psychiatric Association titles in the 'Depression' series

In recent years, there has been a growing awareness of the multiple interrelationships between depression and various physical diseases. This series of three short volumes dealing with the comorbidity of depression with diabetes, heart disease and cancer provides an update of currently available evidence on these interrelationships.

Depression and Diabetes
Edited by Wayne Katon, Mario Maj and Norman Sartorius
ISBN: 9780470688380

Depression and Heart Disease
Edited by Alexander Glassman, Mario Maj and Norman Sartorius
ISBN: 9780470710579

Depression and Cancer
Edited by David W. Kissane, Mario Maj and Norman Sartorius
ISBN: 9780470689660

Related WPA title on depression:

Depressive Disorders, 3e
Edited by Helen Herrman, Mario Maj and Norman Sartorius
ISBN: 9780470987209

For all other WPA titles published by John Wiley & Sons Ltd, please visit the following website pages:

http://eu.wiley.com/WileyCDA/Section/id-305609.html

http://eu.wiley.com/WileyCDA/Section/id-303180.html

Substance Abuse Disorders

WPA Series
Evidence and Experience

Editors:

Hamid Ghodse

International Centre for Drug Policy, St George's University of London,
London, UK

Helen Herrman

Orygen Youth Health Research Centre, Centre for Youth Mental Health,
The University of Melbourne, Melbourne, Australia

Mario Maj

Department of Psychiatry, University of Naples SUN, Naples, Italy

Norman Sartorius

Association for the Improvement of Mental Health Programmes,
Geneva, Switzerland

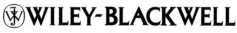

A John Wiley & Sons, Ltd, Publication

This edition first published 2011, © 2011 by John Wiley & Sons, Ltd.

Wiley-Blackwell is an imprint of John Wiley & Sons, formed by the merger of Wiley's global Scientific, Technical and Medical business with Blackwell Publishing.

Registered Office: John Wiley & Sons, Ltd, The Atrium, Southern Gate, Chichester, West Sussex, PO19 8SQ, UK

Other Editorial Offices:
9600 Garsington Road, Oxford, OX4 2DQ, UK
The Atrium, Southern Gate, Chichester, West Sussex, PO19 8SQ, UK
111 River Street, Hoboken, NJ 07030-5774, USA

For details of our global editorial offices, for customer services and for information about how to apply for permission to reuse the copyright material in this book please see our website at www.wiley.com/wiley-blackwell

Library of Congress Cataloging-in-Publication Data

Substance abuse disorders : evidence and experience / editors, Hamid Ghodse . . . [et al.].
    p. cm.
  Includes index.
  ISBN 978-0-470-74510-6 (cloth)
  1. Substance abuse.   2. Substance abuse–Etiology.   3. Substance abuse–Treatment.   I. Ghodse, Hamid.
  RC564.S83155   2011
  616.86–dc22

                                       2010033338

A catalogue record for this book is available from the British Library.

This book is published in the following electronic formats: ePDF: 978-0-470-97507-7; Wiley Online Library: 978-0-470-97508-4; ePub: 978-0-470-97594-7

Set in 10/12 Times by Aptara Inc., New Delhi, India.
Printed and bound in Singapore by Markono Print Media Pte Ltd

First Impression   2011

Contents

List of Contributors

Steve Allsop
National Drug Research Institute, Curtin University of Technology, GPO Box U1987, Perth WA 6845, Australia

Adriana Blanco
Pan American Health Organization, 525 23rd St NW, Washington, DC 20037, USA

Helen Fung-Kum Chiu
Department of Psychiatry, Faculty of Medicine, The Chinese University of Hong Kong (CUHK), China

Nicolas Clark
Institute for Health Services Research, Monash University, Melbourne, Australia

Ilana B. Crome
Academic Psychiatry Unit, Keele University Medical School, St George's Hospital, Corporation Road, Stafford ST16 3SR, UK

Vera da Costa e Silva
Rua Pinheiro Guimarães, 149 casa 145, 22281-080 Rio de Janeiro, Brazil

Pim Cuijpers
Department of Clinical Psychology, Vrije Universiteit, Amsterdam, The Netherlands

David A. Deitch
University of California, San Diego, CA, USA

Colin Drummond
National Addiction Centre, Institute of Psychiatry, King's College London, London SE5 8BB, UK

Griffith Edwards
National Addiction Centre, Institute of Psychiatry, King's College London, London SE5 8BB, UK

Nady el-Guebaly
Addiction Division, Department of Psychiatry, University of Calgary, Calgary, Alberta, Canada

Waleed Fawzi
Ministry of Health, Egypt

Susanna Galea
Community Alcohol & Drug Services, Auckland, Pitman House, 50 Carrington Road, Point Chevalier, Auckland, New Zealand

Coral Gartner
School of Population Health, University of Queensland, Brisbane, Queensland, Australia

Abdu'l-Missagh Ghadirian
McGill University, Faculty of Medicine, Montreal, Quebec, Canada

Wayne Hall
School of Population Health, University of Queensland, Brisbane, Queensland, Australia

Igor Koutsenok
Department of Psychiatry, University of California San Diego School of Medicine, 5060 Shoreham Place, Suite 200, San Diego, CA 92122, USA

Noeline C. Latt
Area Drug and Alcohol Service, Herbert Street Clinic, Royal North Shore Hospital, St Leonards, Sydney, NSW 2065, Australia

Nasser Loza
Ministry of Health, Egypt

Neil McKeganey
University of Glasgow, Glasgow, UK

Maria-Elena Medina Mora
Division of Epidemiology and Psychosocial Research, National Institute of Psychiatry Ramón de la Fuente Muñiz, Calzada México Xochimilco 101, Tlalpan, México D.F. 14370, Mexico

Ahmad Mohit
Department of Psychiatry, Iran University of Medical Science, Tehran, Iran

Maristela Monteiro
Pan American Health Organization, 525 23rd St NW, Washington DC 20037, USA

Marcus R. Munafò
School of Experimental Psychology, University of Bristol, 12a Priory Road, Bristol BS8 1TU, UK

Filippo Passetti
Division of Mental Health, St George's University of London, London SW17 0RE, UK

Jayadeep Patra
Centre for Addiction and Mental Health, 33 Russell Street, Room T-508, Toronto, Ontario, M5S 2S1 Canada

Vladimir B. Pozynak
Training and Research Centre, Belarussian Psychiatric Association, Minsk, Belarus

Mark Prunty
Respond (Community Substance Misuse Service), Surrey and Borders Partnership NHS Foundation Trust, Leatherhead, Surrey, UK

Rebeca Robles
Division of Epidemiology and Psychosocial Research, National Institute of Psychiatry Ramón de la Fuente Muñiz, Calzada México Xochimilco 101, Tlalpan, México D.F. 14370, Mexico

Duncan Raistrick
Leeds Addiction Unit, 2150 Century Way, Thorpe Park, Leeds LS15 8ZB, UK

Tania Real
Division of Epidemiology and Psychosocial Research, National Institute of Psychiatry Ramón de la Fuente Muñiz, Calzada México Xochimilco 101, Tlalpan, México D.F. 14370, Mexico

Kylie D. Reed
National Addiction Centre, Institute of Psychiatry, King's College London, London SE5 8BB, UK

Jürgen Rehm
Centre for Addiction and Mental Health, 33 Russell Street, Room T-508, Toronto, Ontario, M5S 2S1 Canada

Robyn Richmond
School of Public Health and Community Medicine, University of New South Wales, Kensington NSW 2052, Australia

Pedro Ruiz
Department of Psychiatry and Behavioral Sciences, University of Miami Miller School of Medicine, Miami, Florida, USA

Andriy V. Samokhvalov
Centre for Addiction and Mental Health, 33 Russell Street, Room T-508, Toronto, Ontario, M5S 2S1 Canada

John B. Saunders
Centre for Youth Substance Abuse Research, Faculty of Health Sciences, University of Queensland, Herston Qld 4029, Australia

Fabrizio Schifano
University of Hertfordshire, School of Pharmacy, College Lane Campus, Hatfield AL10 9AB, UK

John Strang
National Addiction Centre, Institute of Psychiatry, King's College London, London SE5 8BB, UK

Joshua Tsoh
Department of Psychiatry, Faculty of Medicine, The Chinese University of Hong Kong (CUHK), China

Robert West
Department of Epidemiology and Public Health, University College London, 2-16 Torrington Place, London WC1E 6BT, UK

James White
Department of Primary Care and Public Health, School of Medicine, Cardiff University, 4th Floor Neuadd Meirionnydd, Heath Park, Cardiff CF14 4YS, UK

Yu Xin
Institute of Mental Health, Peking University, Beijing, China

Preface

This book offers a comprehensive review of substance abuse disorders that, it is generally recognized, have proved to be very difficult problems for medical and psychiatric practice over the last century. It has three sections, one each for tobacco, alcohol and 'drugs'. Each section contains three reviews: epidemiology, treatment and management and prevention. Whole books have previously been dedicated to the subject of each section and indeed to each chapter within each section. This book does not seek to achieve that level of detail; instead, by standing back and taking a broader perspective, it highlights the differences and the similarities between the areas of study and emphasizes the importance of prevention, health-care delivery, policy formation and academic research. The authors of each chapter are internationally renowned in their respective fields and their chapters are complemented by commentaries from world-class authorities in research, teaching and clinical practice.

The misuse of tobacco, alcohol and of licit and illicit drugs is one of the greatest health challenges in the world today. It affects not just the health of those using these substances, but also all other aspects of their life as well as their families, their colleagues and the wider society. It lies behind a high proportion of all crime, costing nations billions of dollars each year in prevention and treatment programmes, in law enforcement and other economic costs. This imposes a heavy burden on the social infrastructure of developed and developing countries. Valuable human and financial resources have to be diverted away from productive activities contributing to development and prosperity, while drug trafficking foments corruption that is one of the most formidable obstacles to good governance.

The young people of today live in a world that is very complex. It provides them with tremendous opportunities as well as difficult challenges, with many benefits and many risks. The influence of their peers and their surroundings upon them and their behaviour, their life style and their health is greater than ever before. Peer influences no longer emanate solely from school or the local neighbourhood but can come from thousands of miles away. Indeed, adolescents' ideals and role models may be in another continent; their problems may start from under the same roof or from far away. The provision of a healthy environment has thus become more difficult and the sociocultural control of behaviour less predictable. These complex societal changes might have contributed to the increase of mental and behavioural problems of children and adolescents. Indeed, the scale of misuse of tobacco, alcohol and drugs is such that practioners are likely to see its impact on patients on most days. In comparison, the control of traditional diseases now appears relatively simple.

Smoking remains the single biggest preventable cause of ill health – and the smoking epidemic has yet to peak in low- and middle-income countries where the majority of the world's smokers now live. Tobacco use is strongly correlated with and can be a substantial contributor to social disadvantage. If current trends continue, it will kill 1000 million people prematurely during this century. According to the World Health Organization, three out of every five young people who experiment with tobacco will become dependent smokers into adulthood and half of them will die prematurely. However, studies demonstrate that no single youth-focused intervention will be effective if society as a whole does not address tobacco use as a social problem. Therefore, the main recommendation for public-health decision makers and activists is to concentrate efforts on changing the environment in parallel with any youth-orientated strategy in order to ensure adherence of this population to the concept that the best life option is to be or become a nonsmoker.

An instructive comparison can be made between the control regimes for illicit drugs and tobacco. Although it is both psychoactive and addictive, nicotine was never put under a drug-control regime like those of the International Conventions for the control of narcotic and psychotropic drugs. The recent World Health Organization Framework Convention on Tobacco Control adopts a very different approach. It emphasizes interlinked strategies for harm reduction, demand reduction, denormalization of tobacco use and regulation of the tobacco industry. Tobacco markets are relatively unregulated, relying on taxation, advertising and age-related controls on consumption. In this context, it is interesting that the annual prevalence of tobacco use is about one quarter of the world population (age 15+) – some 1.7 billion people – while the annual prevalence of use of any illicit drug is only 5% of the world population (age 15–64) – some 200 million people. The prevalence of tobacco consumption is thus eight times that for illicit drugs. Tobacco also claims 25 times as many lives as illicit drug abuse. In the early twentieth century and prior to any international drug control, the prevalence of drug dependence in many parts of the world was very high indeed. In China alone there were 10 million opium addicts out of a total estimated population of 450 million and in the United States according to a government report 90% of narcotics were used for nonmedical purposes.

Had there been no drug-control system, the size of the drug-using population, as well as the burden of disease associated with it, would have been much greater – perhaps even at levels close to tobacco. It can be argued therefore that the multilateral drug-control system has helped to contain the problem at 5% of the world population (age 15–64) or <1% if only problem drug use is considered. This is an achievement that should not be underrated and provides a useful perspective within which more recent developments can be analysed.

It is evident from the chapter on the epidemiology of drug abuse that in some parts of the world the abuse of prescription drugs has already surpassed the abuse of traditional illicit drugs such as heroin and cocaine. For example, in the United States, the abuse of prescription drugs, including pain killers, stimulants, sedatives and tranquillizers, exceeds that of practically all illicit drugs, with the exception of cannabis. The unregulated market for pharmaceuticals, particularly through the internet, exposes people to serious health risks through the delivery of often poorly documented, unsafe, ineffective or low-quality medicines. An additional concern is that the gains of the past years in international drug control may be seriously undermined by this ominous development, if it remains unchecked.

The epidemiological data that have been reviewed show that the most salient issue is the global nature of drug abuse, including the changing geographical location of crops and drug production, and the density and malleability of trafficking routes. Changes in drug use or policies within one country inevitably impact on others, emphasizing the need for international collaboration on a problem that knows no borders. A global view of the problem shows that knowledge of changes in the prevalence rates in one country or modification of the trafficking routes or oversupply of drugs in the illicit market allows some prediction of potential problems in other countries. This global view also facilitates international collaboration in relation to the interchange of information, evidence of best practice, coordination of activities and mutual support.

The importance of this type and level of collaboration is emphasized when it is realized that hundreds of preventive programmes were implemented around the world at various times without any attempt to evaluate their effectiveness or cost effectiveness. Under increasing pressure from governments and funding agencies to demonstrate the effectiveness of drug prevention interventions, several reviews have been undertaken during the past decade and the number of methodologically sound studies is now growing. Similarly, with regard to treatment, currently available evidence does not support any single treatment approach as yielding better outcomes for the chronic, relapsing nature of addiction, with all its correlates and consequences. Indeed, it seems likely that the most promising results come from a combination of pharmacotherapeutic and psychosocial treatment approaches that take account of the local sociocultural environment.

Worldwide, of course, alcohol consumption is one of the most important risk factors in the global burden of disease, ranking fifth, behind underweight (from malnutrition and underfeeding), unsafe sex, high blood pressure and tobacco use. In addition, it is important to remember that alcohol abuse contributes to some of the other risk factors for disease – for example to the prevalence of unsafe sex. The prevalence and severity of alcohol-use disorders depend on many factors, such as the amount and quality of alcohol consumed on a daily basis and the frequency of drinking. This is reflected in the distribution of alcohol-use disorders in different world regions. Although aggregate alcohol consumption is escalating fast in the developing world, limited research data are available on the regional prevalence and patterns of alcohol use in a vast number of countries. Such data would aid in the formulation of cost-effective treatment strategies within the medical and social infrastructures of those countries because most of the currently recommended practices for prevention and treatment, together with the supporting evidence, are derived from developed Western healthcare settings. Here, research evidence about effective interventions has not uniquely influenced policy and clinical decisions about responses to alcohol-related problems. Instead, in shaping policy, research evidence competes with: vested interests, such as those of the alcohol manufacturers and retailers; the divergent views of government departments such as treasury, employment, industry and health; and, community and clinician perceptions about the nature and extent of alcohol-related harm. Community views in turn are influenced by an individual's perceived proximity to the adverse outcomes of alcohol consumption and popular perceptions that alcohol problems are resolutely an issue of personal responsibility/individual weakness.

Preventing substance abuse and treating those who suffer from substance abuse disorders is an investment in the health of nations just as much as the prevention and treatment of HIV infection, diabetes or tuberculosis. However, because substance-abuse problems often have associated social problems, the issues have to be addressed by the whole of society. The review carried out within this book will therefore be useful not only to psychiatrists and other medical practitioners, but also to a wide range of professional groups, from health and social services, behavioural and social scientists and practitioners in the judiciary and law enforcement. We hope that it will also contribute to the ongoing debate on some of the controversial issues discussed here.

Hamid Ghodse
Helen Herrman
Mario Maj
Norman Sartorius

Drugs

CHAPTER 1

Epidemiology of Drug Abuse: A Global Overview

Maria-Elena Medina-Mora, PhD, Tania Real, M.S. and Rebeca Robles, PhD

Division of Epidemiology and Psychosocial Research, National Institute of Psychiatry, Ramón de la Fuente Muñiz, México, Mexico

1.1 INTRODUCTION

Public Health is interested in the health condition of the population and in the relation between the health status of groups and the environment. Epidemiology, through the differentiation of healthy individuals from those in poor health, and by the study of biological and social, individual and collective factors related to health and disease, estimates the extension and magnitude of a problem, subgroups of the population affected, trends over time, its determinants and consequences, the proportion of persons exposed to preventive interventions and the treatment demand covered. Its challenge is to describe the problem in a way that provides the evidence required to orientate policy.

Providing a comprehensive view of the drug problem across different cultures poses some difficulties, mainly derived from the availability of accurate information. On the one hand, illicit activities are difficult to evaluate, willingness to report might be affected by social tolerance toward drug use; persons conducting surveys in countries where drug use is defined as a felony and the police are active, might find more difficulties in obtaining an adequate rate of persons accepting to answer a questionnaire and an accurate self-report of use. Also, studies conducted in different countries might reflect differences in methods pursued, populations covered and conceptual definitions of behaviours and consequences, more than variations in rates of use. In spite of these limitations, data available show interesting global trends that can serve as an arena for the discussion of drug policies.

This chapter provides a view of the extension of the problem per type of substance and in different regions of the world; it is introduced by a discussion related to the different approaches epidemiology can follow, it provides evidence on the need to study dimensions of use and problems as separate interacting indicators and of considering the circular nature of the drug problem with epidemic rises, periods when drug use is stable or is reduced,

Substance Abuse Disorders: Evidence and Experience, First Edition. Edited by Hamid Ghodse, Helen Herrman, Mario Maj and Norman Sartorius.
© 2011 John Wiley & Sons, Ltd. Published 2011 by John Wiley & Sons, Ltd.

followed by a new rise, that calls attention to the need to consider replicating studies with a periodicity that allows the description of trends.

Data included in the chapter are drawn from a literature review, from the reports of member countries to the United Nations, from the annual reports of the International Narcotics Control Board, the UNESCO and from statistics and other studies coordinated by the World Health Organization. Regional organizations such as the European Monitoring Centre for Drugs and Drug Addiction (EMCDDA), the Inter-American Drug Abuse Control Commission CICAD, were also visited. This information is completed with data coming from epidemiological studies, household and student surveys, and surveillance systems, when available.

1.1.1   The Scope of Epidemiology

Epidemiology seeks to answer questions such as is there a drug problem? If so, what type of problem? What is its impact at the national and local levels? And depending on the type of problem, what are the more appropriate policies?. To answer these questions it uses surveys and other methodological strategies to assess the prevalence of use and abuse, problems and trends based on conceptual models that provide specific definitions of the problem, the accepted indicators to measure it and the policy to follow. The following section describes the main sources of information available:

A. *Estimates of production and drug seizure.* The availability of drugs in local markets can be derived from studies that assess the cultivation and production of drugs and from seizures that provides information about price and purity of individual drugs and about the type of substances that are available in certain locations, provided it is possible to differentiate quantities aimed for exportation and quantities aimed for local markets, especially in transit countries. In analysing this data caution must be taken as changes in price and purity of illegal substances on the streets do not necessarily indicate changes in prevalence; variations in effectiveness of enforcement and in reporting efforts can also shape this information [1].

B. *Estimating prevalence.* Counting the number of individuals that have used drugs is not enough to determine the scope of the problem in a given society. The impact of the drug problem on public health and thus the type of problem to be faced is modulated by:

    I. The patterns of drug use, that include the type of substances used, the routes of administration, the frequency and quantity of intake, the subgroup of the population using them (i.e. pregnant females, adolescents, etc.) or the circumstances of use (i.e. driving under the influence of drugs).

    II. The likelihood of dependence and of other drug-related problems influenced by variations in the vulnerability of individuals genetic predispositions (i.e. heritability estimates a range between 40 and 60% [2], factors in the development that increase the likelihood of transiting from experimentation to heavy use and dependence (i.e. childhood adversities including exposure to violence), in variations in the proximal environment (i.e. drug availability, drug use amongst siblings and peers, etc.).

    III. Sociocultural factors that include tolerance to use of drugs, *demographic* such as increase in the proportion of young persons with no equivalence in the availability of school and job opportunities, or *social transitions* such as migration. These factors modulate the likelihood of experimenting with drugs and advancing towards dependence as well as its impact in different societies.

IV. Availability of resources to face the problem (i.e. universal or limited access to treatment and other social services) and health and social policies that modulates the availability of resources to cope with the problem. Lower rates of use might result in a greater burden when they occur in contexts of poverty, social inequity or high degree of delinquency, or when there are no resources to identify cases and offer treatment. Formal responses to the problem will affect the availability of drugs on the streets and the number of persons imprisoned for drug use or possession. Special features of the *illegal production, diversion from legal sources* and *traffic of drugs* and organized crime will also affect the problem, influencing the rate of violence and drug availability.

C. *Mortality and morbidity.* Mortality studies focus on the most serious forms of drug abuse, causes being numerous from direct causes such as overdose, to indirect accidents or murder; they can relate to the route of administrating drugs or specific lifestyles such as HIV, hepatitis B or C. Mortality information can be driven from national causes of death statistics, examinations from the medical examiner, police or hospital records, amongst other sources [1]. The accuracy of information varies from country to country. According to Single *et al.* [3] illicit drugs have been implicated as a sufficient or contributory factor in at least 90 causes of death and disease. For each of these causes it is possible to estimate the excess mortality of persons with an addiction as compared to the general population controlled by age and sex [4], it is also possible to estimate aetiologic fractions or attributable proportions and estimate the numbers of deaths and admissions to hospital that can be causally attributed to illicit drugs.

D. These indicators can be resumed in a concept known as *burden of disease,* that includes premature mortality attributable to the disease and days lived without health. Substance-attributable burden is usually estimated by combining relative risk data with exposure prevalence data and disease-related mortality and morbidity information, from national databases [5].

The extent of drug use and the *social perception* of the extent of the problem does not always show the same trend, for instance a stabilization in drug use and even a reduction of new cases after a period of rapid increase can be accompanied by an increase in problems and of the demand for treatment as a result of chronic use by a proportion of those that started experimenting some time back. This trend can be accompanied by more visibility if an increase in murders occurs as a result of modifications in the drug cartels organization and their fight for markets, or if public policies change, or if the mass media focuses more closely on an old problem, modifying the social perception. The challenge of epidemiology is to assess the problem from a scientific perspective and to deliver knowledge in a way that is understood by the population, especially those that are in charge of public policies.

In summary, knowledge about the number of persons that use, abuse or become dependent and the trends over time is an important base for policy, but might not be enough to understand the impact of the problem in a given society. Approaches that evaluate the problem on two axes, substance use on the one hand and problems on the other, and that analyse their interrelation in the sociocultural context can provide a more accurate view of the problem by integrating in the analysis of prevalence, drug supply, individual and contextual variations, social perceptions of the problem and policies [6].

1.1.2   Conceptual Framework

Paradigms underlying epidemiological studies are also central because they define the basic suppositions upon which the problem is constructed, the aetiological explanations that are provided, indicators that are accepted as valid for its study and as such it is closely related to the way policies are conceived and actions are taken to counteract the problem [7].

The paradigm of *infectious diseases* conceives disease as a result of the interaction of a host with different degrees of susceptibility, exposed to an agent, in defined modes of transmission and environments; this model has been extended to study behavioural disorders such as drug abuse. The paradigm is mechanical biological and determinist in nature and follows a logical lineal causal mode. Public health interventions derived from this explanation seeks to block the casual link by eliminating the agent and by protecting the host, reducing the level of exposure to the agent and modifying the environmental conditions that facilitate exposure. The epidemiological tools are surveys to determine the proportion of the population exposed and that using drugs, the notification systems and the follow up of individuals to determine the routes of contact.

In accordance with the disease model, the more salient policy during the last century was the *reduction of supply*. It was assumed that the expansion of the problem could be prevented by reducing the opportunities of exposure that in turn depended on drug availability.

This notion of the individual as a passive host affected by an agent if exposed gave way to a more complex formulation that conceived an individual actively seeking for the agent. The resulting *psychosocial paradigm* considers the multifactor nature of the phenomenon; replaces the concept of a unique casual agent for the exposure to a wide variety of risk or protecting factors that affect the likelihood of an individual to experiment with drugs or to develop dependence.

Actions derived from this paradigm place less emphasis on the control of the agent, instead it aims at the reduction of risk factors and the enhancement of factors that make the individual less vulnerable or more resistant to the risks present in his environment; promotes healthy lifestyles and health protection through education. Interventions were then aimed at increasing the resilience of individuals to drugs. This model shares the linear causal model of the infectious diseases model and fails to explain variations derived from more distant contextual factors such as the role of affluence or extreme poverty and unemployment.

The tradition in *psychiatric epidemiology*, by definition more interested in substance-abuse disorders than in their use, includes *symptoms* as indicators. The use of this approach has made important contributions in the determination of treatment needs and the proportion covered, but provides information on only one of the elements of the drug phenomenon, this is dependence.

A *phenomenological model* considers that behaviour is mediated by cognitive processes through which the individuals construct the meaning of the world in which they live. *Alternative models* consider that public policy in itself plays a causal role in the shaping of the problem and in the social response.

The increase in problems in different regions, globalization and perhaps also the claim of drug-producing developing nations that the demand of drugs in the developed world was eliciting supply, turned to the recognition of the need of a more balanced approach in the efforts and budgets aimed at reducing both supply and demand. This conception has gone even further, by considering that only an integrated approach that combines components of supply and demand could make a difference.

A model based on *drug markets* [8], has also gained recognition, it considers supply and demand mediated by factors such as the needs of users, their priorities and lifestyles. The market approach considers drug use as a complex behaviour determined by the individual himself, his environment and the drugs available. It considers that markets are affected by the interaction between the demand for drugs and their availability, which in turn are influenced by the sociocultural environment and by political forces.

It acknowledges that supply satisfies and creates demand that supports existing drug supply or creates a new one. This continuum is affected by factors such as the emergence of alternative substances and sources for obtaining them, new markets of users, relapse rates, social ideology and the situation of the economy.

Illicit drug markets might be considered as new (emerging) or well established (mature): they vary by type of substances involved and by the number and type of users. Emerging markets are formed by a large proportion of abusers who consume smaller volumes of illicit drugs, with stimulant-type amphetamines being a paradigmatic example. Mature markets, on the other hand, are formed by small proportions of heavy drug users who consume large volumes of drugs, a typical example being the heroin market. Both markets can coexist side by side [9].

Whatever the paradigm chosen, or the combination of several of them, they will determine the methods and indicators followed to study and the recommendations on strategies to face the problem.

Most epidemiological evaluations of the problems around the world use a combination of indicators coming from the paradigms we have described. Room [10] has characterized epidemiological studies in four traditions: i) *medical epidemiology,* interested in patterns of drug use as risk factor for health problems; the outcome variable can be chronic disease such as heart disease, or infectious diseases such as HIV of Hepatitis B and C. The role of epidemiology being the elucidation of the circumstances under which the association between use and consequences occur (i.e. injuries derived from driving under the influence of drugs) and the proportion of the disease is attributable to substance use; ii) an alternative *tradition interested in the substances* by themselves, with little interest in assessing consequences; it has two ramifications aimed on the one hand at assessing variations in exposure and on the other to study different patterns of substance use; ii) a third tradition, *psychiatric epidemiology*, defines its outcome as harmful use, abuse or dependence defined through diagnostic criteria; iii) a fourth tradition: *social epidemiology,* is interested in the study of problems derived from abuse; uses the term problematic use more than dependence and is interested in patterns of use as the predictor variable and social problems as outcome. A fifth tradition of *psychosocial research* not considered by Room in his paper, focuses on the individual and is interested in the study of the relative impact of risk and protective factors in drug initiation, continuous use, development of dependence, remission and relapse.

Following this traditions, some countries started assessing the problem by tracking drug-related deaths and hospital and treatment centre registers of cases; others followed a tradition by conducting surveys having as the main indicator *ever use of drugs* and *use in the last 12 months.* Some assessed different patterns of use as a predictor variable of health or social consequences; others pay more attention to the role of psychosocial variables on the individual and in its immediate environment. And still others are interested only in cases diagnosed as having a *substance abuse* problem in the American Psychiatric Association DSM IV tradition or *harmful use* in the World Health Organization ICD 10 tradition and dependence disorders, similarly conceptualized in both systems.

Today it is more often recognized that approaches are complimentary and help understand the impact of the problem in the health and social welfare of the population. The tradition of counting the number of persons exposed to drugs, later evolved to accept the multifactor nature of the problem and epidemiology included amongst its objectives and thus as indicators in questionnaires, the search for risk and protective factors for drug experimentation, continuous use, dependence and remission and included risk behaviours (i.e. syringe sharing) health (i.e. infections resulting from injecting procedures) and social consequences (i.e. delinquency), and the assessment of similarities and differences across cultures. A later recognition that dimensions of supply and demand are necessary in the assessment of the problem has led to more global approaches in data recollection and interpretation.

To end this first part of the chapter, we consider it important to analyse the *cyclical nature* of the problem. Trends in drug abuse frequently follow a cycle whereby individual, drugs or consumption patterns re-emerge at different times and or in different regions. These cycles are influenced by opportunities for illicit cultivation, diversion or trafficking, and of changing public attitudes and patterns of consumption.

According to Musto [11] the cocaine epidemic in the United States at the beginning of the last century predicted the outbreak observed in the 1970s with cycles of tolerance and intolerance responding to cultural and political strains. Aspects initially considered as beneficial such as euphoria and stimulation of the central nervous system, were later seen as seductive risks and the drug considered as a threat to society.

These trends have also been observed in the case of several substances including opium, morphine and cannabis [11]. Mäkelä *et al.* [12] have described the same phenomenon for alcohol consumption that crosses political systems and cultures of drinking.

Following this conceptualization, low levels of problems coincide with public attitudes of tolerance, this phase gives rise to an increase in rates of use and consequences and to the modification of public attitudes that become less tolerant and to more restrictive policies, which in turn diminish the problems and along with it, public attitudes become more tolerant and policy less restrictive, in an ongoing cycle, that according to Musto [11] lasts a generation.

These historical moments have implications in the effect of programs aimed at reducing use and consequences: in periods of increase the aim should be to maintain and accelerate the diminishment of problems, and to control or reduce this trend, the same prevention program could have very different results depending on the historical moment. These cycles vary from one place to another. Today, market economies are experiencing a reduction of the problem, and the more disadvantaged countries an increase [13].

Epidemiology aimed at informing public policies should take into consideration this phenomenon when interpreting results. This evidence calls attention to the convenience to conduct studies in a continuous form, and to include as variables for study public attitudes toward drug use and policy.

1.1.3   The Scope of the Problem

The twentieth century ended with the conviction that drug abuse was a global problem and thus global solutions were required. The apparently neat boundary between producer, transit and consumer countries has clearly broken down. Drugs are illegally produced in developed and developing regions, and precursors required for the manufacture of drugs from the raw products are usually distributed from more industrialized countries to usually less-developed regions where drugs are produced.

Globalization has diminished geographical barriers making drugs more available throughout the globe, yet the level of development, geography and drug markets play an important role in drug problems.

As to *production,* marijuana grows in most countries of the world and is today the most widely consumed substance; amphetamine-type stimulants can be produced inside countries provided precursors are available: since 1990, 60 countries have reported to the United Nations illegal production of this substance [13]; in contrast, 99% of the cocaine is grown in the Andean region in South America and the large majority of opium is cultivated in Afghanistan (93% of the world production) with Myanmar, Pakistan and Lao People's Democratic Republic contributing in a lesser proportion; in the Americas, Colombia, Mexico and more recently Guatemala cultivate small quantities of this drug [13], mainly for the United States market estimated in 1.3 million users [14].

Drugs produced in these limited number of countries are trafficked and made available to drug users around the world, it is possible to track changes in traffic routes and in local rates of drug use and problems. As an example, we describe the changes in the routes of cocaine in the Americas to the US market and to Europe, and the modifications of drug-use rates in the same periods.

In the 1970s, the Colombian cartels preferred the Caribbean corridor, *interdiction* success produced a change in routes. These modifications have affected significantly the rates of drug use in the region. By 1998, UNODC estimated that 59% of the cocaine went via Central America/Mexico and 30% via the Caribbean; by 1999, flows of drugs passing though the Central American/Mexico corridor dropped to 54%, while flows through the Caribbean increased to 43%; in 2000, the proportions shifted to 66% and 33%, respectively; the rates for 2003 were 77%, 22% and in 2006, 90% was said to have transited trough the Central America/Mexico corridor [14].

In Mexico, the cumulative incidence or number of cases that have used the drug and survived to the moment of the survey of cocaine use were as low as 0.33% amongst the urban population 12–65 years of age [15]; by 2002, it had increased to 1.23% [16] and in 2008 it reached 2.37% of the adolescent and adult urban population [17].

A more recent example is the increase in the amount of cocaine shipped to West Africa from South America. It has been estimated that in 2007, 35% of the cocaine shipped from the coasts of Colombia, Venezuela, Brazil and the Guyanas is trafficked through this corridor [14]; in parallel, a resulting increase in the amount of drug use in these regions has been observed [13], for example, in Brazil the annual prevalence rate of cocaine changed from 0.4% in 2001 to 0.7 in 2005 [18].

The increase in drug availability is a contributing factor to the enlargement of the population that uses drugs if other variables in the social context that facilitate drug use, co-occur.

The *number of countries that report use of different substances* provides useful information on the extension of use of different type of substances. From this indicator we know that cannabis (marijuana and hashish) is the most extended drug in the world, by 2000 it was used in 96% of countries that report to the United Nations, followed by opiates (heroin, morphine and opium: 87% and derivates from the coca leaf (81%). The use of these natural products is followed by amphetamine-type stimulants (73%), benzodiazepines (controlled psychotropic that has a depressant effect on the central nervous system) (69%), various types of solvent inhalants (69%) and hallucinogens (60%) [19].

There are important variations within the countries in the *proportion of the population that has been exposed to the substances*. The United Nations estimated that in 2006/2007; around 5% of the population 15–64 years of age had used drugs at least once in the last 12 months and that problem use reached 0.6% of the population. The most widely consumed drug was cannabis with 3.9% of users, followed at a considerably lower extent by amphetamines with 0.6% of the world's population (with use of ecstasy reaching 0.2%), opiates were reported by 0.39% of which 0.28% was heroin, and 0.38% had used cocaine [20].

Globally, the United Nations has estimated that in 2007 between 172 and 250 million people took drugs at least once in the last 12 months and that there are between 18 and 38 million problem drug users aged 15–64 years. Of the total persons that used drugs in the previous year, between 134 and 190 million correspond to marijuana and other forms of cannabis, between 16 and 51 million to amphetamine group and between 12 and 24 million are ecstasy and ATS users in East and South East Asia, of methamphetamines in North America, of amphetamines in Europe and in the Near and Middle East. As for opiates, between 15 and 21 million reported their intake with higher rates found along the trafficking routes close to Afghanistan, in 2006 it was estimated that some 11 million were taking heroin, with an increase in Asia, and no differences in other parts of the world. In 2007 between 16 and 21 million reported the intake of cocaine [13].

As not all the population exposed become heavy consumers and develop dependence, it is important to consider rates of *drug abuse and dependence*. From the tradition of psychiatric epidemiology, the World Mental Health Initiative, reports rates of substance abuse without dependence and dependence with abuse (dependence was estimated only for those that reported having experienced problems) for seven developing countries, Nigeria [21], two sites in China (Beijing and Shangai) [22], Colombia [23], South Africa [24], Ukraine [25] Lebanon [26] and Mexico [27] and two countries from the developed world, United States [28] and New Zealand [29].

Results from this initiative show interesting differences in lifetime prevalence. The highest rates were observed in the United States (7.9% abuse and 3% dependence) and in New Zealand (5.3% abuse and 2.2% dependence), and the lowest in Lebanon (0.5% abuse and 0.1% dependence), China (0.5% abuse), Nigeria (1.0% abuse) and in Ukraine (0.9% abuse and 0.5% dependence); from the developing world, South Africa (3.9% abuse and 0.6% dependence), Mexico (2.7% abuse and 0.8% dependence) and Colombia (abuse 1.6%, dependence 0.6%) ranked relatively high.

Treatment demand has been used to describe geographical differences in the type of drug problem that countries are phasing. This indicator [13] shows that in South-America the highest demand is derived from cocaine (52% of all treatment demand) it is also the main drug of abuse amongst people in treatment in North America (33.5%); in contrast, in Europe and Asia, opiates occupy the first place (60% and 65%, respectively), and cocaine represents a small proportion, 8.4% in Europe and only 0.3% in Asia. In Africa, cocaine is gaining importance representing 7.2% of treatment demand, but cannabis remains as the main reason for seeking treatment (63%); this is also true in Oceania (47% in Australia and in New Zealand); cannabis is playing a more important role in Europe (19.5% of treatment demand is due to the use of this drug). In North America (Canada, US and Mexico) after cocaine (33.5%) cannabis (23.3%) occupies second place of importance in treatment demand; opiates on average in the North American region occupy the third place (20.7%), but in México only 7% of patients in treatment have reported heroin use [30], opiates are rarely seen amongst patients in treatment in South America (1.7%) but represent 16.5% of treatment demand in Africa. Amphetamine-type stimulants were more prominent in Asia (18%), Oceania (20%) and in North America (18%) and are responsible for an increasing proportion of treatment demand, in South America (10.9%) [13].

It is well known that not all persons with drug dependence reach treatment, the WHO World Mental Health Survey [31], documents a *treatment gap* amongst persons with substance-abuse disorders in the year previous to the surveys in developed and developing countries, in the United States, for example, 51.5% of the population 18 years of age and older received any treatment [28], the rate for Mexico was only 17% [32].

Overall, only a small proportion of cases had contact with treatment during the first year of onset of the substance-abuse disorder, including alcohol, ranging from 0.9% in Mexico to 2.8% in Nigeria and China. In the developed world, the proportion was larger but still low, 6% in New Zealand and 11.3% in the United States. By age 50, a larger proportion had been treated in these countries, an average of 22% of cases in the developing countries and 62% in the countries from the developed world [33].

Drug use is related to an important number of health outcomes (morbidity), that include infectious diseases such as HIV Hepatitis B and C, suicide, neuropsychiatric conditions, complications for the offspring of addicted mothers, overdoses, accidents and poisoning and suicide [5]. Injecting drug use, reported in 148 countries and territories [34] has been a behaviour of special concern due to the frequency in which contaminated injection equipment is used and because the lifestyles of this group are often related to high-risk sexual behaviour. Furthermore, poor living conditions and stigmatization are important barriers for accessing services.

HIV infection amongst people who inject drugs has been reported in 120 countries and it has been estimated that there are approximately 16 million injecting drug users worldwide, 3 million of which are infected with HIV. The largest numbers of HIV positive people who inject drugs are in Eastern Europe, East and Southeast Asia and Latin America; it has been estimated that up to 40% of some groups in these regions are HIV positive. China, the United States, the Russian Federation and Brazil have the largest populations of injectors and account for 45% of the total estimated worldwide population of people who inject drugs [35]. Hepatitis C is a related disorder, estimated to affect over 80% of injecting drug users [36]. Other forms of drug use, particularly amphetamine and methamphetamine have also been associated to risk of developing the immunodeficiency syndrome [35].

Overall, it has been estimated that in 2000, 0.4% (0.6% for males and 0.2% for females) of the *mortality* in the world was attributable to illicit drugs, when days without health are included, using a measure known as *Burden of Disease*, the estimated proportion increases to 0.8% (1.1% for males and 0.4% for females) [5].

Rehm *et al.* [5] estimated that the global burden, measured in disability adjusted life years attributable to illicit drugs, was higher in the developed world 1.8% (2.3% for males and 1.2% for females) followed by low mortality in developing regions or emerging economies, 0.8% (1.2% for males and 0.3% for females) and only 0.5% (0.8% for males and 0.2% for females) in high-mortality developing regions. This measure includes death by murder but does not include other indicators of the social impact of *drug-related violence* that affect societies [37]. For instance, the people of the Latin America region identify economic issues and crime as their two greatest problems [37].

Illegal production and trafficking routes are factors related to availability of substances, and thereby have an impact on the variations in rates of use described above, as well as on different sociocultural factors that validate certain forms of use in well-defined social groups. There are certain individual characteristics that make a person more vulnerable to experimenting and going on to abuse and depend on drugs (for example emotional problems, low self-esteem or low perception of risk associated to the use of different drugs). There are also characteristics of the proximal environment where individuals develop (for example whether or not their close friends use drugs) and those of the more distal context such as social inequality, lack of employment opportunities for youth and access to treatment, that impact on this vulnerability. But availability of substances is a necessary precondition for drug use [33, 38, 39].

The rate of problems is modulated by Illicit production increasingly focuses either on the territory of unsuccessful or geographically marginalized states, not necessarily wedded to the production of illegal drugs, but more likely, where drug production has become a symptom of wider structural problems [40]. According to the United Nations, particularly vulnerable to drug-trafficking organizations are states with a weak social and institutional fabric, or in which political events, domestic instability and conflict have contributed to the collapse or weakening of state structures and controls [41]. And those more attractive for the establishment of new markets are those where drugs are produced or trafficked. The rate of problems is also determined by the access to treatment and by availability of treatment options for the dependence to different substances.

In the following sections particularities of the different substances are discussed.

1.1.4   Cannabis

Marijuana is a greenish-grey mixture of the dried, shredded leaves, stems, seeds and flowers of the hemp plant *Cannabis sativa*. Its main active chemical is THC (delta-9-tetrahydrocannabinol), which causes the mind-altering effects of intoxication. The amount of THC (which is also the psychoactive ingredient in hashish) determines the potency and, therefore, the effects of marijuana. As THC enters the brain, it causes a user to feel euphoric – or 'high' – by acting on the brain's reward system, areas of the brain that respond to stimuli such as food and drink as well as most drugs of abuse. THC activates the reward system in the same way that nearly all drugs of abuse do, by stimulating brain cells to release the chemical dopamine [42].

Cannabis is produced in all regions and in almost all latitudes of the world. In the last decade, 120 countries reported illegal cultivation in their territories. The main region of production is located in the north of Africa and there is evidence that the cultivation in Latin America has diminished, while an increase is observed in Europe, Asia and Africa. Indoor production has enlarged in some areas of Europe and North America and in the east of Europe, increasing the concentration of THC from 3 to 7% registered in the 1990s to 10 to 30% [19].

According to the UNODC [20] the estimated global number of cannabis users ranges from some 142.6 to 190.3 million persons, equivalent to a range from 3.3 to 4.4% of the population aged 15–64 who used cannabis at least once in 2007.

The World Mental Health Initiative [31] included not only substance-use disorders, aetiological factors and the analysis of the treatment gap in different countries, but also the cumulative incidence or history of drug involvement of those individuals from a defined cohort that have survived to the moment of the study, it is also defined as the proportion of cases that have ever been exposed or prevalence of ever use. It is considered as a good measure to study the risk of becoming a drug user as is not limited to time frames as is the case of other commonly used measures of prevalence such as annual use and current prevalence (use in the 30 days before the surveys).

Results from this initiative show that the market-economy countries have higher rates of cannabis use, the first seven places from higher to lower cumulative incidence are occupied by developed countries, ranging from 42% of the adult population in the United States to 6.6% in Italy; in the developing countries the rates varied from 10.8% in Colombia to 0.3% in China.

The American hemisphere produces more than half the world's cannabis herb [43], several studies have been conducted but direct comparison are difficult due to the differences in methods outstandingly the urbanicity status of the sites included in the surveys, nonetheless some interesting trends can be derived.

The highest prevalence rates are found in the United States, where almost half (46.1%) the population aged 12 years and older has tried this drug and 14.4% (35.6 million people) reported having used it in 2007 [44]. Chile is next in accumulated incidence with 27% of the urban population of 91 cities with more than 30 000 inhabitants, reporting having experimented [45], while the rate for Argentina in studies of urban areas of more than 80 000 inhabitants is 16.7%, and 12.2% in Uruguay (urban areas of more than 20 000 inhabitants) [46].

Surveys conducted in Peru in urban areas of more than 20 000 inhabitants [47], and in Mexico in a national sample of both rural and urban areas, showed similar rates with 4% of their population reporting ever use of cannabis. Rates for use in the past year range from 7% in Chile and Argentina to 0.7% in Ecuador and Peru.

School surveys conducted in selected countries in Central America show rates ranging from 7% in Panama to 2.2% in Nicaragua [48], lower than that reported for college students in the US, which totalled 10%, 24% and 32% amongst 8th, 10th and 12th grade students, respectively, in 2007 [49].

Except for the United States – where cannabis use was reported as stable after a reduction from 18%, 33% and 35% amongst 8th, 10th and 12th grade students, respectively, observed in 1996 [49], in other countries where surveys are available, use is increasing. In Brazil, ever use increased from 6.9 to 8.8%, and annual use from 1 to 2.6% in the same period. Argentina showed an even stronger increase in the annual prevalence rate of cannabis use, rising from 1.9% of the population ages 16 to 64 in 2004 to 6.9% of the population aged 12 to 64 in 2006 – reversing a previous downward trend. In Uruguay, annual prevalence of cannabis use increased amongst the population ages 15 to 65, from 1.3% in 2001 to 5.3% in 2007. In Mexico, ever use grew from 3.48% in 2002 to 4.19% in 2008, with rates for annual use being 0.6 and 1.03%, respectively [43].

In contrast, in Europe there is a clear downward trend. In England and Wales cannabis use fell from a prevalence rate of 10.9% amongst the population aged 16–59 in 2002/03 to 7.4% in 2007/08. This trend was first observed amongst school population, annual prevalence of cannabis use amongst people aged 16–24 fell from 28.2% in 1998 to 17.9% in 2007/08.

In Spain, considered as the door for Morocco's cannabis production to Europe, household survey data showed a moderate decline, reversing the previous rising trend, from a peak of 11.3% of the population aged 15–64 in 2003, to 10.1% in 2007.

A similar trend of rising cannabis use in the 1990s followed by some decline in recent years can be also noticed in recent household surveys from a number of other European countries. Cannabis use seems to have remained stable in the Netherlands (5.5% in 2001 and 5.4% in 2005). Following increases in the 1990s, cannabis use levels also remained quite stable in some of the new Central European EU member states, including Poland (2.8% in 2002; 2.7% in 2006), the Czech Republic (10.9% in 2002; 9.3% in 2004) and Slovakia (7.2% in 2000; 6.9% in 2006). Finally, from a total of 21 African countries reporting cannabis use trends for 2007, 7 countries saw use levels rising and 4 countries reported a decline. The rest show a downward trend in a number of countries. [13].

1.1.5   Opium and Heroin

The most abused and the most rapidly acting of the opiates is *heroin*. It is processed from morphine, a naturally occurring substance extracted from the seed pod of certain varieties of poppy plants. Soon after its injection or inhalation, heroin crosses the blood/brain barrier and is converted to morphine to bind rapidly opioid receptors [42].

Heroin is a matter of special concern due to its abuse and dependence liability. Abuse of this and other substances used intravenously is now a major vector for the transmission of infectious diseases, in particular the immunodeficiency virus (VIH) and the acquired immunodeficiency syndrome (AIDS), hepatitis and tuberculosis. Drug injecting has been identified in more than 136 countries, of which 93 report HIV infection amongst injecting drug users. The joint United Nations Program on HIV/AIDS [35] estimates that the global proportion of HIV infections due to contaminated injection equipment was from 5 to 10% in 1996.

During the 1990s Afghanistan became the world's largest producer of *illicit opium* from where heroin is extracted. The United Nations Drug Control Program [40] reports that in 1999, 79% of global illicit opium was produced in this country and that though in 2000, this proportion was reduced, it was still 70%, by 2007, Afghanistan alone accounted for 92% of global production, producing 82000 mt. of opium at an average opium yield of 42.3 kg/ha; 82% of their global area was under opium poppy [50].

Opium has been traditionally a crop in Afghanistan since the eighteenth century, but it began to emerge as a significant producer of illicit opium in the period of protracted war that started in 1979 and unfortunately is likely to persist for some time in the future; from 1986 until 2000 illegal production showed an annual growth rate of 23%.

This growth in production occurred in a background of economical, political and geostrategic factors, mainly, a lack of effective government control over the whole country, the degradation of agriculture and most economic infrastructures due to more than twenty years of civil war that made opium poppy cultivation a livelihood strategy for many rural households. At the same time, the abolition of production in neighbouring countries such as Turkey in 1972 and Iran in 1979 made Afghanistan an alternative source of world supply [40].

Afghanistan and Myanmar produced in 2002, 86% of the illegal world opium, in the latter country it was reduced by 23% in 2004, while in the former it grew by 16%. This is a change from the situation observed in 2000 when the Taliban imposed a prohibition in the production of opium. Nonetheless great quantities from illicit existences were placed in the market and thus the supply continued to be considerable [51]. In 2007, the total area under illicit opium poppy cultivation increased by 17%, fuelled by both Afghanistan and Myanmar; but overall, global cultivation remains below 1998 levels. In Myanmar, for example, although opium cultivation increased by 29% (by 46% to 460 mt.) it is still 65% lower than a decade ago [50].

As a result of the wide availability of opiates in the region, consumption, injecting and HIV in West Asia has increased. In Pakistan, the UNODCs Global Assessment Programme on Drug Abuse, (GAP) published in 2002, indicated high rates of drug abuse, in urban and rural areas. The prevalence rates were estimated at 3.5 million drug users of which 500 000 were heroin users. More recently, an increase in dependence to buprenorphine has been reported [9].

Opiate global consumption remains relatively stable in Europe and in some cases it declined, especially in North America, whereas some countries produce this substance mainly for local markets. By the end of the 1990s, 65% of the heroin seized in the United States came from Colombia [19], and in Mexico, use of heroin seems to concentrate in regions close to the border with the United States, where more than 25% of treatment demand is due to this substance, as compared to a national average of 5% [52].

According to the 2008 World Drug Report, The total number of opiate users is now estimated at around 16.5 million people. Then, global consumption of opiates shows only a marginal increase in annual prevalence: from 0.37% of the population age 15–65 years in 2005, to 0.39% in 2006. However, in certain consumer markets in and bordering Afghanistan and along trafficking routes, expansion of injecting drug use has been noticed and could pose a future challenge to resource-strapped public services [50].

The largest number of opiate users are in Asia (more than half of the world's opiate-using population), especially along the main drug-trafficking routes out of Afghanistan. In the South-West Asia subregion the average prevalence rate is the highest, at 1% of the population age 15–64 years old. In 2006, Europe remain the second largest consumer market for opiates, with an annual prevalence of 0.7% of the population age 15–64, but stable to declining consumption levels in West and Central Europe. Finally, in the Americas (North, central and South America and the Caribbean) overall use of opiates was found to be fairly stable, affecting only 0.4% of the population age 15–64 (13% of all opiate users in 2006) [50].

1.1.6   Cocaine

Cocaine is extracted from the leaf of the *Erythroxylon* coca bush, which grow primarily in the Andean region. It is a powerfully addictive stimulant because it directly affects the brain regions that are stimulated by all types of reinforcing stimuli such as food, sex, and many drugs of abuse [53].

There is evidence that during the Spanish Conquest in the sixteenth century cultivation and use of *coca leaf* had extended to Central America up to Nicaragua and to the Caribbean to the territories of today's Dominican Republic and Haiti and along the Atlantic cost to Venezuela and Guyan. Though the major concentration remained in Peru and Bolivia. After the alkaloid was isolated in 1859/1860, as the market of coca expanded so did the cultivation of the leaf to a number of Asian territories colonies of the British, Dutch and Japanese Colonies; between the turn of the century and 1912 Peru and the Dutch colony of Java emerged as the world's largest producers and exporters of coca leaf. Peru's export of coca leaf, which amounted to 8 tons in 1877, rose to 610 tons in 1901. Peru's total production of coca leaf in 1901 was estimated at around 2100 tons.

Exports peaked at 1490 tons in 1900. Exports from Java grew from 26 tons in 1904 to 1353 tons in 1914 that supplied Europeans and later Japanese manufacturers, while coca exports from Peru was destined for the US and Europe mainly Germany. Musto [19] estimates that there were 250 000 addicts to cocaine and morphine at that time, equivalent to 0.5% of the total population age 15 and above at the beginning of the twentieth century. Nowadays, world coca production takes place in Colombia (55% of coca bush cultivated), Peru (30%) and Bolivia (16%) [50]. In 1999, cultivation dropped in two thirds in Peru and in Bolivia coca cultivation and trafficking were almost completely wiped out from the Chapare region [41]. But by 2004, cultivation in these two countries started to rise again [56]. In 2007, Colombia had 99 000 ha of coca bush, an increase of 27% (21 000 ha) compared to 2006, for example [50].

Cocaine is distributed to the world through the Caribbean Sea and through Mexico by the Pacific Coast. At the beginning of the 1990s Mexico became a supplier of cocaine for the south-western states of the United States [19]. In this decade, the rate of experimentation amongst Mexican adolescents increased 400% [54] and close to 300% amongst the adult population between 18 and 65 years of age [55]. The rates of ever use of powered cocaine (1.5%) were similar to those observed in Colombia (1.6%). This estimate does not include the use of coca paste or 'basuco' that is rare in Mexico and is used by an additional 1% of the population of Colombia [40], rates rose in Colombia 2004 [56] and in Mexico [57].

According to World Drug Report 2008 [50], more than 80% of cocaine is seized in the Americas, with 45% for South America, where most cocaine is manufactured, but this region is not the largest cocaine market. Both Central America and the Caribbean have 19% of the total cocaine users (3.1 million people) compared with North America with 24%, (that represents 7.1 million people). The only large market outside Americas is West and Central Europe (24% or 3.9 million people). By contrast, abuse of cocaine in the Asia region or in Eastern Europe is still at relatively low levels.

Trends of world use in the United States, Canada and Colombia are stable, in Peru and Bolivia use is decreasing, while in Mexico, some European countries and in Africa it is increasing [50].

1.1.7   Inhalants

Inhalants are volatile substances that produce chemical vapours that can be inhaled to induce a psychoactive effect, such as volatile solvents, aerosols, gases, and nitrites. *Volatile solvents* include paint thinners and removers, dry-cleaning fluids, degreasers, gasoline, glues, correction fluids, and felt-tip marker fluids; *aerosols* are sprays that contain propellants and solvents (i.e. spray paints, deodorant and hair sprays, vegetable oil sprays for cooking, and fabric protector sprays); *gases* include medical anesthetics (i.e. ether, chloroform, halothane, and nitrous oxide) as well as gases used in household or commercial products (i.e. butane lighters, propane tanks, whipped-cream dispensers, and refrigerants); finally, *nitrites* that act primarily to dilate blood vessels and relax the muscles and are used as sexual enhancers, include cyclohexyl nitrite, isoamyl (amyl) nitrite, and isobutyl (butyl) nitrite [42].

Inhalants constitutes a special group of drugs as due to their wide industrial and domestic use they have a considerably availability. Their use is a widespread practice mainly amongst children and adolescents in the developed and developing world, predominantly by poorest ones. In Mexico, for example, it is still the drug of choice of children that work in the streets, a phenomenon that results from economical crises when all eligible members within the household, including children go out to work as a survival strategy observed amongst poor families [58, 59]. In a survey conducted at Mexico City, 4.4% of high school students had used inhalants in the last year [60]. In Alberta, Canada, 2.5% reported use of glue and 5.8% solvents [61]. Chile's annual prevalence amongst students is 3.3% [45], and in Colombia 10th and 11th grade students reported 1.1% prevalence [62]. These rates increase dramatically in the United States with 19.7%, 30.7% and 38% amongst 8th, 10th and 12th graders, respectively [63].

In 2006, inhalants lifetime prevalence's in the United States and Brazil were high, (with 9.3 and 6.1% of population aged 12 years or more that had used it, respectively), compared with 2.6% in Panama [66], 2% in Canada [67], 1% in Spain and Peru [68,69].

Amongst secondary students (14 to 17 years of age) Ireland and Brazil reported high prevalence of inhalant use: 18% and 15.3%, respectively [64,65], which are considerably higher than those in Bulgaria (3%), Colombia (3.5%), Argentina (2.6%) or Ecuador (2.3%) (23). the lowest rates in these group were reported by Peru (1.8%), Uruguay (1.5%) Paraguay (1.5%) and Bolivia (1.2%) [70].

In general terms, trends remained stable. However, the rate of past-year inhalant use amongst females showed an important increment. In United States, for example, increased from 4.1% in 2002 to 4.9% in 2005 [11].

1.1.8   Amphetamine-type stimulants ATS

In contrast to the long history of abuse of plant-based drugs such as heroin and cocaine, over the past decade the synthetic drug phenomenon has re-emerged linked to lifestyles and group identity of young people. The first wave was linked to the production of synthetic hallucinogens, mainly LSD in the second half of the last century, and the second wave, to the production of *amphetamine-type stimulants (ATS)*, a group of substances comprised of synthetic stimulants.

Methamphetamine is a very addictive stimulant that is closely related to amphetamine. It acts by increasing the release of dopamine in the brain, which leads to feelings of euphoria. It can be taken orally or by snorting or injecting, or a rock 'crystal' that is heated and smoked. Methamphetamine increases wakefulness and physical activity, produces rapid heart rate, irregular heartbeat, and increased blood pressure and body temperature. Methamphetamine alters the brain in ways that impair decision making, memory, and motor behaviours, and causes structural and functional deficits in brain areas associated with depression and anxiety, long-term use can cause mood disturbances, confusion, insomnia, dental problems and violent behaviour. In addition, methamphetamine use is related with HIV, hepatitis C and other sexually transmitted diseases due to risky sexual behaviour and the use of contaminated injection equipment.

MDMA (ecstasy) is a synthetic psychoactive drug that is similar to the stimulant methamphetamine. It is taken orally as a capsule or tablet. Primary effects include feelings of mental stimulation, emotional warmth, enhanced sensory perception, and increased physical energy. Adverse health effects of MDMA can include nausea, chills, sweating, teeth clenching, muscle cramping, blurred vision and also can produce confusion, depression, sleep problems, drug craving and severe anxiety [71].

In geographical terms, ATS abuse gradually spread from a few countries to neighbouring countries within the same region and then to other regions of the world. Since the mid-1990s abuse of ATS has been perceived as a global phenomenon, although different substances predominate in different parts of the world. Abuse of ATS has been estimated to affect 6 of each thousand people age 15–64 years in the world [50]. Prevalence rates differ significantly from country to country. About half the users are found in Asia, the Americas and Europe account for one third, and its use has also been reported in South America and in Africa.

In 2001, about 0.1% of the global population (age 15 and above) consumed the methamphetamine form known as 'ecstasy'. According to the United Nations Drug Control Program [40], 60% of the global consumption was concentrated in Europe, Western Europe and North America, together accounting for almost 85% of global consumption. In Australia and in most countries of Western Europe, ATS are the second most widely consumed group of illegal drugs after cannabis. In Japan about 90% of all seizure cases and of all drug-related arrests in 1998 involved methamphetamines. In Thailand this substance displaced heroin as the most heavily abused drug in the late 1990s [41].

Into the 2006/2007 period, ATS reported an overall stabilization [50]. In Germany and London, for example, from 2003 to 2006, lifetime prevalence of ecstasy use remained close to 2% (2.5 and 2.2%; 1.9 and 1.6%, respectively) [72]. Also, during 2006 and 2007 the United States population age 12 or above reported 5% lifetime and 0.9% last year prevalence's of *ecstasy* use [73].

In addition, potential for increases in near and Middle East region (South Arabia) and in some South America countries (Argentina, Peru, Guatemala, El Salvador and Dominican Republic) has been reported [50].

Illicit production of ATS has taken place in the United States and Western Europe since the 1960s after it extended to the East in the 1980s, and in the 1990s to almost all regions. According to the World Drug Report 2008 [50], methamphetamine manufacture is growing in many other regions, particularly in Oceania, Central and Eastern Europe, East and South-East Asia, and in South Africa.

While trafficking in most drugs is interregional, trafficking of amphetamine-type stimulants is largely intraregional, that is, production and consumption are usually within the same region, often within the same country. The exception is *'ecstasy'* that is still produced in Europe and in the 1990s trafficking from Europe to America and other countries increased significantly [19]. Seizures of this substance increased by four times between 1990 and 1998, while seizures for heroin and cocaine increased by only 50% [19]. In 2006, the amphetamines group constituted 91% of ATS seizures, while ecstasy ones accounted for just 9%, and for the first time, growth in amphetamine seizures outpaced that of methamphetamine [50].

1.1.9 Abuse of Prescription Drugs

Prescription drugs commonly nonmedical used or abused include three main groups of substances: i) *Opioids,* which are most often prescribed to treat pain because they act on the brain and body by attaching to specific proteins called opioid receptors, which are found in the brain, spinal cord, and gastrointestinal tract [74]; ii) Central nervous system (CNS) *depressants* sometimes referred to as sedatives and tranquilizers (i.e. barbiturates, benzodiazepines). Most of them act on the brain by affecting the neurotransmitter gammaaminobutyric acid (GABA) and are mainly used to treat anxiety and sleep disorders [74]; iii) CNS *stimulants* (i.e. dextroamphetamine, such as Dexedrine and Adderall, and methylphenidate like Ritalin and Concerta) that have chemical structures similar to a family of key brain neurotransmitters *monoamines* (including noradrenaline and dopamine) are prescribed to treat the sleep disorder narcolepsy and attention-deficit hyperactivity disorder (ADHD). As its name suggests, stimulants increase alertness, attention, and energy, as well as elevate blood pressure and increase heart rate and respiration [74].

Amphetamines were first introduced as medicines perhaps because stopping their use after prolonged periods did not produce the obvious withdrawal symptoms associated with opiates withdrawal. For several decades it was widely believed that they were not addictive.

Immediately after their introduction into medical practice in the 1930s, amphetamine and methamphetamine, considered to be the parent drug of the ATS group began to be used for nonmedical purposes.

When *Benzedrine* became available in tablet forms it began to be used for nonmedical purposes, reports of abuse in 1947 in a USs prison, the nonmedical use of these substances spread rapidly in the 20 years after the second world war when they were seen as relatively safe and effective medicines or harmless stimulants despite reports indicating dangers associated with their use. Despite warnings they were used in large quantities in the US for both medical and nonmedical use throughout the world thorough the 1970s and 1980s.

Methanphetamine was widely available on prescription as *Damphetamne* through the post-war period marketed for narcolepsy and obesity, the first epidemic of intravenous use started in California in the 1960s and was triggered by the inappropriate prescribing of the drug for heroin dependency. Speed began to replace hallucinogenic drugs such as LSD. In the 1980s another form of a new and highly pure form of *DMethamphetamine* known as ice became available in Hawaii initially imported from the Far East.

In the United States of America, since 2004–2007, around 20% of the population age 12 and above reported lifetime nonmedical use of psychotropic medication [75]. In 2007, last-year prevalence was 6.6%, showing an increment with respect to those reported in 2004 (6.2%). According to the 2005 Drug Policy Alliance: Africa [76], this region is reported to hold the largest market for methaqualone in the world.

In general, drug abuse appears to be more prevalent in males. Between 70 and 80% of users are male, a proportion that is higher than that observed in developed countries and slightly lower than the observed in traditional Asian societies. Women appear to participate primarily in the consumption of psychotropic drugs. The majority of users are between the ages of 18 and 25, with the cocaine and heroin being used primarily by those at the high end of the age bracket [56]. Overconsumption of internationally controlled drugs is more frequent in the elderly population [74]. The reason might be that such medication is more frequently administered and therefore available than in their younger counterparts.

1.2   THE CASE OF VULNERABILITY POPULATIONS

Social vulnerability could play an important role to explain the rapid spread of psychoactive substance use and abuse. People in disadvantage social position might use drugs like a coping mechanism in dealing with adverse situations they face, and need urgent attention. Poverty, political instability, social unrest and refugee problems are some of variables suggested to explain the increase of the problem in some regions. According to Odejide [77], poor funding, insufficient skilled health personnel, poor laboratory facilities, inadequate treatment facilities, and lack of political will are some of the impediments to controlling substance use/abuse in Africa, for example. In this kind of context, *street children* (and also adults who live or work on the street) have to be treated as a special group, because they are more likely to use psychoactive substances that are readily available and relatively cheap, such as solvents or cannabis [78].

1.3   DISCUSSION AND CONCLUSIONS

This chapter reviewed in its first section the scope of epidemiology, paradigms indicators and methods available to study the drug phenomenon; in the second section it described the problem as derived from the use of epidemiological approximations. Epidemiology has evolved from focusing mainly on one side of the problem, availability and interest in the substances by themselves, to more complex approaches that combine factors in the individual, both in the immediate and in the more distal environments within specific cultural contexts. The cyclical nature of the problem with periods of increase and decrease in the rate of problems that change along with public attitudes and social policies, has also been recognized and thus the convenience of conducting studies in a periodical form, and to include as variables for study public attitudes toward drug use and policy.

Epidemiology uses a combination of indicators coming from the paradigms described, today it is more often recognized that approaches are complementary and help understand the impact of the problem in the health and social welfare of the population. The tradition of counting the number of persons exposed to drugs, evolved to accept the multifactor nature of the problem and epidemiology included the search for risk and protective factors for drug experimentation, continuous use, dependence and remission, as well as risk behaviours such as syringe sharing, health (i.e. infections resulting from injecting procedures) and social consequences (i.e. delinquency), and access to treatment. A later recognition that dimensions of supply and demand are necessary in the assessment of the problem, has led to more global approaches in data re-collection and interpretation focusing in individuals immersed in drug markets.

Still, an important proportion of the information available outside the developed world is obtainable through the efforts of international organizations. For some countries the information is limited to prevalence estimates and in many cases it relies on the opinion of experts; more research, including surveys and rapid assessment approaches, is needed not only limited to counting people affected but including the analysis of problems faced by users and communities and of the contexts where the problem occurs. Efforts aimed at supporting developing countries to access local research results in international journals must be recognized and supported.

The data shown in this chapter illustrates the diversity and complexity of drug problems around the world; forms of use with a long tradition in some cultures emerge in others, availability of drugs and changes in the sociocultural context playing a major role. Data reviewed also suggest that countries are not equally affected by this problem, an important mediating factor being the availability of resources to cope with the problem.

Marijuana grows in most countries of the world and is today the most widely consumed substance, in contrast, 99% of the cocaine is grown in the Andean region in South America and a large majority of opium is cultivated in Afghanistan (93% of the world production). Amphetamine-type stimulants have been reported by 60 countries since 2000. Drugs are trafficked from producing country to different parts of the world and in this transit they impact the local drug problem; Increases in drug availability contributes to the enlargement of the population that uses drugs if other variables in the social context that facilitate drug use co-occur.

From the number of countries that report use of different substances we know that cannabis (marijuana and hashish) is the most extended drug in the world, by 2000 it was used in 96% of countries that report to the United Nations, followed by opiates (heroin, morphine and opium) (87%), and derivates from the coca leaf (81%) [19].

As for the number of users within countries where use has been reported, the United Nations estimated that around 5% of the population 15–64 years old has used drugs at least once in the last 12 months and that problem use reached 0.6% of the population. A total of 3.9% reports use of cannabis, use of other substances is considerable lower, amphetamines is used by 0.6% of the world's population (with use of ecstasy reaching 0.2%), opiates were reported by 0.39% of which 0.28% was heroin, and 0.38% had used cocaine [20].

Ecstasy and ATS use is more extended in East and South East Asia, methamphetamines in North America, and amphetamines in Europe and in the Near and Middle East. The highest rates of opiates are found along the trafficking routes close to Afghanistan and in Europe and Asia they occupy the first place of treatment demand; cocaine is more widely used in the Americas, the continent where it is produced. Cannabis remains as the main reason for seeking treatment in Africa and in Oceania [13, 79].

In injecting drug use, because the high risk of blood-borne infections including HIV is of high concern, the largest numbers of HIV positive people among those who inject drugs are in Eastern Europe, East and Southeast Asia and Latin America [35].

Overall, it has been estimated that in 2000, 0.4% (0.6% for males and 0.2% for females) of the mortality in the world was attributable to illicit drugs, when days without health are included, (Burden of Disease), the estimated proportion increases to 0.8% (1.1% for males and 0.4% for females), it is higher in the developed world 1.8% followed by low-mortality developing regions or emerging economies, 0.8% and by high-mortality developing regions, 0.5% [5].

Level of development affects both the likelihood of the problem and the impact made on societies, with higher rates and fewer problems among the highly developed societies. The treatment gap among persons with substance-abuse disorders is high in developed and developing countries with a bigger proportion in the latter [33].

Epidemiological data reviewed suggest some avenues for policy, perhaps the most salient issue is the global nature of the problem, geographical situation of crops, density and malleability of traffic routes, and international impact on changes in drug use or policies within one country, supports the need of international collaboration and the convenience to manage the problem within regional and global organizations. Interchange of information, evidence of best practices, coordination of activities and mutual support are required to phase a problem that does not recognize borders.

A global view of the problem allows some prediction of possible emerging problems within countries, changes in the prevalence rates in one country, modification in the traffic routes, and oversupply of drugs in the illicit market, might result in increases of problems in neighbouring countries or among those in the new traffic routes, thus supporting efforts to gather accurate information internationally and making it available to policy makers.

From the data, it is also evident that a global approach that includes actions aimed at regulating both supply and demand are required and that cultural adaptations to local contexts and ways in which the problem manifests are also important. In this sense, Odejide [78] further suggests that well-coordinated civil society participation is necessary in the control of drug problems in order to achieve a balance between supply and demand reduction efforts.

Research aimed at collecting more accurate and comparable data, especially among countries that do not gather routinely information should receive more international support. The efforts made to support publication of local studies in international journals is recognizable, such efforts must be continued and strengthened.

REFERENCES

1. Ghodse, H. (2002) *Drugs and Addictive Behavior. A Guide to Treatment*, 3rd edn, Cambridge University Press, United Kingdom.
2. Reich, T., Edenberg, H.J., Goate, A. *et al.* (1998) Genome-wide search for genes affecting the risk for alcohol dependency. *American Journal of Medical Genetics*, **81**, 207–215.
3. Single, E., Rehm, J., Robson, L. *et al.* (2000) The relative risks and etiologic fractions of different causes of death and disease attributable to alcohol, tobacco and illicit drug use in Canada. *Canadian Medical Association Journal*, **162** (12), 1669–1675.
4. Ghodse, H., Sheehan, M., Taylor, C. *et al.* (1985) Deaths of drug addicts in the United Kingdom 1967-81. *British Medical Journal*, **290** (9), 425–428.
5. Rehm, J., Taylor, B. and Robin, R. (2006) Global burden of disease from alcohol, illicit drugs and tobacco. *Drug and Alcohol Review*, **25** (6), 503–513.
6. Room, R. (1989) Cultural changes in drinking and trends in alcohol problems indicators: recent U.S. experience. *Alcologia*, **1** (2), 83–89.
7. Hartnoll, R. (1993) Epidemiological research on drugs. *T. Alc. Drugs*, **19** (4), 218–237.
8. Caulkins, J. and Reuter, P. (2006) Illicit Drug Markets and Economic Irregularities. *Socio-Economic Planning Sciences*, **40** (1), 1–14.
9. International Narcotics Control Board (2004) *Reports 2001-2004*. United Nations, Vienna.
10. Room, R. (2000) Concepts and items in measuring social harm from drinking. *Journal of Substance Abuse*, **12** (1–2), 93–111.
11. Musto, D. (1992) *Pautas en el abuso de drogas y la respuesta en Estados Unidos. En: El combate a las drogas en América*, Peter H. Smith, compilador. Fondo de Cultura Económica, México.
12. Mäkelä, K., Room, R., Single, E. *et al.* (1981) *Alcohol Society and the State: 1. A Comparative Study of Alcohol Control*, Addiction Research Foundation, Toronto.
13. United Nations Office on Drugs and Crime (UNODC) (2009) *World Drug Report 2009*. Vienna, Austria.
14. United Nations Office on Drugs and Crime (UNODC) (2008) *The Threat of Narco-Trafficking in the Americas*, Vienna.
15. Medina-Mora, M.E., Cravioto, P., Villatoro, J. *et al.* (2001) *Estudios en población general: Encuestas de Hogares*, En Observatorio Epidemiológico sobre Adicciones. SSA, México.
16. Villatoro, J., Medina-Mora, M.E., Cravioto, P. *et al.* (2003) *Uso y abuso de drogas en México: Resultado de la Encuesta Nacional de Adicciones 2002. En Observatorio Mexicano en Tabaco,

Alcohol y Otras Drogas 2003. Ed. Secretaría de Salud. Editorial: Consejo Nacional contra las Adicciones, CONADIC.

17. Consejo Nacional contra las Adicciones, Instituto Nacional de Psiquiatría Ramón de la Fuente, Instituto Nacional de Salud Pública, Secretaría de Salud. *Encuesta Nacional de Adicciones, 2008.* México: Instituto Nacional de Salud Pública, Cuernavaca, Morelos, México, 172 páginas.

18. Barros, H. (2008) Report on the State of the Drug Situation in Brazil, Proceedings from the Meeting of the Red Latinoamericano de Investigadores sobre Drogas (REDLA).

19. United Nations Office for Drug Control and Crime Prevention (2000) *World Drug Report 2000.* United Nations Office for Drug Control and Crime Prevention, Great Britain.

20. United Nations Office on Drugs and Crime (UNODC). *World Drug Report 2007.* Vienna, Austria.

21. Gureje, O., Adeyemi, O., Enyidah, N. *et al.* (2008) Mental disorders among adult Nigerians: risks, prevalence, and treatment, in *The WHO World Mental Health Surveys: Global Perspectives on the Epidemiology of Mental Disorders* (eds. R.C. Kessler and T.B. Ustun), Cambridge University Press, New York.

22. Huang, Y., Liu, Z., Zhang, M. *et al.* (2008) Mental disorders and service use in China 447, in *The WHO World Mental Health Surveys: Global Perspectives on the Epidemiology of Mental Disorders* (eds. R.C. Kessler and T.B. Ustun), Cambridge University Press, New York.

23. Posada-Villa, J., Rodríguez, M., Duque, P. *et al.* (2008) Mental disorders in Colombia: Results from the world mental health survey, in *The WHO World Mental Health Surveys: Global Perspectives on the Epidemiology of Mental Disorders* (eds. R.C. Kessler and T.B. Ustun), Cambridge University Press, New York.

24. Herman, A., Williams, D., Stein, D.J. *et al.* (2008) The South African stress and health study (SASH): A foundation for improving mental health care in South Africa, in *The WHO World Mental Health Surveys: Global Perspectives on the Epidemiology of Mental Disorders* (eds. R.C. Kessler and T.B. Ustun), Cambridge University Press, New York.

25. Bromet, E.J., Gluzman, S.F., Tintle, N.L. *et al.* (2008). The state of mental health and alcoholism in Ukraine, in *The WHO World Mental Health Surveys: Global Perspectives on the Epidemiology of Mental Disorders* (eds. R.C. Kessler and T.B. Ustun), Cambridge University Press, New York.

26. Karam, E.G., Mneimneh, Z.N., Karam, A.N. *et al.* (2008) Mental disorders and war in Lebanon 265, in *The WHO World Mental Health Surveys: Global Perspectives on the Epidemiology of Mental Disorders* (eds. R.C. Kessler, T.B. Ustun), Cambridge University Press, New York.

27. Medina-Mora, M.E., Borges, G., Lara, C. *et al.* (2008) The Mexican national comorbidity survey (M-NCS): overview and results 144, in *The WHO World Mental Health Surveys: Global Perspectives on the Epidemiology of Mental Disorders* (eds. R.C. Kessler and T.B. Ustun), Cambridge University Press, New York.

28. Kessler, R., Berglund, P., Chiu, W.T. *et al.* (2008) The national comorbidity survey replication (NCS-R): Cornerstone in improving mental health and mental health care in the United States 165, in *The WHO World Mental Health Surveys: Global Perspectives on the Epidemiology of Mental Disorders* (eds. R.C. Kessler and T.B. Ustun), Cambridge University Press, New York.

29. Oakley-Browne, M.A., Wells, E. and Scott, K.M. (2008) The New Zealand mental health survey 486, in *The WHO World Mental Health Surveys: Global Perspectives on the Epidemiology of Mental Disorders* (eds. R.C. Kessler and T.B. Ustun), Cambridge University Press, New York.

30. Sistema de Vigilancia Epidemiológica SISVEA. (2007) *Informe 2007. Subsecretaría de Prevención y Promoción de la Salud*, Dirección General Adjunta de Epidemiología. Secretaría de Salud, México.

31. Kessler, R. and Ustun, T.B. (2008) *The WHO World Mental Health Surveys: Global Perspectives on the Epidemiology of Mental Disorders*, Cambridge University Press, New York.

32. Medina Mora, M.E. (2008) El papel del género en la demanda de atención por problemas asociados al consumo de alcohol en México. *Revista Panamericana De Salud Pública*, **23** (4), 231–236.

33. Wang, P., Angermeyer, M., Borges, G. *et al.* (2007) Delay and failure in treatment seeking after first onset of mental disorders in the World Health Organization's World Mental Health Survey Initiative. *World Psychiatry*, **6** (3), 177–185.

34. Mathers, B.M., Degenhardt, L., Phillips, B. *et al.* (2008) Global epidemiology of injecting drug use and HIV among people who inject drugs: a systematic review. *The Lancet*, **372**, 1733–1745.

35. UNAIDS (2009) HIV prevention among injecting drug users 24th Meeting of the UNAIDS. Programme Coordinating Board UNAIDS/PCB, Geneva, Switzerland.

36. Magis-Rodríguez, C., Lemp, G., Hernandez, M.T. *et al.* (2009) Going North: Mexican migrants and their vulnerability to HIV. *Journal of Acquired Immune Deficiency Syndromes*, **1** (51), 1:S21.

37. United Nations Office on Drugs and Crime UNODC (2007) Crime and Development in Central America: Caught in the Crossfire. *Mesoamerica*, United Nations Publication.

38. Medina-Mora, M.E., Villatoro, J., López, E. *et al.* (1995) Los factores que se relacionan con el inicio, el uso continuado y el abuso de sustancias psicoactivas en adolescentes mexicanos. *Gaceta Médica de México*, **131**, 383–387.

39. Borges, G., Medina-Mora, M.E., Philip, S. *et al.* (2006) Treatment and adequacy of treatment of mental disorders among respondents to the Mexico national comorbidity survey. *American Journal of Psychiatry*, **163**, 1371–1378.

40. United Nations Office on Drug Control and Crime Prevention (UNODCCP) (2001) *Global Illicit Drug Trends 2001*, New York.

41. Commission on Narcotic Drugs (2000). First biennial report of the Executive Director on the implementation of the outcome of the twentieth special session of the General Assembly, devoted to countering the world drug problem together, Geneva.

42. National Institute on Drug Abuse (2005) Research Repport Series. Marijuana. Research Repport Series. Heroin. Research Repport Series. Inhalant Abuse, National Institute on Drug Abuse.

43. United Nations Office on Drugs and Crime (UNODC) (2008) *The Threat of Narco-Trafficking in the Americas*. This report has not been formally edited.

44. Substance Abuse and Mental Health Services Administration (2008) *Results from the 2007 National Survey on Drug Use and Health: National Findings* (Office of Applied Studies, NSDUH Series H-34, DHHS Publication No. SMA 08-4343), Rockville, MD, p. 28.

45. Consejo Nacional para el Control de Estupefacientes (CONACE) (2006) Ministerio del Interior Gobierno de Chile Sexto estudio nacional de drogas en población escolar de Chile, 2005 8o básico a 4o medio.

46. Comisión Interamericana para el Control del Abuso de Drogas (CICAD) (2006) Primer estudio comparativo sobre uso de drogas en población escolar secundaria. www.cicad.oas.org/oid/NEW/Statistics/siduc/InfoFinal_Estudio_Comparativo.pdf [Accessed July 2009].

47. Encuesta Nacional sobre Prevención y Consumo de Drogas (2002). *Población urbana de 12 a 64 años. Perú.* www.opd.gob.pe/cdoc/_cdocumentacion/estadistica_opd/demanda.pdf [Accessed July 2009].

48. Dormitzer, C.M. and Gonzalez, G.B. (2004). The PACARDO research project: Youthful drug involvement in Central America and the Dominican Republic. *Rev Panam Salud Publica*, **15**, 400–416.

49. Johnston, L.D., O'Malley, P.M., Bachman, J.G. *et al.* (2008) *Monitoring the Future National Results on Adolescent Drug Use: Overview of Key Findings 2008, National Institute of Drug Abuse*, National Institute of Health, Bethesda, MD.

50. United Nations (2008) *World Drug Report 2008*, United Nations, Office on Drugs and Crime. Viena.

51. International Narcotics Control Board (2001) *Annual Report 2001*, United Nations.

52. Centros de Integración Juvenil (CIJ) (2001) *Demanda de tratamiento en: Observatorio Epidemiológico en Adicciones*, SSA, México.

53. National Institute on Drug Abuse (NIDA) (2009) Research Report Series. Cocaine: Abuse and addiction. National Institute on Drug Abuse.

54. Villatoro, J., Medina-Mora, M.E., Cardiel, H. *et al.* (1999) La situación del consumo de sustancias entre estudiantes de la Ciudad de México: medición otoño 1997. *Salud Mental* **22** (1), 18–30.

55. Secretaría de Salud (1998) Subsecretaría de Prevención y Control de Enfermedades, Instituto Mexicano de Psiquiatría, Dirección General de Epidemiología, Consejo Nacional Contra las Adicciones. *Encuesta Nacional de Adicciones*.

56. United Nations Office on Drugs and Crime (2005) *Coca Cultivation in the Andean Region. A Survey of Bolivia, Colombia and Peru*, Viena.

57. Encuesta Nacional de Adicciones (2008) Secretaría de Salud, Instituto Nacional de Salud, Pública, Instituto Nacional de Psiquiatría Ramón de la Fuente Muñiz.

58. Medina-Mora, M.E., Villatoro, J. and Fleiz, C. (1999) Uso indebido de sustancias. En: Estudio de niños, niñas y adolescentes entre 6 y 17 años. *Trabajadores en 100 ciudades*, **7**, 369–374.

59. Medina-Mora, M.E. (2000) *Estudio de Niñas, Niños y Jóvenes Trabajadores en el Distrito Federal. Capítulo de Abuso de Sustancias*, DIF/UNICEF, México.

60. Villatoro J., Medina-Mora, M.E., Fleiz, C. *et al.* (2001). *Estudios en estudiantes de enseñanza media y media superior. Ciudad de México*, en Observatorio Epidemiológico en Adicciones, SSA, México.

61. Alberta Alcohol and Drug Abuse Commission. Canadian Addiction Survey 2004, Alberta report. 2006 Edmonton, Alberta, Canada: http://www.aadac.com/documents/cas2004_alberta_detail.pdf [Accessed July 2009].

62. Martínez Mantilla, J.A., Amaya-Naranjo, W., Campillo, H.A. *et al.* (2007) Consumo de substancias psicoactivas en adolescentes, Bucaramanga, Colombia, 1996–2004. *Revista de Salud Pública*, **9** (2), 215–229.

63. SAMHSA The NSDUH report (2007) Patterns and Trends in Inhalant Use by Adolescent Males and Females: 2002–2005. http://www.oas.samhsa.gov/2k7/inhalants/inhalants.htm [Accessed July 2009].

64. Wu, L.T. and Ringwalt, C.L. (2006) Inhalant use and disorders among adults in the United States. *Drug Alcohol Depend*, **15; 85** (1), 1–11.

65. Carlini, E.A. (2005) *II Encuesta domiciliaria sobre uso de drogas psicotrópicas en Brasil: estudio en 108 ciudades del país, 2005. Brasilia*: Centro Brasileño de Información sobre Drogas. Secretaria Nacional Antidrogas. 2006, 468 p. http://www.unifesp.br/dpsicobio/cebrid/lev_domiciliar2005/index.htm [Accessed July 2009].

66. Organización de Estados Americanos (OEA), Comisión Interamericana para el Control del Abuso de Drogas (CICAD), Observatorio Interamericano sobre Drogas (OID), Sistema Interamericano de Datos Uniformes Sobre Consumo de Drogas (SIDUC) (2003) Informe Comparativo 7 Países, encuestas escolares a nivel nacional: El Salvador, Guatemala, Nicaragua, Panamá, Paraguay, República Dominicana y Uruguay 2003.

67. Adalaf, E. and Paglia-Boak, A. (2007) Drug use among Ontario Students 1997–2007. www.camh.net/Research/Areas_of_research/Population_Life_Course_Studies/OSDUS/OSDUHS2007_Drug Detailed_final.pdf [Accessed August 2009].

68. Observatorio Español sobre Drogas (2004) *Informe 2004. Situación y tendencias de los problemas de drogas en España.* http://www.pnsd.msc.es/Categoria2/publica/pdf/oed-2004.pdf [Accessed August 2009].

69. Dormitzer, C.M. and Gonzalez, G.B. (2004). The PACARDO research project: Youthful drug involvement in Central America and the Dominican Republic. *Revista Panamericana de Salud Pública*, **15**, 400–416.

70. United Nations Office on Drugs and Drug Conrol (UNODC), the Inter-American Drug Abuse Control Commission (CICAD/OAS) (2006) *Youth and Drugs in South American Countries: A Public Policy Challenge. First Comparative Study of Drug Use in the Secondary School Student Population in Argentina, Bolivia, Brazil, Colombia, Chile, Ecuador, Paraguay, Peru and Uruguay,* Lima, Peru.

71. National Institute on Drug Abuse (2006) Research Report Series. Methamphetamine: Abuse and Addiction. National Institute on Drug Abuse.

72. European Monitoring Center for Drugs and Drug Addiction (2006) Annual report 2006: the state of the drug problem in Europe. www.emcdda.europa.eu/publications/searchresults [Accessed August 2009].

73. National Survey on Drug Use and Health (2008) The NSDUH Report. http://www.oas.samhsa.gov/2k8/hallucinogens/hallucinogens.htm [Accessed August 2009].

74. National Institute on Drug Abuse (2005d) Research Repport Series. Prescription Drugs: Abuse and addiction. National Institute on Drug Abuse.

75. Substance Abuse and Mental Health Service Administration (SAMHSA) (2007). Results from the 2007 National Survey on Drug Use and Health: National Findings. http://oas.samhsa.gov/nsduh/2k7nsduh/2k7Results.pdf [Accessed August 2009].

76. Drug Policy Alliance: Africa (2005) www.drugpolicy.org/global/drugpolicyby/africa [Accessed August 2009].

77. Odejide, A.O. (2006) Status of drug use/abuse in Africa: a review. *International Journal of Mental Health and Addiction*, **4**, 87–102.

78. Morakinyo, O. and Odejide, A.O. (2003) A community based study of patterns of psychoactive substance use among street children in a local government area of Nigeria. *Drug and Alcohol Dependence*, **71**, 109–116.

79. Degenhardt, L., Chiu, W.T., Sampson, N. *et al.* (2008) Toward a global view of alcohol, tobacco, cannabis, and cocaine use: findings from the WHO World Health Surveys. *PLoS Medicine*, **5**, 141.

CHAPTER 2

Drug Abuse: Prevention

Vladimir B. Poznyak[1], MD, PhD, James White[2], PhD and Nicolas Clark[3], MBBS, MPH, MD

[1] *Training and Research Centre, Belarussian
Psychiatric Association, Minsk, Belarus*
[2] *Research Associate in Social Epidemiology,
Cardiff University, United Kingdom*
[3] *Institute for Health Services Research, Monash University,
Melbourne, Australia*

2.1 INTRODUCTION

In the context of this chapter the term 'drug' mainly refers to illicit drugs such as cocaine, cannabis, amphetamine-type stimulants and heroin, and to the nonmedical use of psychoactive medications, such as benzodiazepines or opioid analgesics. The psychoactive effects of cannabis, opiates and coca leaves have been known for centuries, but only recently have drug use and related problems become a threat to global public health and a security and development problem. The prevalence, patterns and contexts of drug use vary significantly across countries, but there are many similarities in health and social problems caused by different drugs that are mainly determined by their psychoactive properties, ways of administration and behavioural manifestations of the drug-dependence syndrome. According to UNODC estimates, in 2007 between 172 and 250 million people aged 15–64 have used illicit drugs at least once during the past year, and the most commonly used drugs in the world are cannabis and amphetamine-type stimulants. The global estimates of 'problem drug users' range from 18 to 38 million [1]. A significant proportion of 'problem drug users' are individuals suffering from drug dependence.

Following advances in international epidemiological research, new data has become available on cross-country comparisons of drug use and drug-use disorders. Data from the WHO World Mental Health Surveys indicate that the estimated cumulative incidence of cannabis use is as high as 42% in the US and New Zealand, whereas in China and Japan it is less than 2% in populations. Similar differences are observed in estimated cumulative incidence of cocaine use [2]. The prevalence of drug-use disorders (i.e. abuse and dependence) in populations is significantly lower than prevalence of drug use *per se*,

Substance Abuse Disorders: Evidence and Experience, First Edition. Edited by Hamid Ghodse, Helen Herrman, Mario Maj and Norman Sartorius.
© 2011 John Wiley & Sons, Ltd. Published 2011 by John Wiley & Sons, Ltd.

though up to now very few countries have good epidemiological data on prevalence of drug-use disorders based on the data from representative surveys. One of the large-scale epidemiological studies conducted in the Unites States of America reported an overall lifetime prevalence of illicit drug abuse and dependence, including prescription drug-use disorders, of 6.2% [3] and results of a more recent survey report the lifetime prevalence of drug abuse and dependence at 7.7 and 2.6%, respectively [4]. Reported past-year prevalence of drug-use disorders was 2.8% in one of the recent surveys conducted in the United States of America [5]. During recent years there is a growing concern over the increasing rates of nonmedical use of psychoactive medications [6].

2.2   HEALTH AND SOCIAL CONSEQUENCES OF DRUG USE AND DRUG-ATTRIBUTABLE BURDEN

For many drugs even a single episode of use may be associated with increased risk of negative health consequences, including perceptual distortions or impairment of thinking and judgement in acute intoxication, respiratory depression in overdose, injury, or infection with HIV or HCV (in the case of injecting drug use or high-risk sexual behaviour under the influence of drugs). Repeated exposure to drugs is associated with increased levels of health risks and may result in the development of drug dependence. From the public-health perspective, of particular importance is injecting drug use (with its associated high risk of transmission of blood-borne viruses and infectious diseases), opioid overdoses, drug-related injuries (including suicides) and drug dependence. Injection drug use continues to be the major risk factor for HIV transmission in many countries, particularly in Asia and Eastern Europe [7].

The WHO comparative assessment of 24 global risk factors to health included alcohol, illicit drugs and tobacco use. In the recent 2008 update (based on 2004 data) illicit drug use occupies the 19th position amongst 24 leading risk factors to global health based on the proportion of disease burden expressed in disability-adjusted life years (DALYs) lost and attributable to these risk factors [101]. According to the global estimates for 2004, 245 000 deaths globally, or 0.4% of all deaths, and 0.9% of the global disease burden expressed in DALYs were attributable to illicit drug use (Table 2.1). This is an underestimate of the real burden attributable to drug use as the analysis included only heroin, cocaine and amphetamine-type stimulant use. In the structure of the disease burden attributable to drugs the majority (about 65%) of the disease burden is due to drug-use disorders *per se*, followed by HIV/AIDS, self-inflicted injuries and road-traffic accidents due to drug use. The disease burden attributable to illicit drugs is significantly lower that the disease burden attributable to alcohol or tobacco [8], which is also related to the lower prevalence of drug use.

Drug use and drug-use disorders are associated with numerous social consequences such as crimes, road-traffic accidents, violence, decreased productivity at work, absenteeism and unemployment. The national economic cost of drug use can be substantial, accounting for almost 2% of GDP in [9], similar to that of tobacco and alcohol and is largely determined by the costs associated with drug-related crimes and productivity losses, followed by road accidents and health-care costs [9, 10]. Prevention of drug abuse and drug-related harm has become a priority area for the international community and national governments around the world.

2.3   TARGETS FOR PREVENTION

There are different conceptual approaches to the prevention of drug use and drug-related harm, and none of them is fully satisfactory. A common approach to reducing drug-related problems encompasses supply-reduction strategies, which are beyond the scope of this chapter, demand-reduction strategies, and these two approaches are often complemented by the approach of harm reduction that is focused on reduction of drug-related harm, while not necessarily addressing the demand for psychoactive substances. Recent developments in epidemiology of drug use and psychosocial and biological determinants of drug use and dependence further inform the process of target setting for preventive efforts in this area.

2.4   REDUCING THE BURDEN ATTRIBUTABLE TO DRUG USE

In order to reduce drug-attributable burden it is important to address the major causal factors of premature deaths and disability associated with drug use. One of the key targets is prevention of drug dependence *per se*, which is often associated with substantial impairment and disability, also due to extended periods of severe intoxication and withdrawal. The neurobiological basis and clinical signs of drug dependence determine particular high-risk behaviours of significant public-health importance, such as impaired capacity to control drug-taking behaviour, neglect of associated risks, and persistence with drug use despite obvious negative consequences to health and social functioning.

Prevention of HIV and other blood-borne pathogen transmission attributable to drug use involves preventing and reducing injection drug use, reducing the health risks associated with injecting, such as, for example, through making available sterile injecting equipment, and preventing drug-related high-risk sexual behaviour. As a rule, repeated drug injecting is associated with drug dependence, and effective treatment of dependence is one of the key prevention strategies. Prevention of acute intoxication due to use of drugs is also an important prevention target in view of the role of intoxication in road accidents, violence and high-risk sexual behaviour.

Overall, at the population level, reduction of health and social burden attributable to drug use requires multisectoral and multilevel actions with different targets [11], and effective prevention strategies should address levels of exposure to drugs in populations, patterns and context of drug use amongst drug users, and broad socioeconomic and other environmental factors associated with increased risk of drug use and drug-related harm (Figure 2.1).

2.5   TRAJECTORIES OF DRUG USE: PRIMARY, SECONDARY AND TERTIARY PREVENTION

Incidence and prevalence of drug use varies significantly in populations, reflecting the diversity and complexity of factors influencing drug use in populations. Of those who start to use drugs in adolescence about half develop drug abuse or dependence [13]. Repeated exposure to drugs with known dependence-producing properties is always associated with the risk of drug dependence, and for some vulnerable individuals and population groups this risk could be well above the average population level. Animal models of drug dependence

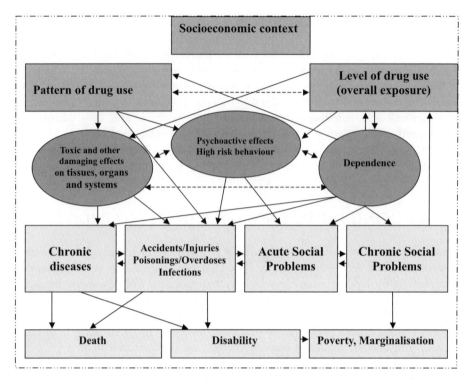

Figure 2.1   Mechanisms of drug-attributable health and social burden. Based on [12].

and drug-taking behaviour, demonstrated in different animals of the mammalian family and for the same drugs that are abused by people, indicate intrinsic and universal (across different mammalian species) biological mechanisms of vulnerability to drug dependence [14].

From the perspective of trajectories of drug use from its first episode through repeated drug use to particular patters of drug use within the frame of the dependence syndrome with potential numerous health and social consequences, the traditionally used distinction of primary, secondary and tertiary prevention [15] is a useful conceptual approach (Figure 2.2).

Within this approach primary prevention of drug-use disorders would include prevention of initiation of drug use and prevention of repeated and frequent drug use and facilitation of its cessation. At the population level effective primary prevention efforts are expected

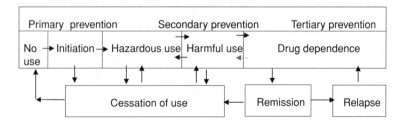

Figure 2.2   Trajectories of drug use and prevention continuum. Based on [102].

to reduce the levels of exposure of population to illicit drugs and reduce the incidence of drug-use disorders. Controlling the level of exposure to drugs protects individuals and population groups with high vulnerability to drug dependence, particularly important are those with genetic predisposition to substance dependence [16]. Primary prevention activities usually include health promotion and the activities addressing a broad range of social determinants of health [17], which are relevant for drug use and drug-related harm: from drug-policy frameworks to inequities and inequalities in health between and within countries. Sometimes such broad, nonspecific and primarily sociopolitical preventive strategies are distinguished from primary prevention interventions targeting specific causal factors and are conceptualized as primordial prevention aimed at 'avoiding emergence and establishment of the social, economic and cultural patterns of living that are known to contribute to an elevated risk of disease' [18].

Secondary prevention, involves early identification and management of disorders in order to reduce their prevalence in populations. Secondary prevention has particular importance for health-care professionals and health-care systems, and within the context of drug-use disorders it is important that this concept includes not only early identification and management of harmful use of drugs or drug abuse and drug dependence, but also repeated drug use that is associated with increased risk of health consequences even in the absence of harmful use and dependence syndrome. Data on the effectiveness and cost effectiveness of brief interventions for hazardous and harmful use of alcohol [19] and emerging evidence of effectiveness of similar approaches for illicit drug use [20] suggest a significant public-health importance of this approach if implemented in health-care settings. Secondary prevention also includes early identification and treatment of drug dependence, including pharmacological approaches such as, for example, opioid agonist pharmacotherapy for opioid dependence with its well-documented profile of effectiveness [21], although drug-dependence treatment is discussed elsewhere in the book. In the context of clinical practice, secondary prevention should also be considered to include treatment of co-morbid conditions that have a significant impact on the clinical course and outcomes of drug-use disorders [22, 23].

Tertiary prevention aims at reducing disability and health and social consequences of an established disease or a disorder. In the context of drug-use disorders tertiary prevention can include harm-reduction interventions, including those aimed at prevention of infectious diseases amongst drug-dependent injecting drug users, as well as the efforts aimed at restoring at the highest possible level social functioning of affected individuals.

2.6 PREVENTIVE INTERVENTIONS: UNIVERSAL, SELECTIVE AND INDICATED

A significant advancement in the development of evidence-based drug prevention programs was Hawkins, Catalano and Miller's [24] review of risk and protective factors for alcohol and drug abuse during adolescence. It was suggested that prevention programs should have a dual focus: 1) they should attempt to mitigate factors associated with the onset or progression of drug and alcohol use (risk factors) and 2) they should enhance factors associated with drug abstinence or a reduction in drug use (protective factors). More recent reviews of risk and protective factors have confirmed major findings from the previous reviews, but also added a developmental perspective by grouping risk and protective factors for different stages of development, from the period prior to birth to school age, adulthood and old age and not distinguishing specific risk factors for different types of psychoactive substances [25]. Amongst the risk factors identified for drug use at different stages of individual development are the following [11]:

- Prior to birth:
  - extreme social disadvantage and family economic deprivation;
  - maternal drug use in pregnancy.
- Infancy and preschool:
  - early school failure;
  - child neglect and abuse;
  - conduct disorder;
  - aggression.
- Secondary-school period:
  - low involvement in activities with adults;
  - perceived and actual levels of community drug use;
  - community disadvantage and disorganization;
  - availability of drugs within the community;
  - positive media portrayal of drug use;
  - parent–adolescent conflict;
  - favourable parental attitudes to drug use;
  - parental alcohol and drug problems;
  - parental rules permissive of drug use;
  - peer drug use;
  - delinquency;
  - sensation seeking and adventurous personality;
  - favourable attitudes to drug use.

Protective factors for development of drug use and drug-use disorders at school period include:

- social and emotional competence;
- religious involvement;
- family attachment;
- low parental conflict;
- parent-adolescent communication.

Advances in indentifying risk and protective factors for drug use prompted new conceptual approaches to drug prevention. The Institute of Medicine report [26] classified preventive interventions in the area of mental health into: a) 'universal' that target whole population or the general public with an aggregate average level of risk; b) 'selective' interventions that target population groups with the risk significantly above the average and c) 'indicated' interventions that target high-risk individuals with early signs of emerging disorders. Later 'targeted' interventions were added to this typology, which refer to a combination of selective and indicative interventions [25]. This theoretical framework facilitated the development of prevention programmes designed for particular populations. Selective and indicated preventive interventions, which are also relevant to prevention of drug use include: improving parenting and family functioning; enhancing child development, including social competence; enhancing academic achievement and school behaviour; increasing skills to resist social influences regarding substance use; promoting social norms against drug use; enhancing marital relationships; improving coping skills following divorce or job loss or death of a spouse; enhancing the personal development of new mothers; providing social support to caregivers of chronically ill family members [27]. As a rule, the prevalence of illicit drug use in populations is much lower than alcohol or tobacco use, and drug use and drug-use disorders tend to concentrate in population groups and individuals with a combination of different risk factors, and the balance of universal and targeted interventions for prevention of illicit drug use should be different to those for licit substances.

2.7   LEVELS OF INTERVENTIONS

Prevention of drug use implies several levels of activities that were described in the public health system model of prevention of alcohol and drug problems suggested by Lenton [28]. Prevention activities can be developed and implemented at the following levels:

- international;
- national;
- state (province);
- local community;
- organizational/institutional;
- group/individual/collective.

At the international level there are three main international treaties, which were negotiated and adopted for regulating supply and availability of psychoactive substances to prevent drug abuse and at the same time to ensure availability of drugs under international control for medical and scientific purposes:

- Single Convention on Narcotic Drugs, 1961, as amended by the 1972 Protocol Amending the Single Convention on Narcotic Drugs;
- Convention on Psychotropic Substances, 1971;
- Convention Against Illicit Traffic in Narcotic Drugs and Psychotropic Substances, 1988.

In implementation of the conventions it is critical to guarantee the availability of narcotic drugs, regulated under the Single Convention on Narcotic Drugs and Psychotropic Medicines, regulated under the Convention on Psychotropic Substances, for Medical and Scientific Purposes. Several drugs under the international control are included in the WHO Model List of Essential Medicines such as codeine, methadone and morphine that are regulated under the Single Convention of 1961 and buprenorphine, diazepam, lorazepam and phenobarbital that are regulated under the Convention on psychotropic substances of 1971 [29]. Coordination of prevention and treatment policies at the international level is discussed at the sessions of the Commission on Narcotic Drugs (CND) held each year in Vienna. In 2009 a new Political Declaration and Plan of Action on International Cooperation towards an Integrated and Balanced Strategy to Counter the World Drug Problem was adopted. The Political Declaration emphasizes the need for a comprehensive approach to demand reduction and related measures and highlights key approaches for action, including the emphasis on human rights and dignity, scientific evidence, availability and accessibility of demand-reduction services, and the targeting of vulnerable groups and conditions [30].

At the national and state/province levels prevention of drug use and drug-use disorders involves a range of measures in the following domains of preventive actions:

- National and subnational policies, plans and regulations, which involve specific drug policies and plans, those that correspond to legal obligations under the international treaties, as well as those that address socioeconomic determinants of health, risk and protective factors for drug use and drug-related harm, law enforcement, general health care and education.
- Policies and regulations with regard to psychotropic drugs and other medicines with abuse potential that reduce the risk of diversion from licit channels and nonmedical use, while ensuring their availability for medical and scientific purposes for all those in need and their rational use within health-care systems.
- Development of appropriate coordinating mechanisms and structures for implementation of the relevant policies, plans and regulations according to the national context and epidemiological situation with drug use and drug-use disorders.
- Ensuring the access to information and public awareness programs with regard to health and other risks associated with drug use and national/state policies and regulations avoiding the stigmatization of people with drug-use disorders, and raising awareness of information on treatment and care alternatives for affected individuals and their families.
- Developing and maintaining the capacity of health-care and social-welfare sectors to provide effective prevention and treatment interventions, particularly at the early stages of development of drug-use disorders, treatment of drug dependence and co-morbid conditions and rehabilitation of affected individuals.
- Developing supportive policy frameworks and implementation mechanisms for effective prevention of drug use and drug-related harm in prisons and other closed settings, also ensuring implementation of diversion schemes from law enforcement to public health and social welfare systems.
- Developing sustainable national and subnational systems of monitoring and surveillance of drug use and drug-use disorders in order to assess and monitor the levels, patterns and contexts of drug use and the magnitude and nature of drug-related harm in societies to inform policy and programme development. Effective monitoring and surveillance mechanisms are essential for evaluation of implemented policies, programmes and regulations and the results of evaluation should guide further prevention activities at the national and subnational levels.

At the community level preventive interventions can take into consideration the specific local determinants and community risk and protective factors for drug use and drug-use disorders. Communities have a particular role in supporting local cultural norms discouraging drug use and creating a health-promoting environment. Communities have the capacity to mobilize societal responses at the local level to such problems as drug use, but it is the responsibility of authorities to ensure that community responses are ethical, orientated towards public-health goals and supportive of people affected by drug dependence. Adequate information and education campaigns facilitate the acceptance by communities of their responsibilities in reducing drug-related harm. Successful community prevention programs build upon the existing community networks, sustain their actions by institutionalization of prevention activities and have a strong perception of ownership of the programs by the target communities [31, 32].

Prevention policies and programs at the organizational/institutional level usually include the workplaces, educational institutions, health- and social-care organizations and institutions. A 'zero-tolerance' approach is often being implemented and enforced in workplaces and military settings, particularly when the work is associated with security and safety concerns. With advances in relevant technologies, drug testing is becoming a commonly used approach to detect recent use of drugs amongst employees, military servicemen, students and clients of health-care settings, particularly emergency rooms and programs for treatment of substance-use disorders [33]. Drug testing in educational and health-care institutions raises ethical and programme questions with regard to, amongst others, informed consent, individual autonomy, risk of breaching confidentiality and utility of testing results [34, 35]. Prevention of drug use at schools involves the provision of a caring, supportive and safe environment, high expectations of academic achievements by students, clear standards and rules for appropriate behaviour, and participation and involvement of students in school tasks and decisions [36, 37].

At the group/individual/collective level prevention activities may include promotion and support of involvement with positive peer-group activities and norms and resistance to negative pressures from peers who use drugs and engage in other forms of problem behaviour [24, 38]. Peer education and outreach is one of the key components of a harm-reduction approach amongst injecting drug users aimed primarily at prevention of HIV and other health consequences of injection drug use [39]. Family settings are the key in promoting the health of children and adolescents and reducing the risk of drug use and drug-use disorders. The most important preventive factors in family settings include: developing and maintaining high levels of family attachment and warmth and an absence of severe criticism; clear family rules and expectations, including high expectations, for children; low parental conflict; disapproval and discouragement of drug use; active involvement of children in family life and responsibilities; and an absence of alcohol and drug problems in a family [25, 40–42].

2.8   PRINCIPLES FOR DRUG PREVENTION

To be effective, activities aimed at the prevention of drug use and drug-use disorders should address levels, patterns and context of drug use in populations and different populations groups as well as socioeconomic determinants of drug use and drug-related harm. The maximal reduction of drug-attributable disease and social burden requires not only minimization of the health consequences of drug use, but also reducing, to the extent possible, nonmedical use of dependence-producing substances. Integrated approaches to the prevention of health and social consequences of licit and illicit drug use are recommended [43]. Based on the reviews of available evidence on the origins of drug use behaviour and effectiveness of prevention programs, the National Institute of Drug Abuse (NIDA) in the USA developed a set of prevention principles in order to guide planning and implementation of drug prevention programs at the community level with a focus on children and adolescents [44] (Table 2.2).

2.9 EVIDENCE ON EFFECTIVENESS OF PREVENTION INTERVENTIONS

Hundreds of programs have been implemented around the world to prevent drug use and drug-use disorders without attempts to evaluate their effectiveness and cost effectiveness. The majority have been implemented amongst adolescents in school-based and other settings. With increasing pressure from the governments and funding agencies to demonstrate effectiveness of drug-prevention interventions, several reviews of the evidence of effectiveness of different interventions have been undertaken in the past decade [11, 25, 42] and the number of methodologically sound studies on effectiveness of drug-prevention interventions is growing. At the same time the evaluation of broad prevention efforts at the population level continues to present significant challenges and very little data is available for policy makers to evaluate the effectiveness of the wide range of interventions. Besides, the available research data comes predominantly from very few developed countries, and the generalizability of findings to other societies with different cultural norms and levels of development remains in question. In this section we summarize the evidence on primary and secondary drug-prevention programs.

2.10 CONTROL OF AVAILABILITY OF DRUGS AND JUDICIAL PROCEDURES

There is convincing data on the importance of regulating the availability of alcohol for reducing the harm attributable to the use of these substances [45].

With regard to illicit drugs the actions to reduce their availability at the community level usually involves policing and law-enforcement interventions that are aimed at reducing supply and, therefore, increasing street prices of drugs and diminishing their physical and economic availability [46]. Research data in this area is very scarce, and very often it is not possible to quantify policing interventions in a way appropriate for research projects, but available data indicates that law-enforcement actions have an impact on the market of illicit drugs, but do not result in eradication of drug supply. Besides, controlling availability of drugs by appropriate law-enforcement measures sends a message of social disapproval of drug use, reinforces social norms against drug use and may indirectly encourage dependent drug users to enter treatment. However, the enforcement of a 'zero-tolerance' approach or application of criminal sanctions for drug use and possession for personal use may have unintended consequences of public-health importance such as transitions to drug injection, more risky drug-taking behaviours, avoidance of drug treatment and other health care facilities, and increased number of arrested and incarcerated persons with drug-use disorders [42, 47, 103]. Besides, there is a growing awareness of the ineffectiveness of incarceration alone for addressing drug-use disorders. To prevent drug-related crimes and associated recidivism in drug-dependent individuals, the application of criminal sanctions alone is largely ineffective unless the underlying drug dependence is properly addressed by treatment and rehabilitation strategies. From the public-health perspective, significant societal benefits can be achieved by the implementation of diversion schemes from the criminal justice system to health-care and social-welfare systems. The accumulated experience of functioning of drug-treatment courts in several jurisdictions shows promising results [48, 49].

2.11 MASS MEDIA INTERVENTIONS

Mass media interventions, as a rule, receive broad support from communities, policy makers and the population at large. Often, mass media interventions are based on the assumption that providing education and information about, for example, health risks associated with substance use, will change the behaviours and reduce drug use in populations. The available evidence indicates that media campaigns have little effect on substance use behaviour, if any [50, 51], but are important for raising awareness of drug-related problems and rendering support of populations to implemented policy measures. To be effective, mass media interventions should have several components: well-defined target groups; undertaking research to understand the target groups and pretest campaign materials; use of messages based on current knowledge of target audiences and meeting the needs and motives of the target groups; a good media plan and a long-term commitment [52, 53].

2.12 PREVENTION PROGRAMS WITH SHORT-TERM AND LONG-TERM EFFECTS ON DRUG USE

Despite the wide range of interventions used in drug prevention, the majority of structured programs can be organized into two categories, 1) school based, 2) nonschool based. As education is mandated in most countries, schools and universities provide a setting to target adolescents and young adults at the population level in a systematic way and reach young people before drug use has occurred [54] or when the risk for drug use is still developing [55]. Nonschool based prevention programs enable preventive efforts to reach individuals who do chose not to attend schools, including older adolescents. These out-of-school settings can include youth clubs, primary care, emergency rooms, colleges, young-offender institutions, the family and the community [56]. The evidence on effectiveness from systematic reviews and meta-analysis of randomized control trials (RCTs) will be presented on programs that showed their impact on drug use over the short-term follow up (up to a year), medium term (1–3 years) and long term (+3 years). The evidence summarized below included studies (1) with a concurrent control with random allocation, (2) delivered to young people (under the age of 25), (3) attempting to prevent drug initiation when drug use at baseline was absent, (4) attempting to bring about a reduction or cessation of drug use, (5) used self-report or biologically validated measures of actual drug use. Control groups ranged from receiving no intervention, another school-based prevention program, or standard treatment (more common in secondary prevention). Any studies that did not report a measure of actual drug use were excluded from the analysis because studies that use attitudes, or behavioural intentions to use drugs as surrogate outcomes, cannot assume these outcomes provide an accurate estimate of changes in drug use. This included programs that attempted to change risk and protective factors including: knowledge about the effects of drugs on the body and mind; self-esteem; self-efficacy; locus of control; social anxiety; peer-pressure resistance; assertiveness; decision-making skills; adult or peer drug use; attitudes towards drugs and intentions to use drugs [57].

2.13   INTERVENTIONS WITH SHORT-TERM FOLLOW-UP (UP TO 1 YEAR)

2.13.1   Nonschool Settings

Several studies identified in this review showed no effect of prevention interventions compared with a control group for some if not all of the outcome measures reported over the short term [58–61]. Four studies provided evidence of a statistically significant benefit in favour of the intervention over controls arm over the short term. McGillicuddy *et al.* [62] reported a small effect ($\eta^2 = 0.8$) on parent reported cannabis use in the past fifty days, using a parenting and coping skills intervention. This effect was not repeated in a delayed intervention condition. Wu [63] reported a statistically significant reduction ($p = 0.04$) in self-report cannabis use over 12 months in the Focus on Kids (FoK) plus the Informed Parents and Children Together (ImPACT) intervention compared to control condition (FoK only). However, the program did not impact upon crack or cocaine use at six (RR = 1.00; 95% CI 0.36 to 2.77) or twelve months (RR = 1.04; 95% CI 0.30 to 3.65).

Two studies using a brief educational or motivational intervention provided evidence of an effect. Oliansky *et al.* [64] reported statistically significant differences in the mean scores on the Substance Use Screening Instrument (SUSI) at 3-month follow-up (intervention = 1.58; control = 7.46; $p = 0.04$), using brief educational content on the consequences of drug use to health provided by nurses in primary care. McCambridge and Strang [65] using brief motivational interviewing (60 min) reported significant decreases in the frequency of self-reported cannabis use in the intervention (15.7 times per week to 5.4) but not control groups (13.3 times per week to 16.9) at three-month follow-up. The intervention group was also less likely to use nonstimulant illicit drugs other than cannabis (OR = 0.32, 95% CI 0.12 to 0.82). There were, however, no differences in the use of stimulant drugs.

2.13.2   School-Based Settings

Four studies provided evidence of a statistically significant benefit in favour of the intervention over control arm over the short-term. Botvin *et al.* [66] reported significantly lower levels of self-reported cannabis use in the past month ($p < 0.05$), at one-year follow-up using the Life Skills Training Program. Also, fewer students reported using cannabis in the last month when booster sessions were delivered by older peers than by teachers. Hansen and Graham [67] reported fewer participants used cannabis in the past 30 days, at a one-year follow-up ($p = 0.009$) who received a normative education than a control or resistance skill training (Adolescent Alcohol Prevention Trial).

Two studies that evaluated the Project Towards No Drug Abuse (PTNDA), based on a health-motivation, social skills, decision-making approach. Dent, Sussman and Stacy [68] reported a large effect on the frequency of hard-drug use (cocaine/crack, hallucinogens, stimulants, inhalants) in the past month ($p < 0.001$), at a one-year follow-up. However, no effect was found for cannabis use. The same pattern of results was found in another study with a significant effect on an index of hard-drug use (SMD $= -0.59$; 95% CI -0.74 to -0.43) but not cannabis use (SMD$= 0.04$; 95% CI -0.11 to 0.19) [69]. This suggests the PTNDA is more effective in the secondary prevention of hard drug than cannabis use.

2.14 INTERVENTIONS WITH MEDIUM-TERM FOLLOW-UP (FROM 1 TO 3 YEARS)

2.14.1 Nonschool Settings

Four studies identified in this review showed no effect of the prevention interventions compared with a control group for some if not all of the outcome measures reported [60, 70–72].

No studies provided evidence of a statistically significant benefit in favour of the intervention over control arm over the medium term.

2.14.2 School-Based Settings

One study provided evidence of a statistically significant benefit in favour of the intervention over control arm over the medium term. Ellickson *et al.* [73] reported fewer individuals initiated cannabis use (RR $= 0.76$; 95% CI 0.66 to 0.88) in the intervention than control condition, using Project ALERT – a program based on improving resistance skills. However, this program did not produce a reduction in the frequency of cannabis use in existing users.

2.15 INTERVENTIONS WITH LONG-TERM FOLLOW-UP (3+ YEARS)

2.15.1 Nonschool Settings

Four studies identified in this review showed no effect of the prevention interventions compared with a control group for some if not all of the outcome measures reported [60, 61, 72, 74].

Two studies provided evidence of a statistically significant effect in favour of the intervention over control arm over the long term. Biglan [75] reported a small effect of a community program in addition to the school-based program on the prevalence of self-reported cannabis use in the past week at a two-year follow-up ($t(14) = 2.22$, $p = 0.04$). This comprehensive program incorporated modules on media advocacy, anti-tobacco, family communication and a module designed to stop stores selling tobacco to minors. Despite this success over two years, the marginal significance between the number of users at four

Table 2.1 Deaths and DALYs attributable to alcohol, tobacco and illicit drug use, and to all three risks together, by region, 2004.

Risk	World	Low and middle income	High income
Percentage of deaths			
Alcohol use	3.6	4.0	1.6
Illicit drugs	0.4	0.4	0.4
Tobacco use	8.7	7.2	17.9
All three risks	12.6	11.5	19.6
Percentage of DALYs			
Alcohol use	4.4	4.2	6.7
Illicit drugs	0.9	0.8	2.1
Tobacco use	3.7	3.1	10.7
All three risks	9.0	8.1	19.2

Source: WHO (2009)

years was small (6.7% versus 8.5%), suggests this program may have limited impact on cannabis use at the population level.

Spoth *et al.* [76] study investigating the Iowa Strengthening Families Program (ISFP), focused on improving parenting skills and parent–child communication, reported a statistically significant difference between control and intervention groups for lifetime (RR = 0.55; 95% CI 0.32 to 0.95) and cannabis use in the past year (RR = 0.44; 95% CI 0.20 to 0.96). The ISFP did not bring about a change in the use of inhalants or other drugs in the past year at the four- and six-year follow-up. Moreover, the difference between control and intervention groups in cannabis use (lifetime and in past year) at four years was nonsignificant. This suggests the effects of the ISFP may be restricted to slowing age-related increases in the prevalence (primary prevention) and frequency of cannabis use (secondary prevention).

2.15.2 School-Based Settings

Three studies identified in this review showed no effect of the school-based prevention interventions compared with a control group for some if not all of the outcome measures reported [77–79].

Two studies provided evidence of a statistically significant effect in favour of the intervention over control arm over the long term. Botvin *et al.* [80] reported a significant effect on the monthly (intervention mean = 0.10 vs. control mean = 0.14; $p < 0.01$) and weekly (intervention mean = 0.05 vs. control mean = 0.09; $p < 0.01$) frequency of cannabis use at a six-year follow-up for high-fidelity participants (i.e. attended 60% of sessions) in the Life Skills Training Program. However, analysis of the full sample, including those with attendance at less than 60% was nonsignificant.

Furr-Holden *et al.* [81] reported fewer participants in a classroom-centred intervention, based on improving classroom management and listening skills, had started using hard drugs (heroin, crack, cocaine) than in a standard education control group after five years. However, this intervention had a nonsignificant effect on preventing the onset of cannabis (RR = 0.68; 95% CI 0.42 to 1.10) and inhalants (e.g. glue, gases; RR = 1.00; 95% CI 0.60 to 1.66).

Table 2.2 NIDA principles of drug prevention [44].

1. Prevention programs should enhance protective factors and reverse or reduce risk factors.
2. Prevention programs should address all forms of drug abuse, alone or in combination, including the underage use of legal drugs (e.g., tobacco or alcohol); the use of illegal drugs (e.g. marijuana or heroin); and the inappropriate use of legally obtained substances (e.g., inhalants), prescription medications, or over-the-counter drugs.
3. Prevention programs should address the type of drug abuse problem in the local community, target-modifiable risk factors, and strengthen identified protective factors.
4. Prevention programs should be tailored to address risks specific to population or audience characteristics, such as age, gender and ethnicity, to improve program effectiveness.
5. Family-based prevention programs should enhance family bonding and relationships and include parenting skills; practice in developing, discussing, and enforcing family policies on substance abuse; and training in drug education and information.
6. Prevention programs can be designed to intervene as early as preschool to address risk factors for drug abuse, such as aggressive behaviour, poor social skills, and academic difficulties.
7. Prevention programs for elementary school children should target improving academic and social-emotional learning to address risk factors for drug abuse, such as early aggression, academic failure, and school dropout. Education should focus on the following skills:
   - self-control;
   - emotional awareness;
   - communication;
   - social problem solving; and
   - academic support, especially in reading.
8. Prevention programs for middle or junior high and high school students should increase academic and social competence with the following skills:
   - study habits and academic support;
   - communication;
   - peer relationship;
   - self-efficacy and assertiveness;
   - drug-resistance skills;
   - reinforcement of antidrug attitudes; and
   - strengthening or personal commitments against drug abuse.
9. Prevention programs aimed at general populations at key transition points, such as transition to middle school, can produce beneficial effects even amongst high-risk families and children. Such interventions do not single out risk populations and, therefore, reduce labelling and promote bonding to school and community.
10. Community prevention programs that combine two or more effective programs, such as family-based and school-based programs, can be more effective than a single program alone.
11. Community prevention programs reaching populations in multiple settings – for example, schools, clubs, faith-based organizations, and the media – are most effective when they present consistent, community-wide messages in each setting.
12. When communities adapt programs to match their needs, community norms, or differing cultural requirements, they should retain core elements of the original research-based intervention.
13. Prevention programs should be long-term with repeated interventions (i.e. booster programs) to reinforce the original prevention goals. Research shows that the benefits from middle school prevention programs diminish without follow up programs in high school.

(Continued)

Table 2.2   (*Continued*)

14. Prevention programs should include teacher training in good classroom management practices, such as rewarding appropriate student behaviour. Such techniques help to foster student's positive behaviour, achievement, academic motivation, and school bonding.
15. Prevention programs are most effective when they employ interactive techniques, such as peer discussion groups and parent role playing, that allow for active involvement in learning about drug abuse and reinforcing skills.
16. Research-based prevention programs can be cost effective. Similar to earlier research, recent research shows that for each dollar invested in prevention, a savings of up to $10 in treatment for alcohol or other substance abuse can be seen.

2.16   INTERVENTIONS WITH EVIDENCE OF LITTLE OR NO EFFECTIVENESS

There were a number of interventions for which there was little or no evidence for the effective prevention of drug use. These included: the social development and school/community intervention [74], Positive Alternatives for Youth [82], Adolescent Decision-Making Program [104] and the Alternatives programs [83]. One intervention, Drug Abuse Resistance Education (DARE), based on enhancing decision making, resistance skills and emphasizing the consequences of drug use, was ineffective in studies with follow-up periods of two [84], five [77] and ten years [79].

2.17   CONTENT AND DESIGN OF PROGRAMS WITH EVIDENCE OF EFFECTIVENESS

There was a lack of evidence that school-based or nonschool-based preventive programs were effective. Two prevention programmes, Life Skills Training Program [80] and the Iowa Strengthening Families Program [76] have received the most evidence of long-term effectiveness in systematic reviews [57, 85]. Additional investigation into more recent RCT evaluation of these programs has found The Life Skills Training Program delayed initiation of cannabis use over five and a half years [86]. Also, a ten-year follow-up of The Iowa Strengthening Families Program was found to significantly delay initiation, slow the rate of increase, and result in fewer users of illicit drugs (cannabis, prescription drugs, amphetamines, barbiturates, cocaine, ecstasy) in early adulthood [87]. Table 2.3 summarizes the components of the LST and ISFP programs.

2.18   EXPERIMENTAL TECHNIQUES

A number of new techniques are currently under development that blur the boundaries between prevention and treatment. Three are discussed here, e-Health, vaccines and depot and implantable medications.

Table 2.3 Components of prevention programs effective over 3+ years.

Program name	Intervention components	Content/elements
Life Skills Training Program	Target: 10–16 year olds Provider: Trained Teachers Setting: Schools Format: Face-to-face Intensity: 24–28 sessions of 40–45 minutes length Duration: a) Age 12–13 (7th grade) 15 sessions over a year; b) Age 13–14 (8th grade) 5–10 booster sessions over a year; c) Age 14–16 (9th–11th grade); 4–5 booster sessions over a year.	Goals: a) Build skills to recognize and resist peer and media pressure to use drugs; b) Teach basic self-management using cognitive behavioural techniques (e.g. managing stress and anxiety, building self-esteem, goal setting); c) Improve social skills (e.g. how to communicate directly, be assertive and develop relationships) Taught using: a) coaching and facilitating; b) role play and modelling; c) feedback and reinforcement; d) homework and out-of-class behavioural rehearsal.
Iowa Strengthening Families Program (ISFP)	Target: 10–14 year olds Provider: Trained program facilitators Setting: Schools in evening Format: Face-to-face, video/DVDs; Intensity: 7 sessions of one-hour length for both parents and children separately followed by a joint parent–child session; Duration: a) 7 consecutive weeks over second semester of 7th grade.	Goals: a) Enhance parenting skills (e.g. clarifying expectations, using appropriate disciplinary practices, managing emotions and communicating effectively); b) Increase family cohesiveness; improve and practise conflict resolution and communication skills. c) Build children's skills to resist peer pressure; d) Teach basic self-management using cognitive behavioural techniques (e.g. managing stress and strong emotions); Taught using: a) Separate and concurrent parent and child sessions; b) A 1-hour parent–child session to practice conflict resolution and communication skills.

2.18.1   'E-Health' and Internet-Based Prevention Approaches

A promising new variation on health promotion, screening and brief interventions and even more substantial treatment is offered by the growing number of 'e-Health' tools.

Consisting of the electronic enablement of public health and individualized health services, predominantly using the internet, individuals receive targeted information, and even treatment. From the perspective of prevention, there are a number of opportunities under development. Information on the risks of substance use can be targeted to individuals based on their internet browsing habits, in the form of advertising. Secondly, individualized feedback can be given on substance use, mimicking the brief intervention provided by health care providers, with regular reminders being provided by mobile phone, email or internet.

E-health fits very well in a client-centred health system. It offers the individual access to a good-quality (evidence-based) intervention, without waiting lists, and (virtually) without confidentiality and embarrassment concerns.

For policymakers, e-Health screening and interventions are attractive as they are of a consistent quality and can be easily be scaled-up, offering a solution when financial and human resources are scarce, while the quality of care is easily controlled.

A specific advantage of e-Health screening and brief intervention is that their validity and effectiveness are relatively easy to investigate. The effectiveness of internet measures in reducing harmful alcohol use has been demonstrated in one randomized trial [88] and real-world implementation [89], with several other studies currently underway. Studies specifically examining the applicability of this principle to reduce harmful drug use are needed.

2.18.2   Vaccines

In theory the impact of taking a drug of addiction can be blocked, or significantly lessened at least, by a vaccination that induces an immune response to that drug. Such vaccine can be produced by binding a large protein molecule with a drug such as cocaine, nicotine or heroin. The large protein molecule prevents the vaccine from crossing the blood/brain barrier and thus from having any central nervous system effects. If sufficiently high anti-body levels are achieved, they can effectively bind to circulating free molecules of psychoactive drugs within seconds, preventing any effect of the drugs. In practice, the immune response from one vaccination is typically not high enough to achieve this effect and multiple vaccinations are required to achieve an anti-body level that diminishes to a significant extent the effects of the drug. Furthermore the levels of circulating anti-bodies reduce over time and so regular booster injections are required. Nonetheless, such vaccines have led to significant reductions in cocaine [90] and nicotine [91] use in clinical trials. At this stage they appear more likely to be developed as treatments than as population-based public-health interventions.

2.18.3   Depot and Implantable Medications

The idea of depot medication as treatment is not new. Depot medications have been used in psychiatry and family planning. Long-lasting depot antagonist medications border the line between prevention and treatment. Currently, the only depot antagonists in clinical use are opioid antagonists. A depot preparation of naltrexone has demonstrated capacity to block opioid use for approximately one month [92]. While there have been attempts to market longer-acting formulations of naltrexone lasting up to one year, and also attempts to formulate other antagonist compounds such as disulfuram (not strictly speaking an antagonist to alcohol, but effectively so) [93] and flumazenil (a benzodiazepine antagonist) [94], to date none have developed into effective medications for prevention or treatment.

2.19 ROLE OF HEALTH-CARE PROFESSIONALS IN PREVENTION OF DRUG USE AND DRUG-USE DISORDERS

Developing comprehensive, effective and sustainable strategies and systems of prevention of drug use and drug-use disorders requires the substantial involvement of health-care professionals. Health professionals have an important role to inform the public and policy makers about the magnitude and nature of public health problems attributable to drug use and to advocate for societal responses to drug-related problems that are guided by research evidence, incorporating a wide range of preventive interventions, including those that aim at reducing harm associated with continued drug use [43,95]. Medical doctors, and particularly psychiatrists, by their professional training, are in a better position to promote the knowledge about the health effects of drug use, the nature of drug-use disorders, mechanisms of drug-attributable health and social burden, as well as effective prevention and treatment strategies, and to inform relevant policy-making processes [96]. Nurses and midwives have a key role in ensuring access to public-health-orientated prevention interventions in health-care settings and communities through assessment, education, brief interventions and community outreach [97]. Health professionals are in a unique position, also in view of confidentiality of medical information, to identify early drug use and drug-use disorders in health-care settings and provide brief interventions, referrals and, whenever necessary, treatment of drug-use disorders and co-morbid conditions. Health professionals play a particularly important role in the prevention of drug-use disorders associated with the nonmedical use of prescribed medicines [98].

New approaches to prevention and treatment of drug-use disorders, including internet-based interventions [99] as well as immunotherapies under development and depot medications present new challenges, including ethical ones [16, 100], but also new potential ways of preventing drug use and drug-related harm. Further developments in this area should be guided by public-health objectives, research evidence and sound ethical principles with sufficient resources allocated for the evaluation of effectiveness of prevention strategies and interventions at different levels.

REFERENCES

1. UNODC (2009) World Drug Report. United Nations Office on Drugs and Crime, Vienna.
2. Degenhardt, L., Chiu, W.-T, Sampson, N. *et al.* (2008) Toward a global view of alcohol, tobacco, cannabis, and cocaine use: Findings from the WHO World Mental Health Surveys. *Public Library of Science Medicine*, **5** (7), e141. doi: 10.1371/journal.

3. Anthony, J.C. and Helzer, J.E. (1991) Syndromes of drug abuse and dependence, in *Psychiatric disorders in America* (eds. L.N. Robins and D.A. Regier), The Free Press/Macmillan, New York, pp., 116–154.

4. Hasin, D.S., Stinson, F.S., Ogburn, E. *et al.* (2007) Prevalence, correlates, disability, and co-morbidity of DSM-IV alcohol abuse and dependence in the United States: results from the National Epidemiological Survey on Alcohol and Related Conditions. *Arch Gen Psychiatry*, **64** (7), 830–842.

5. Hughes, A., Sathe, N. and Spagnola, K. (2008) State estimates of substance use from the 2005-2006 National Surveys on Drug Use and Health. DHHS Publication No. SMA-08-4311, NSDUH Series H-33. Rockwille, MD: Substance Abuse and Mental Health Services Administration, Office of Applied Studies.

6. Compton, W.M. and Volkow, N.D. (2006) Abuse of prescription drugs and the risk addiction. *Drug Alcohol Depend*, **83S**, S4–S7.

7. UNAIDS (2008) Report on the Global AIDS Epidemic. Joint United Nations Programme on HIV/AIDS (UNAIDS).

8. World Health Organization (2009) *Global Health Risks. Mortality and Burden of Disease Attributable to Selected Major Risks*, World Health Organization, Geneva.

9. Collins, D. and Lapsley, H. (2002) *Counting the Cost: Estimate of the Social Costs of Drug Abuse in Australia in 1998–9*, Commonwealth of Australia, Canberra.

10. Rehm, J., Ballunas, D., Brochu, S. *et al.* (2006) *The costs of substance abuse in Canada 2002: Highlights*, CCSA, Ottawa. Available online: http://www.ccsa.ca/2006%20CCSA%20 Documents/ccsa-011332-2006.pdf (Accessed 14 November 2009).

11. Stockwell, T., Gruenewald, P., Toumbourou, J. and Loxley, W. (2005) Preventing risky drug use and related harms: the need for a synthesis of new knowledge, in, *Preventing Harmful Substance Use: the Evidence Base for Policy and Practice*, John Wiley & Sons Ltd.

12. Babor, T. *et al.* (2003) *No Ordinary Commodity: Alcohol and Public Policy*, Oxford University Press, Oxford.

13. Warner, L.A., Canino, G. and Colon HM (2001) Prevalence and correlates of substance-use disorders among older adolescents in Puerto Rico and the United States: a cross-country comparison. *Drug Alcohol Depend*, **63** (3), 229–243.

14. Schuster, C.R. and Johanson, C.E. (1981) An analysis of drug-seeking behavior in animals. *Neurosci Biobehav Rev*, **15**, 35–43.

15. Caplan, G. (1964) *Principles of Preventive Psychiatry*, Basic Books, New York.

16. World Health Organization (2004a) *Neuroscience of Psychoactive Substance Use and Dependence*, WHO, Geneva.

17. CSDH (2008) Closing the gap in a generation: health equity through action on the social determinants of health. Final Report of the Commission on Social Determinants of Health. Geneva, World Health Organization, Geneva.

18. Beaglehole, R., Bonita, R. and Kjellström, T. (1993) *Basic Epidemiology*, World Health Organization, Geneva.

19. Jackson, R., Johnson, M., Campbell, F. *et al.* (2009) Screening and Brief Interventions for Prevention and Early Identification of Alcohol Use Disorders in Adults and Young People. http:// www.nice.org.uk/guidance/index.jsp?action=download&o=45665. (Accessed October 20, 2010).

20. Humeniuk, R., Dennington, V. and Ali, R. (2008) The effectiveness of a brief intervention for illicit drugs linked to the alcohol, smoking and substance involvement screening test (ASSIST) in primary health care settings: a technical report of phase III findings of the WHO ASSIST

randomized controlled trial http://www.who.int/substance_abuse/activities/assist_technicalreport_phase3_final.pdf [electronic resource]. (Accessed October 20, 2010).

21. Mattick, R., Ali, R. and Lintzeris, N. (eds) (2009) *Pharmacotherapies for the Treatment of Opioid Dependence*, Informa Healthcare, Ney York, London.

22. Brooner, R.K., King, V.L., Kidorf, M. *et al.* (1997) Psychiatric and substance use comorbidity among treatment-seeking opioid abusers. *Arch Gen Psychiatry*, **54**, 71–80.

23. Swendsen, J.D. and Merikangas, K.R. (2000) The comorbidity of depression and substance-use disorders. *Clinical Psychology Review*, **20**, 173–189.

24. Hawkins, J.D., Catalano, R.F. and Miller, J.Y. (1992b) Risk and protective factors for alcohol and other drug problems in adolescence and early adulthood: Implications for substance abuse prevention. *Psychological Bulletin*, **112** (1), 64–105.

25. Loxley, W., Toubouru, J. *et al.* (2004) *The Prevention of Substance Use, Risk and Harm in Australia: a Review of the Evidence*, The National Drug Research Centre and the Centre for Adolescent Health, Canberra

26. Mrazek, P.J. and Haggerty, R.J. (eds) (1994) *Reducing Risks for Mental Disorders: Frontiers for Preventive International Research*, National Academy Press, Washington, DC.

27. Mrazek, P.J. (1998) Selective and indicated preventive interventions, in *Preventing Mental Illness: Mental Health Promotion in Primary Care* (eds. R. Jenkins, T.B. Üstun), John Wiley & Sons, Inc., New York.

28. Lenton, S. (1996) The essence of prevention, in *Perspectives on Addiction: Making Sense of the Issues* (eds. C. Wilkinson and B. Saunders), William Montgomery, Perth.

29. World Health Organization (2009a) WHO Model List of Essential Medicines. http://www.who.int/selection_medicines/committees/expert/17/sixteenth_adult_list_en.pdf.

30. United Nations (2009) Political Declaration and Plan of Action on International Cooperation towards an Integrated and Balanced Strategy to Counter the World Drug Problem. Commission on Narcotic Drugs. http://www.unodc.org/documents/commissions/CND-Uploads/CND-52-RelatedFiles/V0984963-English.pdf. (Accessed October 20, 2010).

31. Graham, K. and Chandler-Coutts, M. (2000) Community Action Research: Who does what to whom and why? Lessons learned from local prevention efforts (international experiences). *Substance Use and Misuse*, **35** (1–2): 87–110.

32. Smith, L. (2000) *Take Your Partners! Stimulating Drugs Prevention in Local Communities*, Social Policy Research Centre, Middlesex.

33. DuPont, R.L. and Selavka, C.S. (2007) Testing to identify recent drug use, in *American Psychiatric Textbook of Substance Abuse Treatment*, 4th edn (eds. M. Galanter and H.D. Kleber), American Psychiatric Press, Washington, DC.

34. American Academy of Pediatrics, Committee on Substance Use (1996) Testing for drugs of abuse in children and adolescents. *Pediatrics*, **98**, 305–307.

35. Warner, E.A., Walker, R.M. and Friedmann, P.D. (2003) Should informed consent be required for laboratory testing for drugs of abuse in medical settings? *Am J Med*, **115**, 54–58.

36. Hawkins, J.D., Catalano, R.F. and Associates (1992a) *Communities that Care: Action for Drug Abuse Prevention*, Jossey-Bass Publishers, San Francisco, CA.

37. Elias, M.J., Zins, J.E. and Weissberg, R.P. (1997) *Promoting Social and Emotional Learning: Guidelines for Educators*, Association for Supervision and Curriculum Development, Alexandria, VA.

38. Swisher, J.D. (1992) *Peer Influence and Peer Involvement in Prevention*, Center for Substance Abuse Prevention, Division of High Risk Youth, Rockville, MD.

39. World Health Organization (2004b) *Training Guide for HIV Prevention Outreach to Injecting Drug Users*, WHO, Geneva.

40. Rutter, M. (1979) Protective factors in children's responses to stress and disadvantage, in *Primary Prevention of Psychotherapy: Volume 3. Social Competence in Children* (eds. M.W. Kent and J.E. Rolf), University Press of New England, Hanover, NH.

41. Bernard, B. (1990) *The Case for Peers*, Western Center for Drug-Free Schools and Communities, Portland, OR.

42. Hawks, D., Scott, K. and McBride, N. (2002) *Prevention of Psychoactive Substance Use: a Selected Review of What Works in the Area of Prevention*, World Health Organization, Geneva.

43. World Health Organization (1993) Expert Committee on Drug Dependence. Twenty-eighth report. Geneva, World Health Organization (WHO Technical Report Series, No. 836).

44. NIDA (2003) *Preventing Drug Use among Children and Adolescent. A Research-based Guide for Parents, Educators, and Community Leaders*, 2nd edn, National Institutes of Health. National Institute on Drug Abuse, NIH Publication No. 04-4212 (A).

45. Anderson, P., Chisholm, D. and Fuhr, D. (2009) Effectiveness and cost-effectiveness of policies and programmes to reduce the harm caused by alcohol. *Lancet*, **373** (9682), 2234–2246.

46. Medina-Mora, M.E. (2005) Prevention of substance abuse: a brief overview. *World Psychiatry*, **4** (1), 25–30.

47. Dixon, D. and Coffin, P. (1999) Zero tolerance policing of illegal drug markets. *Drug and Alcohol Review*, **18**, 477–486.

48. Henggeler, S.W. (2007) Juvenile drug courts: emerging outcomes and key research issues. *Curr Opin Psychiatry*, **20** (3), 242–246.

49. Werb, D., Elliott, R., Fischer, B. *et al.* (2007) Drug treatment courts in Canada: an evidence-based review. *HIV/AIDS Policy Law Rev*, **12** (2–3), 12–17.

50. Makkai, T., Moore, R. and McAllister, I. (1991) Health education campaigns and drug use: The 'drug offensive' in Australia. *Health Education Research*, **6** (1), 65–76.

51. Proctor, D. and Babor, T. (2001) Drug wars in the post-Gutenberg galaxy: Mass media as the next battleground. *Addiction*, **96**, 377–381.

52. DeJong, W. and Winston, J.A. (1990) The use of mass media in substance abuse prevention. *Health Affairs*, Summer, 30–46.

53. World Health Organization (1997) Prevention approaches for amphetamine-type stimulants, in *Amphetamine-Type Stimulants*, Donoghoe, M. (Ed.) WHO, Geneva.

54. Johnston, L.D., O'Malley, P.M. and Bachman, J.G. (2002) Monitoring the Future: National Survey Results on Drug Use, 1975-2002. Volume 1: Secondary School Students, National Institute on Drug Abuse, Bethesda. MD.

55. Kandel, D. (2002) *Stages and Pathways of Drug Involvement: Examining the Gateway Hypothesis*, Cambridge University Press, New York.

56. Foxcroft, D. (2006) *Alcohol Misuse Prevention for Young People: a Rapid Review of Recent Evidence*, World Health Organization, Geneva.

57. Faggiano, F., Vigna-Taglianti, F.D., Versino, E., *et al.* (2005) School-based prevention for illicit drugs' use. *Cochrane Database Syst Rev.* 2 (Art. No. CD003020).

58. Lindenberg, C.S., Solorzano, R.M., Bear, D. *et al.* (2002) Reducing substance use and risky sexual behavior among young, low-income, Mexican-American women: Comparison of two interventions. *Applied Nursing Research*, **15** (3), 137–148.

59. Palinkas, L.A., Atkins, C.J., Miller, C. and Ferreira D. (1996) Social skills training for drug prevention in high-risk female adolescents. *Preventive Medicine*, **25** (6), 692–701.

60. Spoth, R., Reyes, M.L., Redmond, C. and Shin, C. (1999) Assessing a public health approach to delay onset and progression of adolescent substance use: Latent transition and log-linear analyses of longitudinal family preventive intervention outcomes. *Journal of Consulting and Clinical Psychology*, **67**, 619–630.

61. Wolchik, S.A., Sandler, I.N., Millsap, R.E. *et al.* (2002) Six-year follow-up of preventive interventions for children of divorce: A randomized controlled trial. *JAMA*, **288** (15), 1874.

62. McGillicuddy, N.B., Rychtarik, R.G., Duquette, J.A. and Morsheimer, E.T. (2001) Development of a skill training program for parents of substance-abusing adolescents. *Journal of Substance Abuse Treatment*, **20** (1), 59–68.

63. Wu, Y., Stanton, B.F., Galbraith, J. *et al.* (2003) Sustaining and broadening intervention impact: a longitudinal randomized trial of 3 adolescent risk reduction approaches. *Pediatrics*, **111** (1), e32.

64. Oliansky, D.M., Wildenhaus, K.J., Manlove, K. *et al.* (1997) Effectiveness of brief interventions in reducing substance use among at-risk primary care patients in three community-based clinics. *Substance Abuse*, **18**, 95–104.

65. McCambridge, J. and Strang, J. (2004) The efficacy of single-session motivational interviewing in reducing drug consumption and perceptions of drug-related risk and harm among young people: results from a multi-site cluster randomized trial. *Addiction*, **99** (1), 39–52.

66. Botvin, G.J., Baker, E., Filazzola, A.D. and Botvin, E.M. (1990) A cognitive-behavioral approach to substance abuse prevention: One-year follow-up. *Addictive Behaviors*, **15** (1), 47–63.

67. Hansen, W.B. and Graham, J.W. (1991) Preventing alcohol, marijuana, and cigarette use among adolescents: peer pressure resistance training versus establishing conservative norms. *Prev Med.*, **20** (3), 414–430.

68. Dent, C.W., Sussman, S. and Stacy, A.W. (2001) Project towards no drug abuse: generalizability to a general high school sample. *Preventive Medicine*, **32** (6), 514–520.

69. Sussman, S., Dent, C.W., Stacy, A.W. and Craig S. (1998) One-year outcomes of project towards no drug abuse. *Preventive Medicine*, **27** (4), 632–642.

70. Catalano, R.F., Haggerty, K.P., Gainey, R.R. and Hoppe, M.J. (1997) Reducing parental risk factors for children's substance misuse: Preliminary outcomes with opiate-addicted parents. *Substance Use & Misuse*, **32** (6), 699–721.

71. Perry, C.L., Komro, K.A., Veblen-Mortenson, S. *et al.* (2003) A randomized controlled trial of the middle and junior high school DARE and DARE Plus programs. *Archives of Paediatrics & Adolescent Medicine*, **157** (2), 178.

72. Schinke, S.P., Tepavac, L. and Cole, K.C. (2000) Preventing substance use among native American youth three-year results. *Addictive Behaviors*, **25** (3), 387–397.

73. Ellickson, P.L., McCaffrey, D.F., Ghosh-Dastidar, B. and Longshore, D.L. (2003) New inroads in preventing adolescent drug use: results from a large-scale trial of project ALERT in middle schools. *Am J Public Health*, **93** (11), 1830–1836.

74. Flay, B.R., Graumlich, S., Segawa, E. *et al.* (2004) Effects of 2 prevention programs on high-risk behaviors among African American youth: a randomized trial. *Archives of Pediatrics & Adolescent Medicine*, **158** (4), 377.

75. Biglan, A., Ary, D.V., Smolkowski, K. *et al.* (2000) A randomised controlled trial of a community intervention to prevent adolescent tobacco use. *Tobacco Control* **9** (1), 24–32.

76. Spoth, R., Redmond, C., Shin, C. and Azevedo, K. (2004) Brief family intervention effects on adolescent substance initiation: School-level growth curve analyses 6 years following baseline. *Journal of Consulting and Clinical Psychology*, **72**, 535–542.

77. Clayton, R.R., Cattarello, A.M. and Johnstone, B.M. (1996) The effectiveness of Drug Abuse Resistance Education (Project DARE): 5-year follow-up results. *Preventive Medicine*, **25** (3), 307–318.

78. Ellickson, P.L. and Bell, R.M. (1990) Drug prevention in junior high: A multi-site longitudinal test. *Science*, **247** (4948), 1299.

79. Lynam, D.R., Milich, R., Zimmerman, R. *et al.* (1999) Project DARE: No effects at 10-year follow-up. *Journal of Consulting and Clinical Psychology*, **67**, 590–593.

80. Botvin, G.J., Baker, E., Dusenbury, L. *et al.* (1995) Long-term follow-up results of a randomized drug abuse prevention trial in a white middle-class population. *JAMA*, **273** (14), 1106–1112.

81. Furr-Holden, C.M., Ialongo, N.S., Anthony, J.C. *et al.* (2004) Developmentally inspired drug prevention: middle school outcomes in a school-based randomized prevention trial. *Drug and Alcohol Dependence*, **73** (2), 149–158.

82. Cook, R., Lawrence, H., Morse, C., and Roehl, J. (1984) An evaluation of the alternatives approach to drug abuse prevention. *Substance Use & Misuse*, **19** (7), 767–787.

83. Malvin, J.H. (1985) Evaluation of two school-based alternatives programs. *Journal of Alcohol and Drug Education*, **30** (3), 98–108.

84. Clayton, R., Cattarello, A. and Walden, K. (1991) Sensations seeking as a potential mediating variable for school-based prevention intervention: A two-year follow-up of DARE. *Health Communication*, **3**, 229–239.

85. Gates, S., McCambridge, J., Smith, L.A. and Foxcroft, D.R. (2006) Interventions for prevention of drug use by young people delivered in non-school settings. *Cochrane Database Syst Rev.* (1).

86. Spoth, R.L., Randall, G.K., Trudeau, L. *et al.* (2008) Substance use outcomes 51/2 years past baseline for partnership-based, family-school preventive interventions. *Drug Alcohol Depend*, **96** (1-2), 57–68.

87. Spoth, R., Trudeau, L., Guyll, M., *et al.* (2009) Universal intervention effects on substance use among young adults mediated by delayed adolescent substance initiation. *J Consult Clin Psychol*, **77** (4), 620–632.

88. Riper, R., Kramer, J., Smit, F. *et al.* (2007) Web-based self-help for problem drinkers: a pragmatic randomized trial. *Addiction*, **103** (2), 218–227.

89. Riper, H., Kramer, J., Conijn, B. *et al.* (2009) Translating effective web-based self-help for problem drinking into the real world. *Alcoholism: Clinical and Experimental Research*, **33** (8), 1401–1408.

90. Martell, B.A., Orson, F.M., Poling, J. *et al.* (2009) Cocaine vaccine for the treatment of cocaine dependence in methadone-maintained patients: a randomized, double-blind, placebo-controlled efficacy trial. *Arch Gen Psychiatry*, **66** (10), 1116–1123.

91. Moreno, A. and Janda, K.D. (2009) Immunopharmacotherapy: Vaccination strategies as a treatment for drug abuse and dependence. *Pharmacol Biochem Behav*, **92** (2), 199–205.

92. Comer, S.D., Sullivan, M.A., Yu, E. *et al.* (2006) Injectable, sustained-release naltrexone for the treatment of opioid dependence: a randomized, placebo-controlled trial. *Arch Gen Psychiatry*, **63** (2), 210–218.

93. Johnsen, J. and Mørland J. (1991) Disulfiram implant: a double-blind placebo controlled follow-up on treatment outcome. *Alcohol Clin Exp Res*, **15** (3), 532–536.

94. O'Neil, G., Hulse, G., Chan, C.T., *et al.* (2008) *Outpatient Ambulatory Rapid Benzodiazepine Detoxification*. Paper presented at the Stapleford Conference in Athens, May, 2008.

95. Heather, N., Wodak, A., Nadelmann, E., and O'Hare, P. (eds) (1993) *Psychoactive Drugs and Harm Reduction: from Faith to Science*, Whurr Publishers, London.

96. Poznyak, V.B. (2005) The role of psychiatrists in prevention of psychoactive substance use and dependence: beyond clinical practice. *World Psychiatry*, **4** (1), 31–32.

97. Coles, L. and Porter, E. (2008) *Public Health Skills: a Practical Guide for Nurses and Public Health Practitioners*, Blackwell, Oxford.

98. Ghodse, H. (2002) *Drugs and Addictive Behaviour. A Guide to Treatment*, 3rd edn, Cambridge University Press, Cambridge.

99. EMCDDA (2009) *Internet-Based Drug Treatment Interventions. Best Practice and Applications in EU Member States*, European Monitoring Centre for Drugs and Drug Addiction (EMCDDA).

100. Harwood, H.J. and Myers, T.G. (eds) (2004) *New Treatments for Addiction: Behavioural, Ethical, Legal, and Social Questions*, The National Academies Press, Washington.

101. World Health Organization (2008) *Global Burden of Disease: 2004 Update*, World Health Organization, Geneva.

102. Bonomo Y. and Proimos J. (2005) Substance misuse: alcohol, tobacco, inhalants and other drugs. *British Medical Journal*. 330:777.

103. Loxley, W., Toumbourou, J., Stockwell, T., Haines, B., Scott, K., Godfrey, C. *et al.* (2004) *The Prevention of Substance Use, Risk and Harm in Australia: a Review of the Evidence*. Canberra: Australian Government Department of Health and Ageing.

104. Snow DL, Tebes JK, Arthur MW, Tapasak RC. Two-year follow-up of a social-cognitive intervention to prevent substance use. *Journal of Drug Education*. 1992;**22** (2):101–114.

CHAPTER 3

Drug Abuse: Treatment and Management

Fabrizio Schifano, MD, MRCPsych

*University of Hertfordshire, School of Pharmacy, College Lane Campus,
Hatfield, UK*

3.1 INTRODUCTION

Drug addiction is a chronic relapsing disorder characterized by the compulsion to seek and take the drug, the loss of control in limiting intake and the emergence of a negative emotional state when access to the drug is withdrawn. Despite individual variation in the liability to abuse psychoactive substances, there is substantial commonality shared by drugs of abuse [1]. This chapter will try to reflect on some updates that have been recently published providing further indepth knowledge on pharmacological and nonpharmacological intervention for drug misusers as a component of drug misuse treatment. In particular, comments on issues related to the treatment and management of opiates; stimulants (cocaine; amphetamine and amphetamine-like substances); ecstasy and ecstasy-like drugs; and benzodiazepines will be offered here. Particular focus will be on medications available and possible promising future agents for the treatment and management of most drug misuse conditions. Furthermore, an update of the most recent literature papers regarding the usefulness of psychosocial treatment, with particular reference to CBT; contingency management; and behavioural approaches will be provided.

3.2 PHARMACOLOGICAL MANAGEMENT OF OPIATE MISUSE; METHADONE

3.2.1 Clinical Pharmacology and Clinical Issues

Methadone is a synthetic opioid that is used mainly for the treatment of opioid dependence. It is widely prescribed in oral liquid formulations and sometimes tablets. Injectable forms are also still fairly common in most EU countries. Methadone dominates the substitute opiate-prescribing market in most western world countries. Such use of the drug has increased over

Substance Abuse Disorders: Evidence and Experience, First Edition. Edited by Hamid Ghodse, Helen Herrman, Mario Maj and Norman Sartorius.
© 2011 John Wiley & Sons, Ltd. Published 2011 by John Wiley & Sons, Ltd.

the years as its advantages have become widely recognized: reducing criminal activity, costs of crime and illicit drug use by opiate addicts; improving social integration and employment prospects; reducing the morbidity and mortality of opiate users [2].

Methadone appears in the blood stream within 30 minutes of being taken orally; it takes 2–4 hours for it to reach peak plasma concentrations. Methadone has a long but variable (15–55 hours) plasma half-life, but it is usually assumed to be 24 hours. In some drug-naïve persons, a single dose can have clinical effects up to 72 hours in duration. The drug is chiefly metabolized in the liver. Care should therefore be taken when administering methadone to patients with hepatic impairment, since methadone plasma levels will be elevated and pose an overdose risk. Methadone takes two to three weeks to induce itself and thus the hepatic enzyme systems (which convert methadone to its metabolites) of new methadone users will therefore take longer to clear methadone from their bodies [2].

There may be genetic variability in the response of a subgroup of individuals to the drug and their metabolism of it, making them more susceptible to overdose. Three types of metabolizers in respect of a genetic polymorphism of cytochrome P450 2D6 that assists in the processing of methadone have been identified: poor, extensive and ultrarapid [2]. The cytochrome P450 3A4 enzyme system (CYP3A4) is the principal agent responsible for metabolizing methadone. The other main enzymes responsible are CYP2D6 and CYP1A2. Any substance that interacts with the CYP3A4 enzyme could precipitate an interaction with methadone.

3.2.2   Precautionary Measures for Administering Methadone; Drug Interactions; Acute Toxicity

It has been suggested that a lethal dose of methadone amongst nondependent subjects is between 0.8 and 1.5 mg/kg of body mass, which may parallel (on average) an intake of 50 mg for adults and 10 mg for children. A serum methadone concentration of over 0.4 mg/L may be enough to cause death from respiratory depression, yet levels of up to 1 mg/L have been found in living patients receiving treatment [2].

The introduction of supervised consumption appears to have helped to reduce the number of fatalities. Despite this, there is still a significant number of deaths to which methadone may have contributed. There is a substantial 'grey'/black market in all forms of diverted methadone. At least three-fifths of deaths associated with methadone in England and Wales are accounted for by the use of methadone that may have been illicitly obtained [3].

Methadone should only be administered following a thorough clinical assessment of opiate/opioid dependence and current level of drug consumption. There is now widespread agreement that for outpatient stabilization the initial dose of methadone will be less than 30 mg; where tolerance is low or uncertain an appropriate dose would be between 10 and 20 mg. Titration of methadone doses is of paramount importance to avoid the risk of overdose [2]. Wolff et al. [4] found that clearance of methadone was significantly lower in opiate addicts at the start of treatment (median elimination half-life 128 h) than in those who had reached the steady-state level (median elimination half-life 48 h). As a consequence, the drug accumulates from one dose to the next, thus posing a risk of overdose during the initial phase of methadone maintenance treatment.

Overdose deaths solely due to methadone are still relatively rare events [5]. It is therefore important to consider the effects of other substances taken concurrently. The concurrent administration of drug inducers such as benzodiazepines, barbiturates and opiates with methadone may result in significantly lower plasma levels of the drug and this in turn may trigger withdrawal symptoms and lead to individuals in maintenance treatment seeking (extra) illicit drugs or prescription drugs especially benzodiazepines to alleviate their symptoms. In this way, although the risk of overdose from methadone may be reduced, the risk of overdose *per se* is not decreased. This risk is further compounded by the fact that the effects of inhibitors are transient and thus plasma levels of methadone will increase again.

The signs of overdose associated with methadone include deep respiratory depression, unusually loud snoring, pin-point pupils, hypotension, circulatory failure, pulmonary oedema and coma. The principal mechanisms for methadone-related deaths are respiratory depression; airway obstruction; pulmonary oedema and bronchopneumonia. Methadone can block nerve conduction through membrane stabilizing activity and this can result in complications such as cardiovascular collapse or cardiac arrhythmias [6].

Respiratory depression develops 12–14 h after ingestion of methadone, particularly in those who have had or have only a weak tolerance to the drug [7]. Tolerance can be rapidly lost through abstinence whilst imprisoned or by having successfully completed inpatient opiate detoxification.

3.2.3 Rapid Reference Check Lists

Opiate users' assessment prior to substitute prescribing; examination and investigations suggested

- Perform urinalysis/other suitable toxicological analysis confirmation (essential).
- Check for injection sites.
- Check for skin infections and/or deep venous thrombosis.
- Check for general health, nutrition and dental health.
- Blood (including liver function) tests to be carried out.
- Pregnancy (to be seen as an emergency/priority situation).

Prescribing methadone maintenance safely

- In the first few days, review regularly/frequently the clinical situation and increase the dosage until no withdrawal symptoms/cravings/heroin in urine is shown.
- Keep on daily supervised consumption for a reasonable amount of time; 3 months is suggested.
- When stable, see every 2–6 weeks.
- Warn re: risks to children if take-home doses are given.
- Warn re: risk of overdose if heroin, alcohol or and benzodiazepines are used as well.
- Warn re: driving; client needs to inform both his/her relevant regulatory/licensing authorities and insurance company.
- Liaise with dispensing pharmacist.
- Take into account the possibility/availability of drug counselling and of other psychosocial support options.
- Retention in treatment is an important indicator of long-term outcome.

- If persistence of morphine/heroin in urine is observed, increase of the dosage may be necessary (daily supervised consumption essential). There is no statutory limit on the dose of methadone although the greater benefits would be achieved with doses of 60–120 mg for those on maintenance [8].
- Stop treatment only for unacceptable behaviour and not in presence of illicit drug use.
- Review persistent use at team meeting for team clinical management plan.
- Referral to inpatient admission for stabilization may be an option.

3.3 PHARMACOLOGICAL MANAGEMENT OF OPIATE MISUSE; BUPRENORPHINE

3.3.1   Clinical Pharmacology Issues

Buprenorphine is a semi-synthetic opioid drug with a partial μ agonist activity. For this reason, when buprenorphine competes with morphine or heroin for μ receptors it can reduce their maximum effect. Buprenorphine binds strongly to μ and κ opiate receptor preparations [9]; it associates with the μ receptor slowly (30 minutes), but with high affinity, low intrinsic activity and slow/incomplete dissociation [10]. The slow dissociation from the receptor probably limits the intensity of withdrawal by preventing the rapid uncovery of the receptor upon discontinuation of buprenorphine treatment [11].

Buprenorphine has a less well-defined effect on the respiratory function than that usually expected for opiates, with a ceiling effect on respiratory depression with increasing doses [12]. Clinically, these issues seem to explain the observation that the desired effects of buprenorphine do not increase in proportion to the administered dose (as happens with full opiate agonists). A ceiling on the respiratory depression is possibly a valuable therapeutic safeguard although the situation is different for sensitive individuals, in which these drugs may cause severe respiratory distress [13].

After sublingual (sl) administration, the peak concentration is reached in 90 minutes–4 hours and the bioavailability is 56% [14]. Conversely, after oral administration the bioavailability is very low (16%; [15]).

High-dose buprenorphine indications are comparable to those of methadone; that is: the medication may be prescribed as an adjunct in the treatment of opioid dependence. However, some have suggested that buprenorphine as sublingual tablets can be used for opiate detoxification in those individuals such as less severe addicts and those who are very well motivated [16].

For patients with severely impaired respiratory function, and for those who are receiving drugs that can cause respiratory depression, buprenorphine is not indicated [17].

Due to its properties as a partial agonist, in those who are administered with high dosages of opiate agonists buprenorphine may precipitate withdrawal effects. Those on methadone should be reduced to a maximum of 30 mg daily before starting buprenorphine [18]. Other centrally acting agents (including alcohol; sedatives-hypnotics; anti-psychotics; clonidine; opiate-containing anti-tussives; H1-receptor antagonists) may potentiate the drowsiness that can be caused by buprenorphine itself. Buprenorphine should be used with caution in patients who are administered with high dosages of benzodiazepines, since both buprenorphine and benzodiazepines are CYP3A substrates [19].

Although the amount of the drug excreted during lactation is very small, it is not advisable to prescribe buprenorphine to lactating mothers; moreover, buprenorphine is not recommended during pregnancy [18]. Use during labour may result in neonatal respiratory depression. Johnson [20] suggested that a neonatal buprenorphine abstinence syndrome may occur in 63% of cases.

Buprenorphine side effects include: drowsiness and sleep disturbances; nausea, vomiting, constipation (less severe than other opiates); sweating, dizziness, fainting (due to orthostatic hypotension); headache; rashes and blurring of vision. Nausea and vomiting may be more frequent with buprenorphine than with other opiates [21]. Potentially fatal respiratory depression is uncommon and is most likely to occur when the drug is administered parenterally.

3.3.2   Clinical Issues

Buprenorphine high dose should be administered in the following dosages; initially, 0.8–4 mg (sl) as a single daily dose, adjusting according to response; maximum 32 mg daily (a gradual withdrawal is advised); in those who have not undergone opioid withdrawal, buprenorphine should be administered at least 4 hours after last use of opioid or when signs of craving appear [18]. Doses of 6–8 mg appear to be equal to 60 mg of methadone as a maintenance agent in drug addiction [22]. As a consequence of buprenorphine being a partial agonist, the drug may have a favourable safety profile. Its limited ability to activate opioid mechanisms results, as said, in a ceiling of the magnitude of its effects. Symptoms of overdose may include: dizziness, nausea, sickness, marked miosis. Respiratory depression is not necessarily part of the clinical picture but, in this case, supportive measures should be instituted and, if appropriate, naloxone in high doses and/or respiratory stimulants can be used.

Mattick [23] compared the efficacy of high-dose buprenorphine with methadone mixture for maintenance treatments in opioid-dependent patients. As soon as adequate induction was achieved, both were equally as effective in reducing opioid use and in drug-craving reports. There were also no differences in retention between the two treatment groups. On the other hand, a number of studies have shown buprenorphine to be: as effective as methadone [24]; more effective [25]; and slightly less effective [26].

A meta-analysis comparing buprenorphine to methadone reported that variation amongst trials may be due to differences in dose levels, patient exclusion criteria and provision of psychosocial interventions [27]. The meta-analysis reported that subjects who were receiving a dose of 8–12 mg of buprenorphine were 1.26 times more likely to drop out of treatment than subjects who received 50–80 mg of methadone and they were 8.3% more likely to have a positive urine test for opiates. A further meta-analysis also noted the wide variability in research studies ([28]. There may be a particular subset of individuals who might benefit more than others from buprenorphine. The reverse is also true, with methadone suggested as more useful in those with high levels of dependency. Buprenorphine should not be used simply instead of methadone but as a further treatment option that seeks to increase access to services for a greater number and a more diverse range of clients.

Withdrawal from buprenorphine is thought to be milder and easier than withdrawal from methadone though the evidence is still inconclusive. In fact, a characteristic and long-lasting withdrawal syndrome has been described [29] after abrupt discontinuation of the drug. Its partial agonist characteristics, with slow dissociation from opiate receptors, are considered to be part of the explanation for reports of milder withdrawal symptoms in comparison to other opioids. Some, but not all, reports suggest that treatment with naltrexone could be started within a few days of cessation of low-dose buprenorphine, in contrast to 10 days after cessation of methadone. The possible avoidance of relapse or drop out from services may be quite crucial.

Auriacombe *et al.* [30] computed the death rate from overdose of buprenorphine in France and estimated that the 1994–1998 yearly death rate related to methadone use was at least 3 times greater than the death rate related to buprenorphine use. Kintz [31] examined the files of 117 subjects who died in France between January 1996 and May 2000. Blood levels for buprenorphine were within the therapeutic range: 0.1–76 micrograms per ml. They suggested that IV injection of crushed buprenorphine tablets, a concomitant intake of other psychotropics (especially benzodiazepines and neuroleptics) and the high dosage of buprenorphine formulation available appeared to be the major risk factors for such fatalities. In a number of deaths in which buprenorphine has been implicated, benzodiazepines have also been taken ([32, 33].

Most clinicians suggest the need for supervised dispensing, though there is difficulty with supervision. Sublingual tablets, with an average of 8–12 mg dosage, may take up to 5 minutes to dissolve fully. Anecdotal reports from some services are of crushing the sublingual tablet prior to inhouse dispensing (rather than pharmacy supervision) to avoid any possible diversion or injecting the drug. The drug crushed in this manner is not licensed. Anecdotal reports from patients note some misuse of the drug, either by injecting or dispensing to others, when not supervised for longer periods or not supervised at all.

The recently introduced naloxone/buprenorphine combination seems quite promising in reducing buprenorphine abuse liability (and of its possible IV misuse), although more data are needed to confirm this.

3.4   PHARMACOLOGICAL MANAGEMENT OF OPIATE MISUSE; NALTREXONE

3.4.1   Clinical Pharmacology Issues

Naltrexone is an opioid antagonist; its structure is similar to that of naloxone but it has a higher oral efficacy and a longer duration of action. Both naltrexone and its active metabolite 6-β-naltrexol are competitive antagonists at μ- and κ-opioid receptors. This blockade of opioid receptors is the basis behind its action in the management of opioid dependence; that is: it reversibly blocks or attenuates the effects of opioids. The administration of naltrexone is not associated with the development of tolerance or dependence. In subjects physically dependent on opioids, naltrexone will precipitate withdrawal symptomatology. Naltrexone blocks the effects of opioids by competitive binding at opioid receptors. This makes the blockade produced potentially surmountable, overcoming full naltrexone blockade by administration of very high doses of opiates. Long-term clinical use of naltrexone increases the concentration of opioid receptors in the brain and produces a temporary exaggeration of responses to the subsequent administration of opioid agonists [34]. Although well absorbed orally, naltrexone presents with oral bioavailability of 5–40%. A single oral dose reaches peak plasma concentration in 1–2 hours.

3.4.2 Clinical Issues

The use of naltrexone is indicated as an adjunct to prevent relapse in detoxified formerly opiate-dependent patients who managed to remain opioid-free for at least 7–10 days [18]. Liver function tests are needed before and during treatment. Its use is contraindicated when patients are currently dependent on opiates/opioids and in the case of acute hepatitis or liver failure. Most frequent side effects may include: nausea, vomiting, abdominal pain; anxiety, nervousness, sleeping difficulty, headache, reduced energy; joint and muscle pain; liver function abnormalities. Naltrexone should be initiated in specialist clinics only, at the dosage of 25 mg initially then 50 mg daily; the total weekly dose may be divided and given on 3 days of the week for improved compliance (e.g. 100 mg on Monday and Wednesday, and 150 mg on Friday).

Treatment with naltrexone should not be initiated whenever there is a possibility of opioid use within the past 7–10 days. If there is any question of occult opioid dependence, a naloxone challenge test should be performed. Once the patient has been started on naltrexone, 50 mg once a day will produce adequate clinical blockade of the actions of parenterally administered opioids. As with many nonagonist treatments for addiction, naltrexone is of proven value only when given as part of a comprehensive plan of management that includes some measures to ensure the patient takes the medication.

3.4.2.1 Use of Opioid Antagonists During Rapid Detoxifications; Naltrexone Extended Release Formulations

Naltrexone is sometimes used for a rapid detoxification regime for opioid dependence [35]. The principle of rapid detoxification is to induce opioid-receptor blockade while the patient is in a state of impaired consciousness so as to attenuate the withdrawal symptoms experienced by the patient. The rapid detoxification procedure is usually followed by oral naltrexone daily for up to 12 months. However, the rapid detoxification has been criticized for its questionable efficacy in long-term opioid-dependence management.

Simple but effective naltrexone implants, giving an average blockade of 6–7 weeks, have been available for a number of years [36–38]. Long-acting implantable preparations of naltrexone are, however, licensed only in a few countries.

3.4.2.2 Short-Term Pharmacological Management of Opiate Misuse; the use of Alfa-2 Adrenergic Receptor Agonists

To carry out a detoxification from opiates/opioids, an alternative to methadone and buprenorphine may be given by the administration of a concoction of symptomatic medication. However, there are a few clinical issues that are to be considered when planning such a short-term detoxification procedure. The client to be considered should be young, not pregnant, and presenting with both a short (<2 years) history of addiction and indeed a low level of opiate use. In this case, the prescription of the alfa-2 adrenergic receptor agonists (e.g. lofexidine; clonidine) may be appropriate. The prescription of these agents should facilitate a decrease of the noradrenergic central levels, a feature which is characteristic of the opiate/opioid withdrawal clinical picture. Together with alfa-2 receptor agonists, and only for a short (5–10 days) period, the clinician might take into account the possibility of prescribing other pharmacological agents, including: benzodiazepines, nonopioid analgesics, anti-emetics, anti-diarrhoeal agents and anti-spasmodics. Ideally, these agents should help in alleviating those symptoms that are characteristic of the opiate/opioid-withdrawal syndrome, including: anxiety/sleeping disorders, musculoskeletal pain, diarrhoea and abdominal pain. Due to the possibility of orthostatic hypotension, this procedure should anyway be carried out with a daily/every other day nursing staff clinical supervision and support.

3.5   STIMULANTS (COCAINE; AMPHETAMINE AND METHAMPHETAMINE; ECSTASY AND ECSTASY-LIKE DRUGS)

3.5.1   Clinical and Pharmacological Issues Related to the Management of Cocaine Misuse

Traditionally, cocaine is snorted. However, with crack (which is obtained by heating hydrochloride cocaine with baking soda and water), the user can achieve both a quicker and a stronger 'high', although of a shorter duration. These characteristics can explain the huge potential of dependence liability of the free-base formulation. After the binge (which is characterized by increase in both noradrenalin/NA and dopamine/DA turnover), the beginning of the withdrawal phase is observed. This is schematically divided into three different subphases [39]: crash (characterized by decrease in NA levels); withdrawal properly called (characterized by decrease in both serotonin/5-HT and DA levels); extinction (with a possible rebalance of the neurotransmitter pathways). Crash begins 15–30 minutes after the binge and lasts for a period of 9 hours to 4 days. It is characterized by dysphoria and by different levels of craving. The withdrawal properly called lasts approximately for 1–10 weeks; in the last period of this phase the craving, anxiety and dysphoria levels may be very high and the relapse risk is considerable. If the patient is then able to continue to abstain from cocaine use, the extinction phase begins and both patient's behaviour and mood level gradually revert back to normality. However, if the patient is exposed to environmental stimuli that remind him/her of cocaine, sudden peaks of cravings are observed. With a chronic use of the drug, paranoid ideation is commonly observed; with the free-base formulation, due to its higher frequency of consumption, risk is understandably higher.

3.5.2   Clinical and Pharmacological Issues Related to the Management of Methamphetamines and Other Amphetamine-Like Stimulants ('Speed', 'Meth'; Smokable Forms: 'Ice', 'Crystal') Misuse

Meth is found as a crystal white powder, easily soluble in water and alcohol. It can be snorted, smoked, ingested or injected intravenously. Methamphetamine has both direct (through inhibition of cathecolamines' breakdown) and indirect (through inhibition of catecholamines' presynaptic reuptake) sympathomimetic effects actions. Sympathetic arousal induced by methamphetamine produces rapid and sometimes irregular heartbeat, sweating, pupillary dilation, hypertension, dry mouth, tremor and blurred vision and increased body heat. Occasionally, serious medical complications arise including coronary artery syndrome, seizures and cerebral bleeds [40]. Soon after inhalation or intravenous administration, consumers feel a strong sensation of 'rush', which can last for several minutes. After snorting or ingesting the drug, effects are still euphoriant but both less intense (due to different bioavailability levels) and more delayed (they do appear only after 15–20 minutes). Similar to cocaine, the clinical picture ('tweaking') is characterized by a sort of a 'binge and crash' cycle [41]. After meth intake, hyperactivity, anorexia and arousal increase levels may be observed. Dependence is easily observed with chronic use of the drug. Most frequent psychopathological consequences include violent and bizarre behaviour, anxiety, confusion, sleep disorders, tactile hallucinations (such as the sensation of parasites under the skin), psychotic disorders (paranoid type) and aggressive behaviour. Both suicide and homicide episodes have been described; these high levels of aggression may require significant levels of both physical and chemical restraint [40]. Benzodiazepines (often required in very high doses) should be the first-line medication with anti-psychotics used only where additional tranquilization is required. A diagnosis of a possible underlying or persistent psychotic disorder must be deferred until a reassessment can be made in a drug-free state. These often florid psychoses usually remit within a few days and the user returns to normal functioning. Withdrawal symptoms include depression, anxiety, strong craving and tiredness [41]. Management of withdrawal is largely supportive. The patient should be placed in quiet surroundings for several days. Since anti-depressants have no specific anti-craving effects and the efficacy of anti-depressants in reducing depression is confined to those stimulant users who are depressed, it is useful to wait until after they have stopped using for 2–4 weeks to reassess them for depressive symptoms. The persistence of depressive symptoms beyond 2–4 weeks after stopping amphetamine use may suggest that there is an underlying depressive illness and this should be treated [40] since left unmanaged its presence represents a high risk for relapse.

3.5.3 Pharmacotherapeutic Options

There is currently no widely accepted evidence-based pharmacotherapy regime for the treatment of psychostimulant withdrawal [42]. However, a great deal of resources have addressed the issue of the identification of a suitable medication to address the stimulant, and in particular cocaine, cravings so that the relapse risk can be minimized as much as possible.

Rapid reference checklist; suggested medication to address the cocaine/stimulant cravings

- Amantadine: no effects at all [43] .
- Desipramine: to operate a post-synaptic down-regulation of the NA system. Not a satisfactory retention in treatment has, however, been described [44].
- Levodopa, bromocriptine, lisuride, selegiline, pergolide, mazindol: to operate a post-synaptic down-regulation of the DA system. However, these medications may further predate an 'impoverished' DA system. Agents for subtypes of DA receptors (i.e. D3) and the use of partial agonists may be useful future treatment approaches [45].
- SSRIs: to rebalance the 5-HT system. Useful for the treatment of withdrawal-related depression. Moeller *et al.* [46] carried out a 12-week, double-blind placebo-controlled trial with 76 cocaine-dependent patients receiving either citalopram or placebo along

with cognitive behavioural therapy (CBT) and contingency management (CM). Citalopram-treated subjects showed a significant reduction in cocaine-positive urines during treatment compared to placebo-treated subjects.

- Anti-psychotics: to control cocaine-related acute/subacute psychotic manifestations but are not effective to control cocaine craving [47].
- Carbamazepine/anti-convulsants: controversial use [48].
- Baclofen: the role of GABA-B receptors in addiction has been recently emphasized; the medication, however, might not be effective in humans [49].
- Isradipine: this is a calcium-channel antagonist and as such it should block the cocaine reward effect. Negative evidence in humans, even if administered together with naltrexone [50].
- Amphetamine substitution: risk of amphetamine bingeing behaviours; difficulty in reaching acceptable levels of clinical stabilization. However, very recently Mooney et al. [51] carried out a double-blind, placebo-controlled study to evaluate three treatment conditions in 82 cocaine-dependent individuals: placebo; immediate release (IR) methamphetamine; sustained release (SR) methamphetamine. Both preparation forms of methamphetamine were well tolerated, with similar retention to placebo. Those in the SR condition exhibited consistently lower rates of cocaine-positive urine samples and reported the greatest reduction in craving for cocaine.
- Excitatory amino acid (EAA) antagonists: can prevent neuronal damage that is due to the release of EAA during cerebral ischaemia induced by stimulant use [52].
- Topiramate; Reis et al. [53] carried out a 12-week, open label trial with topiramate 25–300 mg/day. Significant reduction in craving intensity and duration was observed in 25% of the sample.
- Disulfiram: it inhibits DA metabolism. As such, it may exert a direct effect on cocaine use rather than through reducing concurrent alcohol use [54]. Disulfiram increases slightly the cost of methadone treatment, but its increase in effectiveness may be important enough to warrant its addition for treating cocaine dependence in methadone-maintained opiate addicts [55].
- Therapeutic vaccines for substance dependence: a range of immunotherapies, including vaccines, monoclonal anti-bodies and catalytic anti-bodies, have been shown to reduce drug seeking. In human clinical trials, cocaine vaccines have been shown to induce anti-body titers, while producing few side effects [56].

3.5.4 Clinical and Pharmacological Issues Related to Ecstasy and Ecstasy-Like Drugs' Misuse

MDMA (ecstasy; 3,4-methylenedioxymethamphetamine) is only one of a large number of synthetic amphetamine-type drugs possessing varying degrees of stimulant, hallucinogenic and empathogenic effects that are used within the dance scene. Most well-known analogues of MDMA include drugs such as methylenedioxyamphetamine (MDA), N-methyl-1-(1,3-benzodioxol-5-yl)-2-butanamine (MBDB) and methylenedioxyethylamphetamine (MDEA). Regular users will self-administer once or twice a week/month, though there has been increasing recognition of a minority of users who take either very large numbers of tablets (20 or 30) over a single session or extended periods of low-level daily use [57]. Ecstasy is, however, rarely taken in isolation and polydrug use is the norm, with different adjunctive substances taken at different times over the course of a night [57].

After MDMA intake, a number of untoward effects may commonly occur including nausea, vomiting, diarrhoea, tachycardia, arrhythmias, hypertension as well as potentially life-threatening, metabolic acidosis, cerebral haemorrhages, convulsions, coma, rhabdomyolysis, thrombocytopoenia, disseminated intravascular coagulation, syndrome of inappropriate anti-diuretic hormone secretion (SIADH), acute kidney failure, acute liver failure, dehydration and malignant hyperthermia [58]. Dehydration is common and thirsty clubbers naturally tend to replace not sensibly the lost fluids with alcohol. Occasionally, excessive intake of hypotonic fluids, coupled with an increase in vasopressin levels, has led to the occurrence of lethal hyponatraemia. All ecstasy misusers develop a (mild, in most cases) serotonin syndrome after acute drug intake (for a review, see [58]).

3.5.4.1   Clinical Management Issues

Although in the humans relationship between MDMA intake, putative 5-HT neurotoxicity and persistent functional consequences is somewhat controversial, the average single dose size consumed by humans is indeed near to those levels found to be neurotoxic in animals [58]. MDMA is generally considered to be a selective 5-HT neurotoxin. Pathological investigations suggest that 5-HT nerve terminals arising from the dorsal raphe nucleus are specifically involved. The most consistent neuropsychological finding in former MDMA users is a deficit in verbal memory under both immediate- and delayed-recall conditions [40]. Although observations may have been biased by concomitant drug use and/or premorbid functioning, there seems to be an association between MDMA use and increased rates of anxiety, panic, major depressive disorder, prolonged depersonalization, psychosis, flashbacks and even craving for chocolate [40]. History taking should specifically endeavour to identify any pre-existing/persistent depressive/other disorders and to ascertain the functionality of the use of MDMA and the consequences on underlying mood and functioning in days following use. Anti-depressant treatment should usually not be commenced until 2–4 weeks after cessation of MDMA use in order to allow for reassessment and confirmation of any disorder. In prescribing an anti-depressant to a client with a previous history of MDMA use, confining prescribing to only abstinent users is recommended since their effectiveness in a current user would be expected to be poor both as a result of poor compliance and monoamine depletion [40]. In addition, there are at least theoretical causes for concern over potentially fatal interactions between MDMA and selective serotonin reuptake inhibitors (SSRIs) that have very rarely been reported, possibly because some SSRIs (i.e. citalopram) can inhibit the CYP2D6 enzyme [58]. It is conceivable that SSRIs given acutely after MDMA (taken by users to intensify the ecstasy effects) may theoretically increase the risk of precipitating a serotonergic syndrome. Conversely, it is likely that SSRIs and other classes of anti-depressants can be used effectively in this group if a diagnosis of responsive affective/anxiety disorder is confirmed and abstinence is maintained.

3.6   PHARMACOLOGICAL MANAGEMENT OF BENZODIAZEPINE MISUSE

3.6.1   Clinical Pharmacology Issues

Since their introduction over 40 years ago, benzodiazepines have largely replaced older sedative–hypnotic agents in most countries. Benzodiazepine agonists and other agonist ligands at the benzodiazepine site achieve their therapeutic effects by enhancing the actions of the inhibitory neurotransmitter gamma-aminobutyric acid (GABA) at its receptor. Benzodiazepines have a binding site on the GABA receptor, which forms a channel through the membrane and opens and closes to control chloride flow into the cell [51]. When benzodiazepine agonists are on their receptor site, GABA produces a more rapid pulsatile opening of the channel and the flow of chloride is increased. Two GABA receptors have been identified anatomically and pharmacologically. These receptors – variably called type I and type II, benzodiazepine I and benzodiazepine II, or omega I and omega II – are located throughout much of the central nervous system/CNS [59]. Pharmacological studies indicate that the 1,4-benzodiazepines bind with relative nonselectivity to both omega I and omega II sites. The triazolobenzodiazepines (e.g. triazolam) tend to have a greater affinity for omega I and II receptors than do the other benzodiazepines and are more potent. Zopiclone, despite its unusual chemical structure, has a binding profile much like that of the classic benzodiazepines. Zolpidem, however, binds with much greater affinity to the omega I site [59].

The properties of benzodiazepines make them ideally useful for managing anxiety (e.g. diazepam, chlordiazepoxide, lorazepam); insomnia (e.g. temazepam, nitrazepam, flurazepam, lormetazepam); and alcohol withdrawal (chlordiazepoxide) [18].

Used alone or in combination with neuroleptics, benzodiazepines have proved valuable for management of various psychiatric emergencies involving agitation or hostility. However, increased hostility and aggression ('paradoxical effects') following ingestion of these drugs may be observed in vulnerable individuals [41].

3.6.2   Abuse Liability; Management of Benzodiazepine Dependence

Benzodiazepines are usually required for only short periods of treatment; most prescription of these drugs lasts for only a few weeks. However, some disorders for which benzodiazepines are indicated are recurrent or chronic. Therapeutic effects of benzodiazepines are often sustained over months or years, without the need for increased dosage, for the treatment of generalized anxiety disorder and panic disorder. It is of interest that tolerance is not seen to develop in all chronic benzodiazepine users.

Consumption of prescribed medications is higher in certain workplace environments (for a review, see [41]). The onset of withdrawal might be more rapid and the intensity of withdrawal might be greater following discontinuation of short-acting benzodiazepines than after discontinuation of long-acting compounds. Generally speaking, a benzodiazepine dependence condition may be more easily observed if a high-dose, long-term (more than a few weeks/few months), high-potency, compound prescription is made.

Upon abrupt discontinuation of benzodiazepine treatment, dependent patients are likely to experience increased anxiety and/or insomnia (the 'rebound syndrome'). In other words, upon discontinuation of benzodiazepines, the symptoms of anxiety/sleep disturbances for which these compounds were originally prescribed may well reappear. On the other hand, the proper benzodiazepine 'withdrawal syndrome' is characterized by further signs and symptoms, including panic attacks, 'flu-like' syndrome, alterations in taste and smell sensations, tremor, restlessness, gastrointestinal distress, sweating, tachycardia, and mild systolic hypertension. In severe withdrawal states, hallucinations, seizures and deaths have been reported [60]. The syndrome and associated discomfort are usually, but not always, mild reaching peak severity in 2–20 days and abating within 4 weeks after discontinuation. Some recent studies have suggested that symptoms and signs of benzodiazepine withdrawal can persist for many months. Clinical authorities have long recommended that use should be interrupted by occasional 'drug holidays', which would allow reassessment of the need to continue treatment and might also reduce the risk of dependence development. In reducing the benzodiazepine dosage, the *maximum* speed that can be reached is 10% of the previous daily dose (e.g. 100 mg; 90 mg; 81 mg; 73 mg, etc.). If dosages are higher than 30 mg of diazepam, begin to reduce at 5–10 mg/*month* [60]. While reducing the dosage, the use of counselling, support groups and relaxation techniques may be helpful.

Benzodiazepines are relatively safe in overdose if taken alone and rapid reversal of sedation with the receptor antagonist flumazenil is rarely necessary. Even massive overdoses, if taken without other CNS depressants, are almost never fatal. This is because the opening up of the chloride-ion channels depends on the availability of GABA, whose interaction with the receptor is facilitated by benzodiazepines liaising with their GABA receptor portion. This is different from what it happens with barbiturates and alcohol, which interact directly with the chloride ion channels [41]. As a consequence, high dosages of these compounds may facilitate a massive increase of chloride ions inside the CNS cells, thus determining a generalized depression of CNS functions.

3.6.3 Rapid Reference Checklists

How to switch from one benzodiazepine to another [60]:

- If the client is using more than one benzodiazepine, change to one preparation; diazepam is the drug of choice.
- Start with small dosages and increase the dosage to a maximum of 30 mg; doses above 30 mg should be used only occasionally and after appropriate Consultant/senior clinician review.
- Prescribers should take steps to ensure prescribed benzodiazepines are not diverted. Establish with the client at the beginning that this is a short term prescription and that eventually this will be reduced and stopped.
- Divide the daily dose, keeping some of the dose for helping to sleep at night.

Different benzodiazepine dosages equivalent to 10 mg diazepam [59]:

- Temazepam   20 mg;
- Nitrazepam   10 mg;
- Chlordiazepoxide   30 mg;
- Lorazepam   1 mg;
- Oxazepam   30 mg;
- Lormetazepam   1–2 mg;
- Flurazepam   30 mg;
- Flunitrazepam   1 mg.

Management of insomnia in people prone to substance misuse:

- Give sleep hygiene advice.
- Try promethazine 25–50 mg nocte or promazine 25 mg nocte.
- Treat any underlying depression.

Main anecdotal reasons of benzodiazepine use by substance misusers [61]:

- anxiety and insomnia;
- to counteract the noneuphoric effect of methadone;
- depression; many drug users feel benzodiazepines 'help' in lifting their mood;
- to cope with coming down from amphetamines, ecstasy, crack cocaine or cocaine;
- to cope with psychotic disturbances.

3.7 REVIEW OF MOST RECENT LITERATURE ON THE ROLE OF PSYCHOSOCIAL INTERVENTION IN THE TREATMENT AND MANAGEMENT OF SUBSTANCE MISUSE

Methods: The papers here commented were identified with the help of searching databases, including Pubmed (http://www.ncbi.nlm.nih.gov/sites/entrez) and ISI web of knowledge (http://portal.isiknowledge.com/). No studies were excluded due to being written in a language other than English. The literature search was carried out using a combination of the following keywords: psychosocial intervention; substance misuse; drug misuse; cognitive behavioural therapy/CBT; contingency management; motivational interviewing/MI; family therapy. Since the focus was on most recent papers only, articles eligible for inclusion where either review or research papers published between January 2003 and June 2009, with particular attention to those papers published over the last 3 years. References of all retrieved articles were examined for additional studies. In total, some 50 articles were analysed and for 14 of them the focus was felt to be of interest for the present review. To improve their evaluation, identified studies have been grouped here depending on their focus.

3.7.1 Adolescent Substance Misuse and Psychosocial Intervention

Waldron and Turner [62] synthesized findings from 17 studies since 1998 regarding evaluation of outpatient treatments for adolescent substance abuse. They examined 46 different intervention conditions with a total sample of 2307 adolescents. The sample included individual CBT replications; group CBT replications; family therapy replications; and minimal treatment control conditions. According to the meta-analysis carried out, 3 treatment approaches (i.e. multidimensional family therapy, functional family therapy and group CBT) emerged as well-established models for substance abuse treatment.

Youth substance abuse relapse prevention was examined by Burleson and Kaminer [63] as a function of patients' situational self-efficacy (SE), for example their confidence to abstain from substance use in high-risk situations. Eighty-eight adolescent substance abusers were randomly assigned to either CBT or psycho-education (PET) group therapy. Increased SE predicted subsequent abstinence independently from drug urinalysis and treatment condition only during treatment, while previous substance use predicted subsequent self-efficacy. CBT was not differentially effective than PET in promoting SE. Furthermore, Liddle *et al.* [64] examined the efficacy of two adolescent drug-abuse treatments: individual CBT and multidimensional family therapy (MDFT). A total of 224 youths (most being cannabis misusers) were recruited. Although both treatments produced significant decreases in cannabis consumption, significant treatment effects were found favouring MDFT on substance use problem severity and these effects continued to 12 months following treatment termination.

3.7.2 Stimulant Misuse and Psychosocial Intervention

Lee and Rawson [65] carried out a systematic review of CBT and contingency management (CM) for methamphetamine users. Treatment with CBT appeared to be associated with reductions in methamphetamine use and other positive changes, even over very short periods of treatment. CM studies identified a significant reduction of methamphetamine use during application of the procedure, but it was not clear if these gains were sustained at post-treatment follow-up. Baker et al. [66] enrolled 214 regular amphetamine users and found that there was a significant increase in the likelihood of abstinence from amphetamines amongst those receiving two or more CBT treatment sessions. They recommended that clients with moderate to severe levels of depression may best be offered four sessions of CBT for amphetamine use from the outset, with further treatment for amphetamine use and/or depression depending on response. Messina et al. [67] compared the efficacy of 4 study conditions (i.e. CBT, CM, CBT with CM, or methadone maintenance) for the treatment of cocaine dependence amongst methadone-maintained patients with and without anti-social personality disorder (ASPD). They found that personality disorder clients were more likely to abstain from cocaine use during treatment than patients without ASPD and that the strong treatment effect for ASPD patients was primarily due to the CM condition.

Epstein et al. [68] argued whether a combination of contingency management and methadone dose increase would promote abstinence from heroin and cocaine. Participants were randomly assigned to methadone dose (70 or 100 mg/day, double-blind) and voucher condition. Urine-screen results showed that the methadone dose increase reduced heroin use but not cocaine use. The authors suggested that to promote simultaneous abstinence from cocaine and heroin a relatively high dose of methadone appears necessary but not sufficient; an increase in overall incentive amount may also be required. Finally, Knapp et al. [69] carried out a systematic review of all RCTs on psychosocial interventions for treating psychostimulant use disorder. Twenty-seven randomized controlled studies (3663 participants) fulfilled inclusion criteria. The comparisons between different types of behavioural interventions showed results in favour of treatments with some form of contingency management in respect to both reducing drop outs and lowering cocaine use.

3.7.3 Dual Diagnosis and Psychosocial Intervention

Bradley et al. [70] aimed at investigating whether a weekly outpatient group intervention, consisting of MI and CBT, was effective in reducing substance use and improving symptomatology amongst people with psychosis. Those 39 participants who entered the treatment group exhibited significant improvements in terms of substance use, symptomatology and utilization of acute mental health services. Conversely, Baker et al. [71] investigated whether a 10-session intervention consisting of MI and CBT was more effective than routine treatment in reducing substance use in people with a psychotic disorder. There was a short-term improvement in depression and a similar trend with regard to cannabis use amongst participants who received the motivational interviewing/CBT intervention, but overall this was associated with modest improvements.

3.7.4   Cognitive Behavioural Therapy in Substance Misuse

Dutra *et al.* [72] identified a total of 34 well-controlled treatment conditions; 5 for cannabis, 9 for cocaine, 7 for opiate, and 13 for polysubstance users, representing the treatment of 2340 patients. Psychosocial treatments evaluated included CBT, contingency management, relapse prevention and treatments combining CBT and contingency management. Overall, controlled trial data suggested that psychosocial treatments provide benefits reflecting a moderate effect size. Psychosocial interventions turned out indeed to be most effective for cannabis use and least effective for polysubstance use, with the strongest effect being associated with contingency management interventions. Conversely, Carroll *et al.* [73] evaluated the efficacy of a computer-based training in CBT (CBT4CBT) for substance dependence. Seventy-seven outpatients were randomly assigned to standard treatment or standard treatment with biweekly access to the CBT4CBT programme. Participants assigned to the CBT4CBT condition submitted significantly more urine specimens that were negative for any type of drugs and tended to have longer continuous periods of abstinence during treatment. According to Kadden *et al.* [74], however, adding contingency management to cognitive behavioural therapy would be associated with even better abstinence outcomes.

3.8   DISCUSSION AND CONCLUSIONS

This chapter has offered a review related to a number of pharmacological and clinical issues related to the treatment and management of opiates; stimulants (cocaine; amphetamine and amphetamine-like substances); ecstasy/ecstasy-like drugs; and benzodiazepines. Although a particular focus here was on available medications for both treatment and management, an update of the most recent literature papers regarding the use of psychosocial intervention was provided as well.

Beside psychosocial intervention, the evidence-based pharmacotherapeutic approach has become an important factor for the treatment of substance misuse and withdrawal syndromes [75]. For the pharmacological treatment of opiates, the use of methadone, buprenorphine and naltrexone have been more thoroughly discussed here. For opiate dependence, both methadone and buprenorphine treatment seem to be the first-choice pharmacotherapy. However, there are suggestions that buprenorphine might be preferentially offered to individuals such as those who are less severe addicts and who are more motivated [16]. Buprenorphine limited ability to activate opioid mechanisms results, as said, in a ceiling of the magnitude of its effects. As a consequence of buprenorphine being a partial agonist, one could think that the drug may have a more favourable safety profile with respect to methadone. However, some UK data [76] have suggested that only future long-term, controlled, parallel group, naturalistic studies will be able to assess more comprehensively the lethality risk attached to buprenorphine use.

Pharmacological treatment of stimulant misuse still proves to be a challenge. A number of medications, especially targeted at restoring the dopaminergic imbalance resulting from stimulant misuse itself [77] have been tried. However, for cocaine dependence no single medication, or combination of medications, can be recommended so far. Some drugs may seem, however, promising, such as D2/D3 partial agonists; calcium antagonists; disulfiram and the therapeutic vaccines. On the other hand, one could think that although for a long time dopamine has been consistently associated with the reinforcing effects of most drugs of abuse and especially stimulants, recent pharmacological evidence emphasizes the importance of the endocannabinoid system. There seems to be the possibility in fact that the pharmacological management of this system might not only block the direct reinforcing effect of both cannabis and opioids, but also prevent the *relapse* to various drugs of abuse including opioids, cocaine and amphetamine. Preclinical and clinical studies suggest indeed that the manipulation of the endocannabinoid system through the CB(1) receptor antagonists might constitute a new therapeutic strategy for treating addiction across different classes of abused drugs [78]. On the other hand, it is here to be emphasized that rimonabant, likely to be the most well known CB(1) receptor antagonist, was, however, withdrawn from the European market in November 2008 due to medication safety issues. Emerging pharmacogenomics research on addiction to both stimulants and opiates might soon lead to improved clinical outcomes by tailoring the type, dose and duration of treatment to individual patients' genotypes [79]. However, to realize the potential of pharmacogenomics in reducing the burden of addiction, several challenges related to clinical integration of novel treatment strategies will need to be addressed, including the preparedness of primary-care physicians to incorporate pharmacogenetics into clinical practice, patients' willingness to undergo genetic testing, and privacy and anti-discrimination protections sufficient to reassure physicians and patients that genetic testing will not lead to stigmatization and discrimination [79].

Virtually all recreational drugs, including MDMA and methamphetamine, are capable of producing acute adverse psychological experiences in normal users and exacerbating symptoms in those with underlying psychological disorders. Most acute presentations are typically short lived and self-limiting and are only very rarely life-threatening. However, in those who present with acute drug-related psychological symptoms there should be an emphasis on follow-up since in some cases the symptoms will represent the onset of a persistent independent disorder that requires treatment [40].

Taking into account the psychosocial intervention for the treatment of substance misuse, it seems that most of the studies here reviewed were fairly diverse from each other. Furthermore, examining those studies comparing different therapeutic modalities raises important questions about the duration, intensity and type of treatment [80]. Even if these limitations are taken into account it appeared, however, that both CBT and CM approaches emerged as well-established models for substance-abuse treatment, and especially so for substance misuse conditions different from opiate misuse. A number of other models are probably effective as well, with none of the treatment approaches being clearly superior to any others. In terms of stimulant misuse, it is intriguing to note that psychological intervention is likely to be more clinically promising than single pharmacotherapies. In particular, CBT seems to represent a particularly accessible intervention that may be implemented easily within current drug and alcohol services.

According to Knapp et al. [69], however, with the evidence currently available there are no data supporting a single treatment approach that is able to comprise the multidimensional facets of addiction patterns and to significantly yield better outcomes to resolve the chronic, relapsing nature of addiction, with all its correlates and consequences. More than a single treatment approach that is valid for all, it is conceivable that most promising results can be achieved by a combination of both pharmacotherapeutic and psychosocial treatment approaches.

REFERENCES

1. Heidbreder, C.A. and Hagan, J.J. (2005) Novel pharmacotherapeutic approaches for the treatment of drug addiction and craving. *Current Opinion in Pharmacology*, **5**, 107–118.

2. Corkery, J., Schifano, F., Ghodse, A.H., *et al.* (2004) Methadone effects and its role in fatalities. *Human Psychopharmacology Clinical and Experimental*, **19**, 565–576.

3. Ghodse, A.H., Schifano, F., Oyefeso, A., *et al.* (2003) Drug-related deaths as reported by coroners in England, Wales, Scotland, N Ireland and Channel Islands. Annual review 2002 and np-SAD Report no. 11. European Centre for Addiction Studies: London, St George's Hospital Medical School

4. Wolff, K., Rostami-Hodjegan, A., Hay, A.W., *et al.* (2000). Population-based pharmacokinetic approach for methadone monitoring of opiate addicts: potential clinical utility. *Addiction*, **95**, 1771–1783.

5. Ghodse, A.H., Oyefeso, A., Webb, L. *et al.* (2002) Drug-Related Deaths as Reported by Coroners in England and Wales: Annual Review 2001 and np-SAD Surveillance Report no. 9. Centre for Addiction Studies: London, St George's Hospital Medical School.

6. Wu, C. and Henry, J.A. (1990) Deaths of heroin addicts starting on methadone maintenance. The Lancet, **335**, 424.

7. Drummer, O.H., Opeskin, K., Syrjanen, M., *et al.* (1992) Methadone toxicity causing death in ten subjects starting on a methadone maintenance program. *American Journal of Forensic Medical Pathology*, **13**, 346–350.

8. Department of Health: Drug Misuse & Dependence (2007) UK Guidelines on Clinical Management.

9. Hull, C.J. (1985) Receptor binding and its significance. *British Journal of Anaesthesia*, **57**, 131–133.

10. Rosenbaum, J.S., Holford, N.H. and Sadee, W. (1985) In vivo receptor binding of opioid drugs at the mu site. *Journal of Pharmacology and Experimental Therapeutics*, **233**, 735–740.

11. Dum, J., Blasig, J. and Herz A (1981) Buprenorphine: Demonstration of physical dependence liability. *European Journal of Psychopharmacology*, **70**, 293–300.

12. Cowan, A., Doxey, J.C. and Harry, E.J.R. (1977) The animal pharmacology of buprenorphine, an oripavine analgesic agent. *British Journal of Pharmacology*, **60**, 647–654.

13. Ghodse, A.H. (1989) Benefit-risk of agonist-antagonist analgesics. *British Journal of Addiction*, **84**, 455–457.

14. Bullingham, R.E.S., McQuay, H.J., Porter, E.J.B. *et al.* (1982) Sublingual buprenorphine used postoperatively: Ten hour plasma drug concentration analysis. *British Journal of Clinical Psychopharmacology*, **13**, 665–673.

15. McQuay, H.J., Moore, R.A. and Bullingham, R.E.S. (1985) Buprenorphine kinetics, in *Opioid Analgesics in the Management of Clinical Pain* (eds. K. Foley and C. Inturissi), Raven Press, New York.

16. Gilvarry, E. and Schifano, F. (2002) Medical use of buprenorphine in the UK. Special report prepared for the WHO, February 2002, pp. 1–93.

17. Dollery, C. (1999). Buprenorphine hydrochloride. In: *Therapeutic Drugs,* 2nd edn, Edinburgh: Church Livingstone

18. British Medical Association and Royal Pharmaceutical Society of Great Britain (2008) British National Formulary. London.

19. Ibrahim, R.B., Wilson, J.G., Thorsby, M.E. *et al.* (2000) Effects of buprenorphine on CYP3A activity in rat and human liver microsomes. *Life Sciences*, **66**, 1293–1298.

20. Johnson, R.E. and McCagh, J.C. (2000) Buprenorphine and naloxone for heroin dependence. *Current Psychiatry Reports*, **2**, 519–526.

21. Zacny, J.P., Conley, K. and Galinkin, J. (1997) Comparing the subjective, psychomotor and physiological effects of intravenous buprenorphine and morphine in healthy volunteers. *Pharmacology and Experimental Therapeutics*, **282**, 1187–1197.

22. Reisine, T. and Pasternak, G. (1995) Opioid analgesics and antagonists, in *Goodman & Gilman's The Pharmacological Basis of Therapeutics*, 9th edn (eds. J.G. Hardmann, A. Goodmann Gilmann and L.E. Limbird), McGraw Hill, New York.

23. Mattick, R.P., Ali, R., White, J. *et al.* (1999) A randomised double-blind trial of buprenorphine tablets versus methadone syrup for maintenance therapy: efficacy and cost effectiveness. *NIDA Research Monograph Series*, **180**, 77.

24. Ling, W., Charuvastra, C., Collins, J.F. *et al.* (1998) Buprenorphine maintenance of opiate dependence: a multicenter, randomised clinical trial. *Addiction*, **93**, 475–486.

25. Johnson, R., Jaffe, J. and Fudala, P. (1992) A controlled trial of buprenorphine treatment for opioid dependence. *Journal of the American Medical Association*, **267**, 2750–2755.

26. Kosten, T., Shottenfeld, R., Ziedonis, D. *et al.* (1993) Buprenorphine versus methadone maintenance for opioid dependence. *Journal of Nervous and Mental Disease*, **181**, 358–364.

27. Barrau, K., Thirion, X., Micallef, J. *et al.* (2001) Comparison of methadone and high dosage buprenorphine users in French care centres. *Addiction*, **96**, 1433–1441.

28. West, S., O'Neal, K., Graham, C. (2000) A meta-analysis comparing the effectiveness of buprenorphine and methadone, *Journal of Substance Abuse* **12**: 405–414.

29. San, L., Cami, J., Fernandez, T. *et al.* (1992) Assessment and management of opioid withdrawal symptoms in buprenorphine-dependent subjects. *British Journal of Addiction*, **87**, 55–62.

30. Auriacombe, M., Franques, P., Tignol, J. (2001). Deaths attributable to methadone vs buprenorphine in France. *Journal of the American Medical Association*, **285**: 45

31. Kintz, P. (2001) Deaths involving buprenorphine: a compendium of French cases. *Forensic Sciences International*, **121**, 65–69

32. Raynaud, M., Petit, G. and Potard, D. *et al.* (1998) Six deaths linked to concomitant use of buprenorphine and benzodiazepines. *Addiction*, **93**, 1385–1392.

33. Bouley, M., Viriot, E., Barache, D. (2000) Practical reflections on the diversion of drugs. *Therapie*, **55**: 295–301

34. Vickers A P, Jolly A (2006) Naltrexone and problems in pain management. *British Medical Journal*, **332**, 132–133.

35. Carreno, J.E., Alvarez, C.E. and San Narciso, G.I. *et al.* (2003) Maintenance treatment with depot opioid antagonists in subcutaneous implants: an alternative in the treatment of opioid dependence. *Addiction Biology*, **8**, 429–438.

36. Foster, J., Brewer, C. and Steele, T. (2003) Naltrexone implants can completely prevent early (1-month) relapse after opiate detoxification: a pilot study of two cohorts totalling 101 patients with a note on naltrexone blood levels. *Addiction Biology*, **8**, 211–217.

37. Hulse, G.K., Arnold-Reed, D.E., O'Neil, G. *et al.* (2004a) Naltrexone and 6-beta-naltrexol levels following naltrexone implant: comparing two naltrexone implants. *Addiction Biology*, **9**, 59–65.

38. Hulse, G.K., Arnold-Reed, D.E., O'Neil, G. *et al.* (2004b) Achieving long-term continuous blood naltrexone and 6-beta-naltrexol coverage following sequential naltrexone implants. *Addiction Biology*, **9**, 67–72.

39. Schifano, F. (1996). Cocaine misuse and dependence. *Current Opinion in Psychiatry*, **9**: 225–30.

40. Winstock, A. and Schifano, F. (2009) Disorders relating to the use of ecstasy, other 'party drugs' and khat, in *New Oxford Textbook of Psychiatry* (eds. M. Gelder, N. Andreasen, J.J. Lopez-Ibor and J. Geddes). Oxford University Press, Oxford.

41. Schifano, F. (2005) Substance misuse in the workplace, in *Addiction at Work: Tackling Drug Use and Misuse in the Workplace* (ed. A.H. Ghodse), Gower Publishing Ltd., London.

42. de Lima, M.S., de Oliveira Soares, B.G., *et al.* (2002) Pharmacological treatment of cocaine dependence: a systematic review. *Addiction*, **97**, 931–949.

43. Schifano, F. (2009). Stimulant drugs (cocaine; methamphetamine) and recent pharmacological advances in treatment. *SCANbites*, 1–3.

44. McDowell, D., Nunes, E.V., Seracini, A.M. *et al.* (2005) Desipramine treatment of cocaine-dependent patients with depression: a placebo-controlled trial. *Drug and Alcohol Dependence*, **80**, 209–221.

45. Ukai, M. and Mitsunaga, H. (2005) Involvement of dopamine D3 and D4 receptors in the discriminative stimulus properties of cocaine in the rat. *Methods and Findings Experimental Clinical Pharmacology*, **27**, 645–649.

46. Moeller, F.G., Schmitz, J.M., Steinberg, J.L. *et al.* (2007) Citalopram combined with behavioral therapy reduces cocaine use: a double-blind, placebo-controlled trial. *American Journal of Drug and Alcohol Abuse*, **33**, 367–378.

47. Hamilton, J.D., Nguyen, Q.X., Gerber, R.M. *et al.* (2009) Olanzapine in cocaine dependence: a double-blind, placebo-controlled trial. *American Journal of Addictions*, **18**, 48–52.

48. Minozzi, S., Amato, L., Davoli, M. *et al.* (2008) Anticonvulsants for cocaine dependence. *Cochrane Database Systematic Reviews* 2 (Art. No. CD006754).

49. Lile, J.A., Stoops, W.W., Allen, T.S. *et al.* (2004) Baclofen does not alter the reinforcing, subject-rated or cardiovascular effects of intranasal cocaine in humans. *Psychopharmacology (Berl)*, **171**, 441–449.

50. Sofuoglu, M., Singha, A., Kosten, T.R., *et al.* (2003) Effects of naltrexone and isradipine, alone or in combination, on cocaine responses in humans. *Pharmacology Biochemistry and Behaviour*, **75**, 801–808

51. Mooney, M.E., Herin, D.V., Schmitz, J.M. *et al.* (2009) Effects of oral methamphetamine on cocaine use: a randomized, double-blind, placebo-controlled trial. *Drug and Alcohol Dependence*, **101**, 34–41.

52. McCance-Katz, E., Sevarino, K. *et al.* (1999) Pharmacotherapy of stimulant dependence: one of Japan's greatest public health challenges. *Nihon Shinkei Seishin Yakurigaku Zasshi* **19**, 159–186.

53. Reis, A.D., Castro, L.A., Faria, R. *et al.* (2008) Craving decrease with topiramate in outpatient treatment for cocaine dependence: an open label trial. *Revista Brasileira de Psiquiatria*, **30**, 132–135.

54. Carroll, K.M., Fenton, L.R., Ball, S.A. *et al.* (2004) Efficacy of disulfiram and cognitive behavior therapy in cocaine-dependent outpatients: a randomized placebo-controlled trial. *Archives of General Psychiatry*, **61**, 264–272.

55. Jofre-Bonet, M., Sindelar, J.L., Petrakis, I.L. *et al.* (2004) Cost effectiveness of disulfiram: treating cocaine use in methadone-maintained patients. *Journal of Substance Abuse Treatment*, **26**, 225–232.

56. Orson, F.M., Kinsey, B.M., Singh, R.A. *et al.* (2009) Vaccines for cocaine abuse. Human Vaccines Apr 20 [Epub ahead of print]

57. Schifano, F. and Corkery J (2008) Cocaine/crack cocaine consumption, treatment demand, seizures, related offences, prices, average purity levels and deaths in the UK (1990-2004). *Journal of Psychopharmacology*, **22**, 71–79.

58. Schifano, F. (2004) A bitter pill? Overview of ecstasy (MDMA; MDA) related fatalities. *Psychopharmacology (Berlin)*, **173**, 242–248.

59. Hindmarch, I. (2005) Medicines in the workplace: the effects of prescribed and OTC drugs on performance, in *Addiction at Work: Tackling Drug Use and Misuse in the Workplace* (ed. A.H. Ghodse), Gower Publishing Ltd., London.

60. Schifano, F. and Magni, G. (1989) Panic attacks and major depression after discontinuation of long-term diazepam abuse. *Drug Intelligence and Clinical Pharmacy; the Annals of Pharmacotherapy*, **23**, 989–990.

61. Forza, G., Levarta, E., Da Ros, D., *et al.* (1998) Benzodiazepines consumption in a sample of methadone maintained patients: Characteristics of use and psychopathological profile. *European Psychiatry*, **13** (suppl. 4), s15.

62. Waldron, H.B. and Turner, C.W. (2008) Evidence-based psychosocial treatments for adolescent substance abuse. *Journal of Clinical Child and Adolescent Psychology*, **37**, 238–261.

63. Burleson, J.A. and Kaminer, Y. (2005) Self-efficacy as a predictor of treatment outcome in adolescent substance use disorders. *Addictive Behaviour*, **30**, 1751–1764.

64. Liddle, H.A., Dakof, G.A., Turner, R.M. *et al.* (2008) Treating adolescent drug abuse: a randomized trial comparing multidimensional family therapy and cognitive behavior therapy. *Addiction*, **103**, 1660–1670.

65. Lee, N.K. and Rawson, R.A. (2008) A systematic review of cognitive and behavioural therapies for methamphetamine dependence. *Drug and Alcohol Review*, **27**, 309–317.

66. Baker, A., Lee, N.K., Claire, M. *et al.* (2005) Brief cognitive behavioural interventions for regular amphetamine users: a step in the right direction. *Addiction*, **100**, 367–378

67. Messina, N., Farabee, D., Rawson, R. (2003) Treatment responsivity of cocaine-dependent patients with antisocial personality disorder to cognitive-behavioral and contingency management interventions. *Journal of Consulting and Clinical Psychology*, **71**, 320–329.

68. Epstein, D.H., Schmittner, J., Umbricht, A., *et al.* (2009) Promoting abstinence from cocaine and heroin with a methadone dose increase and a novel contingency. *Drug and Alcohol Dependence*, **101**, 92–100.

69. Knapp, W.P., Soares, B.G., Farrell, M. *et al.* (2007) Psychosocial interventions for cocaine and psychostimulant amphetamines related disorders. *Cochrane Database Systematic Reviews*, 18, CD003023.

70. Bradley, A.C., Baker, A., Lewin, T.J. (2007) Group intervention for coexisting psychosis and substance use disorders in rural Australia: outcomes over 3 years. *Australian New Zealand Journal of Psychiatry*, **41**, 501–508.

71. Baker, A., Bucci, S., Lewin, T.J. *et al.* (2006) Cognitive-behavioural therapy for substance use disorders in people with psychotic disorders: Randomised controlled trial. *British Journal of Psychiatry*, **188**, 439–448.

72. Dutra, L., Stathopoulou, G., Basden, S.L., *et al.* (2008) A meta-analytic review of psychosocial interventions for substance use disorders. *American Journal of Psychiatry*, **165**, 179–187.

73. Carroll, K.M., Ball, S.A., Martino, S., *et al.* (2008) Computer-assisted delivery of cognitive-behavioral therapy for addiction: a randomized trial of CBT4CBT. *American Journal of Psychiatry*, **165**, 881–888.

74. Kadden, R.M., Litt, M.D., Kabela-Cormier, E. *et al.* (2007) Abstinence rates following behavioral treatments for marijuana dependence. *Addictive Behavior*, **32**, 1220–1236.

75. Walter, M. and Wiesbeck, G.A. (2009) Pharmacotherapy of substance dependence and withdrawal syndromes. *Therapeutische Umschau*, **66**, 449–457.

76. Schifano, F., Corkery, J., Gilvarry, E. *et al.* (2005). Buprenorphine mortality, seizures and prescription data in the UK (1980-2002). *Human Psychopharmacology: Clinical and Experimental*, **20**: 343–348.

77. Schifano, F. (1998) Cocaine misuse and dependence. *Current Opinion in Psychiatry*, **9**, 225–230.

78. Parolaro, D., Rubino, T. (2008) The role of the endogenous cannabinoid system in drug addiction. *Drug News and Perspectives*, **21**, 149–157.

79. Shields, A.E. and Lerman, C. (2008) Anticipating clinical integration of pharmacogenetic treatment strategies for addiction: are primary care physicians ready? *Clinical Pharmacology and Therapeutics* **83**, 635–639.

80. Denis, C., Lavie, E., Fatséas, M., *et al.* (2006). Psychotherapeutic interventions for cannabis abuse and/or dependence in outpatient settings. *Cochrane Database System Review*, 19; **3**: CD005336.

4.1 Measuring, Preventing and Treating Global Drug Abuse

Kylie D. Reed[1], MA, BMBCh, MRCPsych, Mark Prunty[2], MBChB, MRCPsych and John Strang[1], MBBS, FRCPsych, MD

[1] *National Addiction Centre, Institute of Psychiatry, King's College London, London, UK*

[2] *Respond (Community Substance Misuse Service), Surrey and Borders Partnership NHS Foundation Trust, Leatherhead, Surrey, UK*

Elements of drug abuse and drug prevention strategies tie countries and cultures. As Medina-Mora, Real and Robles explain in their chapter 'Epidemiology of Drug Abuse: A Global Overview', 99% of cocaine is produced in the Andean region of South America, then trafficked illegally throughout the globe; Meanwhile, 'precursors required for the manufacture of drugs from the raw products are usually distributed from more industrialized countries to usually less-developed regions where drugs are produced'. Elsewhere, Babor and colleagues caution against excessive focus on national boundaries, pointing out that the majority of illicit drugs used in the US are actually produced within the US [1]. There is global production of drugs, a global market that is often interconnected and a global problem of drug abuse. Poznyak, in his chapter entitled 'Drugs: Prevention', highlights the health impact, social consequences and economic burden of drug misuse, concluding that 'Prevention of drug abuse and drug-related harm has become a priority area for the international community and national governments around the world'. Schifano in his chapter 'Drugs: Treatment and Management' explores the treatment and management of drugs of abuse, addressing both pharmacological and psychosocial interventions, with clear references to the neurobiological underpinnings of dependence.

CULTURAL DIVERSITY AND ECONOMIC DISPARITY

Under the wide umbrella of the global drug problem resides a complex and varied population: A diverse people, with an extensive breadth of cultural and religious backgrounds,

Substance Abuse Disorders: Evidence and Experience, First Edition. Edited by Hamid Ghodse, Helen Herrman, Mario Maj and Norman Sartorius.
© 2011 John Wiley & Sons, Ltd. Published 2011 by John Wiley & Sons, Ltd.

traditions, social scenarios, economic statuses and geographical circumstances; and alongside this, a diversity of drugs, from plant-based drugs such as heroin and cocaine, to synthetic drugs such as LSD and amphetamine-type stimulants. Measuring global drug abuse and understanding the personal, social and international impact is thus a notable challenge. The purpose, as Medina-Mora *et al.* explain is to 'describe the problem in a way that provides the evidence required to orientate policy'. Poznyak adds, 'Hundreds of programmes have been implemented around the world to prevent drug use... without attempts to evaluate their effectiveness and cost-effectiveness' [1]. He later notes that 'at the population level... very little data is available to policy-makers to evaluate the effectiveness of the wide range of interventions'; while the limited data that is available may not be generalizable to countries with different cultural norms and socioeconomic climates [1]. The recent international science-policy review on 'Drug Policy and the Public Good' goes a considerable way to gather this evidence base [1] but the calls from Medina-Mora *et al.* and from Poznyak for greater attention to conducting and scrutinizing real scientific evidence remain crucial to the future.

Indeed, as Medina-Mora *et al.* emphasize, there are important variations not only between countries but also within countries: 'Variations in rates of use ...are related to sociocultural factors that validate certain forms of use in well-defined social groups'. For example, the Peyote cactus, native to South-western Texas and Mexico and from which the hallucinogen mescaline derives, has a long history of ritual religious and medicinal use by indigenous Americans [2]. This tradition continues to impact acceptability today, with the United States federal law protecting this traditional religious use: 'the use, possession, or transportation of peyote by an Indian for bona fide traditional ceremonial purposes in connection with the practice of a traditional Indian religion is lawful and shall not be prohibited by the United States or any State' [3].

In some cases, despite being governed by the same laws, differing patterns of drug use can be found between culturally different groups living side by side. Cannabis-use patterns of the Maori population of New Zealand have been found to differ from those of the nonindigenous New Zealand population: Compared to other New Zealanders, Maori have been found to begin using cannabis at an earlier age, consume more potent forms and to use it more frequently [4, 5]. A similar picture is found when comparing drug use amongst indigenous and nonindigenous Australians: Clough *et al.* [6] reported that rates of cannabis use amongst Aboriginal males in Australia's Northern Territory were almost double the proportion in the general Northern territory population. Here, we hear echoes of attention to the importance of sociocultural context from earlier decades [7] – and even from more than a century ago [8]. Socioeconomic disadvantage, and social and family adversity have been posited as explanations [5], along with the powerful impact of cultural dislocation following European colonization [5, 9, 10].

Thus, it is worrying that access to health services to tackle drug misuse and associated morbidity is reduced amongst these indigenous populations, most notably amongst those living in remote areas [11]: 24% of the indigenous population of Australia live in remote or very remote localities [12]. Medina-Mora *et al.* also identify poor living conditions and stigmatization as important barriers for accessing services in some areas. Hence 'Lower rates of use might result in greater burden when they occur in contexts of poverty, social inequity ... or when there are no resources to identify cases and offer treatment'.

REDUCING SUPPLY, DEMAND AND HARM

Medina-Mora *et al.*'s explanation of paradigms of drug misuse and dependence provides important background to the models of preventive interventions described by Poznyak: The psychosocial paradigm views the individual within a multifactorial context of risk and protective factors that influence their exposure to and engagement with drug use. This model highlights the reduction of risk factors, such as socioeconomic deprivation, as key; other models draw the focus to a reduction in drug supply; while a model based on drug markets places the onus for interventions across the board, with psychosocial interventions and treatment therapies to reduce demand, and legal and political measures to reduce supply. Poznyak references the 1961, 1971 and 1988 international treaties on narcotic drugs and psychotropic substances that seek to reduce drug supply and availability, while protecting the use of drugs required for therapeutic interventions; and he describes a number of strategies for reducing demand at population and community levels. Poznyak echoes an earlier author [13] in applying Caplan's concepts of primary, secondary and tertiary prevention [14] – primary prevention diminishing exposure to drugs and reducing use of drugs; secondary prevention being early identification of problematic use; and tertiary prevention being the reduction of the health and social consequences of an established drug-use problem. Adding colour to Poznyak's structure, Caplan (2000) likens intervention levels to 'triage programs used by armies to determine the timetables of priorities in treating battlefield casualties. In order to reduce the loss of life, most armies develop the policy of providing immediate treatment for the moderately wounded, who may be expected to be helped to recover by prompt medical and surgical intervention. These are separated from the less-seriously wounded who can recover on their own or with delayed care and the most critically wounded. . .' [15]

TREATMENT AND MANAGEMENT STRATEGIES

Where a drug problem is already established, in addition to implementing tertiary prevention strategies [14] to reduce harm and impact, a strong understanding of the treatment options available is essential for implementation of the most appropriate treatment portfolio. Schifano succinctly describes key practical and safety issues in the use of the current drug treatments in his chapter addressing treatment and management. He highlights the strong evidence base for the use of methadone and buprenorphine as opiate substitutes, and the importance of considering the metabolism of both drugs when managing cases and in assessing the risks of overdose in treatment; he addresses the long-term use of naltrexone, and its neurological impact, and the use of alpha-2 adrenergic receptor agonists. The management of the misuse of stimulants, ecstasy, ecstasy-like drugs and benzodiazepine misuse is also discussed, with an interesting and balanced summary of benzodiazepine abuse liability, as well as detail on subsequent management.

CHANGING TRENDS IN DRUG MISUSE AND IN TREATMENT

While faced with the challenge of developing drug-prevention strategies whose effectiveness can be measured, and modifying these depending on cultural variations, an additional challenge is the changing nature of drug misuse over time, with drug use 'influenced by opportunities for illicit cultivation, diversion or trafficking and of changing public attitudes and patterns of consumption'. Cannabis has been experiencing one such cycle over the past decade: Medina-Mora *et al.* reference the downward trend in cannabis use over this period, from 28.2% in 1998 to 17.9% in 2007/08. Meanwhile, although Medina-Mora *et al.* describe a stabilization in amphetamine-type substance use from 2003 to 2006 in developed countries including Western Europe, increasing reports of the use of new synthetic stimulants may herald the re-emergence of popular stimulant use, possibly again 'linked to life styles and group identity of young people', to use Medina-Mora *at el.*'s phrase: the UK dance magazine, Mixmag, reported in their 2009 survey that 41.7% of respondents had tried mephedrone and 33.6% in the last month [16]. In 2009, Mephedrone, a substituted cathinone with stimulant and MDMA-like properties, was one of a group of so-called 'legal highs' in the UK [17]. In April 2010, mephedrone was brought under the control of the UK Misuse of Drugs Act 1971, classified in April 2010 as a Class B drug [18]. Further illustrating the cyclical phenomenon of drug misuse, the UK Advisory Council on the Misuse of Drugs subsequently reported that many of the websites previously selling mephedrone now purported to be selling naphyrone, through the brand name NRG-1, a drug which bears close structural resemblance to the cathiones [19].

Another growing trend of misuse, apparently enabled by the ease of purchase of prescription and over-the-counter medicines via internet sites, may be particularly hard to measure and monitor (and probably even harder to influence): the National Centre on Addiction and Substance Abuse at Columbia University found a 17% increase in internet sites selling controlled prescription drugs from 2004 to 2006 [20]. Benzodiazepines are the most frequently offered controlled drug on the internet [20]: It is estimated that 89% of the internet supply sites do not require a physician's prescription in order to buy the medications [21]. Internet purchases may further increase the ubiquity of drug abuse, while making it harder still to measure and monitor. Thus, while the internet is shrinking our globe in terms of barriers to communication and accessibility, in the context of drug abuse it is increasing the global problem.

As the catalogue of drugs of abuse grows and evolves, so too must the intervention, management and treatment strategies to tackle them. In his chapter addressing treatment and management, Schifano reviews the range of pharmacological treatments that have been tried in the field of stimulants, including those that have shown little benefit for withdrawal, craving or relapse prevention. He highlights the possible benefits suggested by studies of amphetamine substitution, the use of topiramate, disulfiram and, cocaine vaccines; He discusses too the pharmacological management of ecstasy and ecstasy-like drugs including the potential risks and benefits of prescribing selective serotonin reuptake inhibitors in such cases.

Developing the treatment review beyond psychopharmacology, Schifano assesses current evidence for the impact of psychosocial interventions in drug misuse and dependence. He describes positive, if moderate, effect sizes for a number of different psychosocial interventions and for a range of addictions, while noting the larger effect sizes reported from studies into the use of contingency management. The National Institute for Health and Clinical Excellence (NICE) psychosocial guidelines for drug misuse [22] also stimulated interest in whether these benefits can be sustained over time and across cultures and diverse healthcare settings.

SUMMARY

Medina-Mora *et al.*'s chapter is a mature examination of the diversity and complexity of drug problems around the world, within a context of clearly explained epidemiological paradigms. They note the difficulty of comparing international data, and conclude that research aimed at enhancing the accuracy of such data should be supported. Poznyak provides a framework for the levels at which preventive strategies maybe implemented, highlighting the need for continued evaluation of the effectiveness of prevention interventions, and emphasizing the need for strengthening of the evidence base. Schifano's thoughtful consideration of current and emerging treatment options summarizes the evidence for pharmacological and psychosocial interventions in the treatment and management of addiction, within a clear neurobiological understanding of dependence. He notes the importance of expanding the evidence-based treatment portfolio in the field of drug misuse and dependence, rather than attempting to narrow it to single-solution strategies: 'there are no data supporting a single treatment approach that is able to comprise the multidimensional facets of addiction patterns' [23].

REFERENCES

1. Babor, T., Caulkins, J., Edwards, G. *et al.* (eds.) (2010) *Drug Policy and the Public Good*, Oxford University Press, Oxford, UK.

2. El-Seedi, H.R., De Smet, P.A., Beck, O. *et al.* (2005). Prehistoric peyote use: alkaloid analysis and radiocarbon dating of archaeological specimens of Lophophora from Texas. *The Journal of Ethnopharmacology*, **101** (1–3), 238–242.

3. The United States Code Title 42 > Chapter 21 > Subchapter I > Section 1996 § 1996. Traditional Indian religious use of peyote http://uscode.house.gov/download/pls/42C21.txt (Accessed 26th Feb 2010).

4. Ministry of Health (2007) *Drug use in New Zealand: Analysis of the 2003 New Zealand Health Behaviours Survey-Drug Use*, Ministry of Health, Wellington.

5. Marie, D., David, M., Fergusson, D.M. *et al.* (2008) Links between ethnic identification, cannabis use and dependence, and life outcomes in a New Zealand birth cohort. *Australian and New Zealand Journal of Psychiatry*, **42**, 780–788.

6. Clough, A.R., Lee, K.S.K., Cairney, S. *et al.* (2006) Changes in cannabis use and its consequences over 3 years in a remote indigenous population in northern Australia. *Addiction*, **101**, 696–705.

7. Edwards, G. and Arif, A. (eds.) (1980) *Drug Problems in the Sociocultural Context. A Basis for Policies and Programme Planning*, WHO, Geneva.

8. Kane, H.H. (1882) *Opium-Smoking in America and China: A Study of its Prevalence, and Effects, Immediate and Remote on the Individual and the Nation (1881)*, Kessinger Publishing, USA.

9. Edwards, S., McCreanor, T. and Moewaka-Barnes, H. (2007) Maori family culture: a context of youth development in Counties/Manukau. *Kotuitui New Zealand Journal of Social Sciences Online*, **2**, 1–15. 22.

10. Robson, B. and Harris, R. (2007) Mortality in Hauora Maori standards of health IV. A study of the years 2000-2005. Wellington: Te Ropu Rangahau Hauora a Eru Pomare, School of Medicine and Health Sciences, University of Otago.

11. Bourke, L. (2001) Australian rural consumers perceptions of heath issues. *The Australian Journal of Rural Health*, **9** (1), 1–6.

12. Population Distribution (2006) Aboriginal and Torres Strait Islander Australians. Australian Bureau of Statistics.

13. James, M., Herrell, J.M. and Herrell, I.C. (1984) A lifespan, multimodal matrix for drug abuse prevention. *The Journal of Behavioural Health Sciences and Research*, **11**, 40–42.

14. Caplan, G. (1964) *Principles of Preventive Psychiatry*, Basic Books, New York.

15. Caplan, G., Caplan, R.B. (2000) The future of primary prevention. *The Journal of Primary Prevention*, **21** (2), 131–136.

16. http://www.mixmag.net/mephedrone (Accessed 26th February 2010).

17. Winstock, A. R., Mitcheson, L. R., Deluca, P., Davey, Z., Corazza, O. and Schifano, F., Research report: Mephedrone, new kid for the chop?. Addiction, no. doi: 10.1111/j.1360-0443.2010.03130. (Accessed 13th October 2010).

18. http://www.homeoffice.gov.uk/about-us/home-office-circulars/circulars-2010/010-2010/ (Accessed 13th October 2010).

19. http://www.homeoffice.gov.uk/publications/drugs/acmd1/naphyrone-report?view=Binary. (Accessed 13th October 2010).

20. Levine, D.A. (2007) 'Pharming': the abuse of prescription and over-the-counter drugs in teens. *Current Opinion in Pediatrics*, **19**, 270–274.

21. The National Center on Addiction and Substance Abuse at Columbia University (2006) "You've Got Drugs!" Prescription Drug Pushers on the Internet: 2006 Update. A CASA* White Paper.

22. National Institute for Health and Clinical Excellence (2007) Clinical Guideline 51 Drug misuse: psychosocial interventions.

23. Knapp, W.P., Soares, B.G., Farrell, M. *et al.* (2007) Psychosocial interventions for cocaine and psychostimulant amphetamines related disorders. *Cochrane Database Systematic Reviews* **18** (Art. No. CD003023).

4.2 Epidemiology, Treatment and Prevention of Addictive Disorders

Pedro Ruiz, M.D.

Department of Psychiatry and Behavioral Sciences, University of Miami Miller School of Medicine, Miami, Florida, USA

In this section on 'drugs', three excellent chapters are included. One focuses on 'epidemiology' another on 'treatment and management', and still another on 'drug prevention'. These three topics are of great importance for the field of addiction at large and thus they are very relevant to this textbook.

With respect to the first chapter, Maria Elena Medina-Mora, Tania Real and Rebecca Robles have covered the most essential topics and areas pertaining to the epidemiology of drug use and abuse across the world. In this context, the different cultures that prevail around the world are closely related to the epidemiological data portrayed in this chapter. Also, in this chapter, marihuana (cannabis) is depicted as the most widely used and abused drug worldwide; opium and heroin are also underlined as drugs primarily produced in Afghanistan; cocaine (coca leaf) is also noted as a drug that is predominantly cultivated in the Andean region of Latin America. Besides, other drugs of high use and abuse worldwide were found to be inhalants, amphetamine-type stimulants and prescription drugs.

In this chapter, another very important theme within epidemiology is the cyclical nature of drug abuse with periods of increased use and abuse and periods of decreased use and abuse. These cyclic periods are directly related to prevailing public attitudes, social policies and available resources as well as tools to address and cope with these cyclic situations. This chapter also underlines the interaction that exist in society between the health status of the population groups in question and the environment where these groups lives. This interaction is certainly a part of the public-health interests in the psychical conditions of any population groups. Another factor underlined in this chapter from an epidemiological point of view is the differentiation between healthy individuals and those who are sick, as well as the study of the biological, social, as well as individual and collective factors related to health and disease. Moreover, the study of population subgroups in order to estimate the extension and the magnitude of health-related problems in this population subgroups

Substance Abuse Disorders: Evidence and Experience, First Edition. Edited by Hamid Ghodse, Helen Herrman, Mario Maj and Norman Sartorius.
© 2011 John Wiley & Sons, Ltd. Published 2011 by John Wiley & Sons, Ltd.

overtime and also the health and disease determinants, as well as their consequences, the proportional number of persons exposed to preventive interactions, and the treatment options and demands covered.

Basic to the field of epidemiology, which is nicely depicted in this chapter, is the fact that illicit drug use and abuse is difficult to assess appropriately due to the fact that the users and/or abusers of drugs might not be willing to report their illegal activities. This chapter also addresses the concept of the 'disease model' that leads to the governmental policy directed to the reduction of the supply of drugs as a way of decreasing drug use and abuse in society. In this chapter, the concept of 'emerging marks' are also discussed; that is, the drug use and abuse is based on a complex interaction determined by the individual, his environment and the drug availability; in this context the sociocultural milieu and the prevailing political forces also have great influence in the outcome of this model.

The second chapter, written by Fabrizio Schifano, nicely addresses the 'treatment and management' of illicit drug use and abuse. Special focus is given in this chapter to certain drugs such as opiates; stimulants (cocaine, amphetamine and amphetamine-like substances, ecstasy and ecstasy-like drugs); and benzodiazepines. Attention is also given in this chapter to the clinical pharmacology of the different drugs of misuse and on available medications. Additionally, the clinical usefulness of psychosocial treatments, especially cognitive-behavioural therapy, contingency management, and behavioural approaches, are also addressed in this chapter. Detailed clinical reviews are provided with focus on the clinical management of the most relevant ones.

Focus on some novel treatment approaches are also well discussed in this chapter; for instance, the current role of buphrenorphine on opioid treatment. Also, of naltrexone treatment vis-à-vis opioids. In addition current approaches for the treatment of stimulants, including amantidine, levodopa, bromocriptine, lisuride, selegiline, pergolide and mazindol; others like SSRIs, anti-psychotics, anti-convulsants, baclofen, isradipine, tomiparamate, disulfiram and even vaccinations. The management of benzodiazepine dependence and ecstasy as well as ecstasy-like drugs are all well addressed in this chapter.

In the third chapter, Vladimir B. Poznyak, James White and Nicolas Clark discuss current approaches to drug prevention. In this chapter, the prevention of HIV infection and other blood-borne pathogen transmission related to drug use are emphasized. Factors related to drug dependence as a result of use and abuse is well underlined. Not only prevention from initiation of drug use, but also prevention from repeated utilization are both well addressed. Secondary prevention is also well discussed in this chapter. Tertiary prevention aimed to reduce disability is also noted. Protective factors vis-à-vis drug use and abuse are also well described, as well as it is the level of intervention related to prevention, including the international level, and the national and community levels of prevention.

This chapter also describes principles for drug prevention, evidence on effectiveness of prevention interventions, control of drug availability and judicial procedures, mass-media interventions, and prevention programs aimed at short-term and long-term effects on drug use.

In essence, these three chapters of this drug section are all well conceptualized and addresses well three major topics of the field of addiction.

4.3 The Global Challenge of Illegal Drugs

Neil McKeganey, BA, MSc, PhD FRSA
University of Glasgow, Glasgow, UK

INTRODUCTION

Drug abuse represents one of the great global challenges of the twenty-first century. The harms associated with illegal drug use are multiple, widespread, deep seated and far from easily remedied. Both the prevalence of illegal drug use and the harms that flow from that use have increased steadily in many areas across the globe to the point that there is now barely a country in the world that does not have a drugs problem of at least some degree. The chapters in this section on the epidemiology, on the treatment and management and on the prevention of drugs misuse cover topics that are of enormous importance in enabling an assessment to be made of the scale of the drugs problem we face and the extent of our success in meeting that challenge. On the basis of the contributions from Medina-Mora *et al.*, Schifano and Poznyak, White and Clark should we be optimistic or pessimistic about our ability to tackle effectively the modern day plague of illegal drugs?

Key to any attempt at successfully tackling the problem of illegal drugs use is accurate and up-to-date information on the scale of such use. Important as information on the prevalence of drugs misuse clearly is, it is by no means the case that all countries have well-developed programmes for monitoring changes in drug-use prevalence. Indeed, even within those countries that have a long-standing tradition of research on drugs misuse, such as the UK, we do not have the luxury of a series of drug-misuse prevalence studies with which to chart the growth of the drugs problem over the last thirty years. As a result, we are a long way from having a robust picture of the evolving global epidemiology of drug misuse.

The typical model of drug diffusion is one where illegal substances may be produced in one country then transported along well-defined transit routes to the consumer countries. Historically, the development of distinctive patterns of drug use has taken many years to develop. What we are now seeing, however, is a change in the pattern of drugs diffusion and drugs epidemiology with new drugs being rapidly developed and marketed globally through the Internet to an inexhaustible consumer base. Increasingly, drugs are being designed that can mimic the effects of more traditional drugs of abuse, but that are sufficiently different

Substance Abuse Disorders: Evidence and Experience, First Edition. Edited by Hamid Ghodse, Helen Herrman, Mario Maj and Norman Sartorius.
© 2011 John Wiley & Sons, Ltd. Published 2011 by John Wiley & Sons, Ltd.

in their chemistry to take those drugs outside of the jurisdiction of drugs legislation. In the case of the legal-high drug mephedrone, we have a drug that has gone from being virtually unknown to be being widely consumed within little more than three years. The rapidity with which new drugs are being developed and marketed is severely testing the drugs-legislation system in many countries, which are struggling to cope with the pace of drug development [1].

Increasingly, national prevalence estimates, though useful, will need to be supplemented by research that can chart these new developments in drug marketing and consumption. Just as the Internet has become a tool for rapid drug diffusion there will be a need to explore the epidemiology of drug purchasing and drug use in and through the Internet. Where drug-prevalence studies are being undertaken there is a growing need to ensure that these studies are being replicated on a sufficiently frequent basis to pick up changes in drug-misuse prevalence and that they are using a common methodology thereby enabling us to make meaningful international comparisons ([2, 6]).

The chapter by Schifano outlines current knowledge in the treatment and management of substance misuse, focusing on specific substances in terms of their positive therapeutic effects as well as their risks. The chapter covers the clinical use of methadone, buprenorphine, naltrexone and the management of opiate dependence, cocaine dependence, amphetamine dependence and benzodiazepine misuse. There is much here that will inform the management of substance-misuse problems within both specialist drug-treatment centres as well as in community-based, primary-care services. The chapter also usefully includes information on the application of various psychosocial interventions such as cognitive behavioural approaches in the treatment of substance-misuse problems.

There is no doubt that the therapeutic armamentarium for tackling substance abuse is substantial but that does not mean we can be optimistic in our assessment of the success of treatment. It is still the case that where an individual has an entrenched drug-dependency problem recovery from that problem is hard won and can take many years [3]. It is also the case that some clinicians are of the view that drug dependency, like diabetes, is a life-long condition from which there is no recovery, and for which prescribed substitute medication may need to last a lifetime. A problem that we are going to have to grapple with increasingly is the potential for dependent drug users to become further dependent on the medications that are being prescribed to help them. We know that methadone is a highly addictive substance, widely prescribed to those with an opiate dependency. We are much less clear, however, as to how drug users who have become dependent upon methadone will be helped in due course to become drug free.

Treatment within the substance misuse field is virtually synonymous with treatment for addiction. In other areas of health- and social-care intervention we have begun to see the benefits of early intervention, whereas within the substance misuse field we are only at the earliest stages of thinking about what treatment and the clinical services can contribute for those whose drug use has not yet become addictive but that may still be presenting various problems for the individual, his or her family and the wider community. This is an area that is likely to expand in importance in the years to come and may in due course lead us to rethink the meaning of drugs treatment what it involves and how it is delivered.

The chapter by Poznyak and White takes a very different topic in concentrating on the issue of drug-use prevention, the importance of which is gaining recognition. Within many countries, however, drug-use prevention has been the poor relation of the big spending budgets of treatment and enforcement within government drugs policy.

As drugs misuse has spread across the globe, we have come to realize that its prevention is every bit as important as preventing the spread of HIV infection. Indeed, we no longer have the luxury of choosing between the two. The chapter by Poznyak and White reviews the multiple domains and approaches towards drugs prevention, for each approach reviewing the evidence for its effectiveness in the short, medium and long term. The chapter considers approaches to drug prevention at the national level, at the community level, at the institutional and group level and the level of the individual.

Nobody reading this chapter can be under any illusion that we presently lack the effective means to substantially reduce the likelihood of young people becoming involved in various forms of illegal drug use. Some approaches have proven to be more promising than others. Equally, some of our prevention approaches seem to be more effective with some substances than with others substances. This would be less of a problem were it not for the growth in polydrug use that is occurring in many countries.

We must be cautious that our lack of progress towards developing the means for effective drugs prevention does not breed a kind of pessimism that leads us to believe that drugs misuse itself is an inevitability, which simply has to be accommodated to. Just as the work to develop effective treatments for cancer is not set back by our failure to find a 'cure' nor should the modesty of our efforts in drugs prevention be taken as a reason to give up on this area of work. The goal of effective drugs prevention is simply too important for us to so readily accept failure [4].

One area that the chapter does not mention but that may be important has to do with the possible role of drug testing in schools and workplaces. This is an area that is rife with ethical concerns, including the individual's right of privacy [5]. Drug testing is unique in the realm of drug-prevention methods in being able to reveal the reality of whether or not an individual has used certain drugs. Government policy in relation to drug testing has been blown by fashion rather than hard evidence. We need to ensure that all of the available means of drugs prevention are subjected to rigorous evaluation in order that drug-prevention policy decisions are made on the basis of the best-available evidence. Finally, our efforts to develop better methods of drugs prevention need to be informed by an accurate understanding of the reasons why young people in many countries are increasingly inclined to experiment with various forms of drugs misuse.

Should we be optimistic or pessimistic with regard to our capacity to tackle the global problem of drugs misuse? There is much that we can be optimistic about in the developing fields of drugs epidemiology, drugs treatment and drugs prevention. But just as there are bright minds and committed individuals working in each of these areas so too are there equally bright minds and committed individuals working to facilitate the global production and consumption of illegal drugs. The challenge between these two is every bit as great as the challenge to deal with global warming and global terrorism. There is no guarantee of success in the fight against illegal drugs but there is a guarantee of failure if our efforts are half-hearted, underfunded and poorly evaluated.

REFERENCES

1. Advisory Council on the Misuse of Drugs (2010) *Consideration of the Cathinones*, ACMD, London.

2. European Monitoring Center for Drugs and Drug Addiction (2009) The State of the Drug Problem in Europe, Lisbon.

3. McIntosh, M. and McKeganey, N. (2002) Beating the Dragon The Recovery from Dependent Drug Use Pearson.

4. International Narcotics Control Board (2009) Report of the International Narcotics Control Board for 2009, United Nations.

5. McKeganey, N. (2006) Random Drug Testing: A Shot in the Arm or a Shot in the Foot for Drug Prevention Joseph Rowntree Foundation York.

6. United Nations Office of Drugs and Crime (2009) World Drugs Report.

4.4 Drug Misuse – Lessons Learned Through the Modern Science

Igor Koutsenok, MD, MS

Department of Psychiatry, University of California San Diego School of Medicine, San Diego, CA, USA

This commentary discusses the three chapters – 'Epidemiology of Drug Abuse: A Global Overview' by Maria Elena Medina-Mora, Tania Real, Rebeca Robles; 'Drugs: Prevention' by Vladimir Poznyak, James White and Nicolas Clark, and 'Drugs: Treatment and Management' by Fabrizio Schifano. These chapters represent several of the major perspectives in this emerging and exciting area of addiction science and practice. Each text approaches specific issues in the enormously large area of drug and alcohol misuse and addictive behaviour in ways that are distinctive, comprehensive and interesting. Although each chapter addresses a separate theme, all together they cover the major components of addictive behaviour – biological interventions, psychological vulnerabilities and socioenvironmental factors through epidemiological analysis. They also have several commonalities – a broad view of addiction science, deep knowledge of the current research, thoroughness and presentation that is understandable to and applicable by practitioners.

In reviewing the texts it is important to mention the social context in which current addiction science is unfolding. Drug and alcohol use, misuse and dependence produce dramatic costs to society in terms of lost productivity, a myriad of social consequences, and, of course, multiple and serious health care issues. In response, there has been increased interest in the development and expansion of prevention and treatment programs as a way of dealing with problems directly or indirectly related to drug and alcohol use. Yet, while the large proportion of the public is demanding greater availability and more funding for prevention and treatment, there are others, particularly in governments, insurance industries, health care and the general public who question the efficacy of these activities, and whether or not they are 'worth it'. Such a variety of opinions appears to relate to core public perceptions about substance use in general, and about what would constitute an 'effective' intervention, regardless of its type. Some believe that drug addiction is primarily a 'social problem' requiring a social-judicial solution, rather than a 'health problem'

Substance Abuse Disorders: Evidence and Experience, First Edition. Edited by Hamid Ghodse, Helen Herrman, Mario Maj and Norman Sartorius.
© 2011 John Wiley & Sons, Ltd. Published 2011 by John Wiley & Sons, Ltd.

requiring prevention and treatment. This perception is quite understandable considering the extent and significance of the social problems caused by drug and alcohol abuse. Thus, it is not surprising that many in the policy-making arena and in the public at large rely mostly on law enforcement and interdiction efforts instead of public-health efforts to correct the drug problem. This perception is also related to the widespread scepticism about the effectiveness and value of prevention and treatment for substance use disorders. Many people believe that treatment-orientated approaches send an uncomfortable message that the view of addiction as an illness suggests that the addicted person is not responsible for the disease, nor the addiction-related problems and behaviours. Also, many in the public believe that neither prevention nor treatment 'work'. Specifically, many do not believe that any treatment can get addicted persons 'off drugs and alcohol' and keep them off. This is a view that is apparently shared by many physicians, despite scientific evidence supporting neuronal mechanisms, heritability, treatment responses and a characteristic progressive clinical course of substance use disorders. It has been repeatedly documented over the past three decades that a majority of physicians do not screen for signs of alcohol or drug dependence during routine examinations. The 'failure' of substance-abuse prevention and treatment to reliably produce long-standing abstinence is often seen as confirming the suspicions about the need to continue both efforts. But are these perceptions true? Is there a role for addiction prevention and treatment in public policy aimed at reducing demand for drugs and reducing the social harms and costs associated with drug abuse? If treatment was considered a wise public investment, what treatment –behavioural interventions, medications, or combinations – should be provided? Finally, is there evidence that prevention and treatment can be effective and valuable – not just to the affected patient – but to the society that is expected to support those activities?

One of the important first steps in answering these and many other questions is to get a reliable and comprehensive picture of the extent of the problem both locally and globally. The chapter on epidemiology written by Prof. Dr. Medina-Mora and her collaborators offers the reader exactly that – a comprehensive epidemiological picture of the problem, thus it sets the stage for other chapters and the rest of the book. Although drug and alcohol abuse is definitely a global problem, most of the epidemiological analyses have largely been those of the most affluent and developed countries – United States, Canada, Australia, UK and some other Western European countries. The chapter by Dr. Medina-Mora provides us with very recent data from virtually the entire world. While extremely rich in data and information, there are three very important and unique contributions that I would like to mention. First, the entire epidemiology as science is reviewed from multiple contextual, foundational and cultural perspectives, which largely explains the differences in scientific approaches between different countries, and, quite importantly, emphasizes the issue of scientific tolerance and compatibility between different models. Secondly, the authors emphasize the lesson learned by the entire international community, that in order to better understand the problem and to be more effective in addressing it, an integrated global drug epidemiology information system is essential. Thirdly, it gives a significant rationale for departure from the 'static', 'linear' way of thinking ('works – doesn't work', 'effective – ineffective', etc.), to a more 'circular' conceptual approach considering cultural differences and the circular nature of the drug problem with epidemic rises, periods when drug use is stable or is reduced, followed by a new rise.

The initiation of substance use is primarily an adolescent phenomenon, occurring within the context of great physical and psychological change. During adolescence, individuals typically experiment with a wide range of behaviours and lifestyle patterns as part of the natural process of separating from parents, developing a sense of autonomy and independence, and acquiring some of the skills necessary for functioning effectively in the adult world. Profound cognitive changes occur during the beginning of adolescence that significantly alter the adolescent's view of the world and the manner in which he/she thinks. Also, adolescents tend to have a heightened sense of self-consciousness concerning their appearance, personal qualities and abilities. Furthermore, as children approach adolescence, there appears to be a progressive decline in the impact of parental influence and a corresponding increase in the impact of influence from peer networks. Finally, teens often perceive that they are not susceptible to the hazards presented by risk-taking and health-compromising behaviours. These and other developmental changes occurring during this period increase adolescents' risk of yielding to various direct and indirect pressures to smoke, drink, or use drugs. The authors of the chapter on prevention share the public concern over the issue of drug abuse amongst children and adolescents and present a good review of the science on ways of deterring or delaying onset of this behaviour. This chapter reviews the empirical evidence on the efficacy of substance-abuse prevention efforts and addresses a number of interrelated critical questions: What scientific evidence supports the efficacy and effectiveness of drug-abuse prevention programs and policy in schools, the workplace and communities? What are the associated costs? Are the programs and policies beneficial to those receiving them? How can the practice of prevention be improved by the emerging science of drug-abuse prevention? Practitioners and administrators in the field of drug-abuse prevention programs are seeking science-based answers to these questions in order to plan and implement programs that are high-quality, empirically supported, and cost efficient. These interventions go beyond a simple demonstration of the health consequences of alcohol and drug abuse. They are theoretically based in the fundamental science of human developmental and behavioural psychology. Historically, drug-abuse prevention programs have been founded on the theoretical assumption that children and adolescents used drugs because they are ignorant of the consequences of such use. Failure to recognize negative consequences resulted, according to this theory, in neutral or even favourable attitudes regarding experimentation and/or regular use. During the 1960s, drug-education programs focused on providing information. These programs frequently contained 'fear-arousal messages' regarding the health and social consequences of such use. Available evidence indicates that teaching only about the extreme negative consequences of substance abuse is of marginal value as a prevention strategy. Traditional health-education approaches have been found largely unsuccessful in reducing rates of drug abuse, although certain types of knowledge about the use of tobacco, alcohol and drugs may be a useful component of substance abuse prevention programs. More encouraging results are reported from research studies based on psychosocial models of behaviour from the 1970s, when social scientists had begun to address interpersonal and intrapersonal factors that influenced drug-abuse behaviours amongst children and adolescents. Several studies found drug abuse was associated with attitudes, beliefs and values, as well as other personality factors such as feelings of self-esteem, self-reliance and alienation. These findings have stimulated the development of other approaches to prevention – rather than focusing on drug-abuse behaviours, effective education focused on the factors associated with use, attempting to eliminate the reasons for using drugs by creating a school climate that was supportive of students' social and emotional needs. These programs frequently focused on training the students in effective decision-making skills. Because perceived risk is an important determinant of drug experimentation, the danger of drugs should be conveyed accurately and credibly to our youth. Schools provide a natural setting for these interventions and have the means to identify youth with higher risk. The authors are right in their conclusions that education designed to prevent addiction should be well integrated into our schools and should be further developed with research-based interventions.

In addition to epidemiology and prevention science, research on the neurochemical, molecular and cellular changes associated with drug dependence has led literally to volumes of remarkable findings over the past decade. There is now clear evidence that most addictive drugs have well-specified effects on the brain circuitry that is involved in the control of motivated and learned behaviours. This evidence originated from studies in animals, and with recent developments in brain-imaging techniques, has been confirmed in humans. It is likely that both the direct and sustained physiological changes produced by the drugs themselves and the acquired effects produced by conditioned cues are involved in the ultimate explanation of the continued vulnerability to relapse even amongst motivated and abstinent drug-dependent individuals. The chapter by Dr. Schifano is focused on medications currently available for use by physicians in the treatment of nicotine, alcohol and opioid dependence, and for the treatment of co-morbid psychiatric disorders associated with all forms of substance dependence. These have been tested in multiple trials and have been shown to be effective. Pharmacological strategies are emerging that target specific clinical components of addiction, including drug-induced euphoria, hedonic dysregulation, craving and even denial. The chapter by Dr. Schifano presents a very elegant comprehensive review of the most recent data on a variety of pharmacological options in addiction treatment. It highlights the area of addiction research that illustrates brain involvement and brain dysregulation as one of the core components of substance use disorders, and will definitely stimulate public interest because it is conveyed in a clear and understandable fashion. Furthermore, presented pharmacological options that dramatically improve clinical outcomes should reverse social stigma and justify an expanded care-delivery system. The clinical impact of new treatments also depends on their translation into clinical practice. Even when effective treatments for addiction have been identified, as illustrated by Dr. Schifano's review, they have not always been adequately translated into clinical practice. This can be explained partly by the public attitude toward the problem, briefly mentioned above. Another possible reason is the complexity of neuropharmacological research that is often difficult to understand, let alone apply, even for trained practitioners. So, the author is correct in concluding that there is a need for additional studies on the appropriate use of these medications in 'real-world' treatment of drug-dependence disorders, as well as more translational research. The chapter by Dr. Fabrizio Schifano offers a great example of bridging the gap between academic science and clinical practice by providing clear treatment guidelines and algorithms for different clinical situations, including emergencies. This is particularly important in view of the obvious need for better integration of addiction treatment into mainstream medicine. The role of primary-care physicians and practitioners is essential in both treatment and prevention and they should be provided with the most recent science-based knowledge and skills in pharmacological and nonpharmacological treatment approaches.

The chapters mentioned in this commentary provide a comprehensive scientific analysis of several critically important areas in addiction science. Although very important, perhaps this is not the biggest contribution made by the authors. What is really impressive is the authors' ability to effectively bridge the gap between highly academic science and the realities of daily operations by frontline treatment practitioners. Therefore, I am confident that the entire book will serve the needs of professionals far beyond universities and research laboratories. This will be a great addition to the existing literature in the field.

4.5 An Integrated Approach to Drug-Abuse Treatment: The Role of Prevention

Abdu'l-Missagh Ghadirian, M.D., FRCP(C), DF-APA
McGill University, Faculty of Medicine, Montreal, Quebec, Canada

Medina-Mora and associates in their review of epidemiology of drugs note the diversity and complexity of drug consumption and the cyclical nature of this phenomenon that is characterized by periods of increase and decrease depending on many factors.

Substance abuse varies from culture to culture. A substance that is rejected as illicit in one culture may be accepted in another. Likewise social vulnerability to substance abuse differs from culture to culture. Therefore, epidemiological studies should recognize this cultural variation of attitudes. An alarming increase in nonmedical use of prescription drugs (sedatives, tranquilizers, opioids, amphetamines) is widening [1]. It is estimated that 48 million Americans (ages 12 and older) have made nonmedical use of prescription drugs in their lifetime. This represents approximately 20% of the United States population [2].

Elaborating on the scope of the drug problem, Medina-Mora *et al.* state that by 2000 cannabis was the most widely used illicit drug worldwide followed by opiates and coca-leaf derivatives. Social vulnerability greatly contributes to the rapid spread of drug abuse.

According to the World Drug Report [3], there is encouraging news about reduction in the production of cocaine and heroin. Surveys of drug users in the largest global drug markets for cannabis, cocaine and opioids suggest that these markets are shrinking and cannabis consumption amongst young people is declining in some parts of the world. This underlines the importance of policies for a global approach to regulate supply and demand.

Vladimir Poznyak and associates outline prevention with impressive data and details on preventive measures. Based on the WHO comparative assessment of 24 global risk factors, it is noted that the majority of the disease burden (approximately 65%) is due to drug-use disorders, followed by HIV/AIDS, self-inflicted injuries and car accidents. This estimate reflects the serious economic impact of drug-related disorders worldwide. It also has social consequences, including crime, violence, absenteeism and unemployment.

Prevention of drug abuse is the most crucial approach for eradication of this 'plague' of humanity, yet it is sadly neglected and underfunded. According to the authors, supply

Substance Abuse Disorders: Evidence and Experience, First Edition. Edited by Hamid Ghodse, Helen Herrman, Mario Maj and Norman Sartorius.
© 2011 John Wiley & Sons, Ltd. Published 2011 by John Wiley & Sons, Ltd.

and demand reduction, complemented by harm reduction, are vital in any strategy for prevention. The trajectories of substance abuse comprise primary, secondary and tertiary prevention. To implement these critical stages, however, it is important to integrate a multidimensional paradigm of prevention that encompasses not only biological parameters but also intellectual, emotional, sociocultural and spiritual aspects of human reality with a coherent line of action between prevention, treatment and rehabilitation [4].

The chapter identifies risk and protective factors for substance abuse in different stages of human development [5]. It acknowledges the fact that prevention should begin prior to birth by identifying risk factors for that very early stage, followed by infancy, preschool and secondary-school periods. This view of preventive aspect is laudable but the description of protective factors is far from adequate. It does not explore preventive education during childhood and the role of family and culture in substance abuse prevention. Likewise, the role of learning from social interactions, the concept of socialization and the biopsychosocial approach would have been worth exploring in prevention of drug abuse.

Substance abuse is closely related to learning through social interactions and the influence of peers or family members. Addiction is a type of relationship with a habit-forming drug. This relationship is reinforced by biological factors and genetic predisposition. Culture as a social force plays an important role in human motivation. Culture is defined as a 'system of patterns of belief and behaviour that shapes the world view of the members of society' [6]. Based on cultural attitude and traditional values, each society establishes its code of behaviour that governs an individual's approach to substance abuse [7].

Until recently, the relationship between spiritual beliefs and substance abuse and recovery has received little attention in the literature. But a growing body of research studies in recent years has consistently revealed an inverse relationship between religiosity and substance abuse and dependence [8].

Amongst developmental stages, childhood has not received adequate attention in relation to drug prevention. This is a critical period during which children begin to learn about attitudes toward health and other issues. Home becomes the first place for learning and children are very sensitive to the behavioural attitudes of parents as role models. In the intervention category, the authors identify several important levels in which prevention activities can be implemented. A range of timely educational organizations and programs of prevention and policies are described.

According to the World Drug Report, four types of substance abuse are identified as follows: 1) ritual/cultural; 2) medical/therapeutic; 3) social/recreational; 4) occupational/functional [9]. This classification will readily help to identify target populations for preventive programs. For a comprehensive preventive education against drug abuse, the following three protagonists should be included: individual, family and society [4]. The role of the individual in prevention is often ignored in the literature. It is the individual who becomes the first consumer of illicit drugs and contributes to the rise of demand for supply. There are a number of behavioural qualities that empower individuals to abstain from drug use. These are positive human attributes such as self-esteem and altruism, self-realization and having a sense of purpose in life. In the West, excessive freedom has led to permissiveness and overindulgence in pleasure-seeking behaviour. In today's materialistic society freedom has lost its meaning. True freedom needs to be redefined in relation to personal responsibility. Other exercises of capacity building for healthier lives are conflict resolution and decision making. We have been more preoccupied with combating the pathology of drug abuse than promoting a healthy lifestyle. As Norman Sartorius [10] states, the most important obstacle impeding the task of prevention is low priority attached to a healthy lifestyle.

Family is the foundation of human society and plays a crucial role in prevention of addictive behaviour. A dysfunctional family contributes to vulnerability of children to substance abuse and may weaken their ability to control their impulses. Likewise, society bears a moral responsibility to educate the population on the consequences of drug abuse. Such an education should involve schools, workplaces, sport activities, media and entertainment, universities, religious and all other institutions. The International Labour Organization (ILO) provides a code of practice that emphasizes prevention of substance abuse in the work place [11]. Positive alternatives to drug abuse in the community should have been discussed. Providing positive alternatives as antidotes to stimulate fulfillment of creative potential is vital, particularly for youth. The following are some suggestions on this point: facilities and programs for sport activities, promotion of the arts and development of talents, intellectual stimulation and debates, fostering friendships and a healthy lifestyle, workshops on coping skills and stress management, humanitarian service projects, and activities to help the sick and disabled.

Given the explosion of information and advertising from films, television, internet and other media that glamorize the pleasure of drinking and smoking, children are constantly bombarded by unhealthy messages that influence their impressionable minds. Children and youth need to build capacity to make intelligent choices and to dare to be different when faced with peer pressure. According to Poznyak *et al.*, there have been hundreds of programs implemented for drug prevention intervention without evaluation of their effectiveness. This required several reviews of effectiveness of these interventions. The result of recent reviews of evaluations were not conclusive. Several intervention studies reported little or no statistically significant benefit as compared to the control groups.

These research findings raise questions as to whether there are flaws in the methodology of the research projects. Perhaps the answer lies in a deeper understanding of the relationship between drug use and the purpose of life or an exploration of what drugs are a substitute for. What if drug users are searching for their identity more than seeking pleasure? This may challenge conventional interventions. In contrast, a materialistic concept of life reinforces a pleasure-seeking lifestyle. In my view, prevention or treatment alone will not bring an enduring result until we recognize a deeper meaning in life that would give purpose and hope to existence.

Fabrizio Schifano wrote an indepth review of current clinical pharmacological treatment and management that is aimed at substance abuse. Administration of methadone that is a long-standing medication in treatment of opioid dependence is well elaborated. He also comments on the use of Buprenorphine, a partial agonist that may have a favourable safety profile. Naltraxone, which is an opioid antagonist, provides an effective alternative in the treatment of opioid addiction. It is also sometimes used in rapid detoxification. Clinical treatment and pharmacological issues concerning management of various stimulant misuses are delineated. Likewise, the withdrawal symptoms and pharmacological side effects of opiates and stimulants are discussed.

Misuse of benzodiazepines and other prescribed psychoactive drugs is often frequent in the elderly population. It is to be noted that a high proportion of psychiatric patients, including those with bipolar disorder, use illicit drugs in addition to or in place of prescription medications. Because of chronic pain and other medical or mental disorders, the likelihood of misuse of analgesics with addictive substance as well as tranquilizers is on the rise and so are isolation, loneliness and depression. Therefore, psychopharmacology of late-life addictions should receive more attention. The psychosocial aspects of treatment of substance abuse could have been explored more as therapeutic modalities of nonpharmacological nature described are not adequate. Counselling, individual or family and psychotherapy are very helpful. In particular, cognitive behavioural therapy has been widely used with beneficial effect. Denial is a common factor to reckon with amongst those with drug problems and dealing with this defence mechanism should be part of the therapeutic process.

Another factor in the context of a psychosocial approach to intervention is recognition of the role of spirituality and religious values in implementation of treatment [12]. It was disappointing to note that there was very little included in this chapter as well as in the one on prevention, on the role of Alcoholics Anonymous in prevention and recovery. In assessing the psychosocial aspects of drug misuse the role of culture should not be underestimated. People from different cultures do not readily accept one form of drug as treatment in exchange for another one.

REFERENCES

1. Brook, J.S., Pahl, K. and Rubenstone, E. (2008) Epidemiology of addiction, in *Substance Abuse Treatment*, 4th edn (eds. M. Galanter and H. Kleber), American Psychiatric Publishing Inc., Washington, DC, p. 31.

2. Volkow, N.D. (2004) Prescription drugs – Abuse and addiction (NICA) http://drugabuse.gov/ResearchReports/prescription/prescription.html (Accessed 21 January 2010).

3. United Nations (2009) *World Drug Report: Executive summary*. United Nations Office on Drugs and Crime (UNOCD), New York, p. 9.

4. Ghadirian, A.-M. (2007) *Alcohol and Drug Dependency – a Psychosocial and Spiritual Approach to Prevention*, George Ronald Publisher, Oxford, UK, pp. 113–135.

5. Stockwell, T., Gruenewald, J., Toumbourou, J. and Loxley, W. (2005) Preventive risky drug use and related harms: The need for a synthesis of new knowledge, in *Preventing Harmful Substance Use: The Evidence Base for Policy and Practice*. John Wiley & Sons Ltd.

6. Heath, D.B. (2001) Culture and substance abuse. *Cultural Psychiatry Clin North Am*, **24** (3), 479–496.

7. Abbott, P. and Chase, D.M. (2008) Culture and substance abuse: Impact of culture affects approach to treatment. *Psychiatric Times*, **25** (1), 43–46. http://www.psychiatrictimes.com/substance-abuse/content/article/10168/1147541 (Accessed 21 July 2009).

8. Booth, J. and Martin, J.E. (1998) Spirituality and religious factors in substance use, dependence and recovery, in *Handbook of Religion and Mental Health* (ed. H.G. Koenig), Academic Press, San Diego, p. 175.

9. United Nations (1997) *World Drug Report*, Oxford University Press, Oxford, UK.

10. Sartorius, N. (1986) Putting a higher value on health. *World Health*, 2–3.

11. International Labour Office (ILO) (2006) Coming clean: Drug and alcohol testing in the workplace. *World of Work Magazine*, **57**, 36.

12. Matthews, D.A., McCullough, M.E., Larson, D.B. *et al.* (1998) Religious commitment and health status. *Arch Fam Med*, **7**, 118–124.

4.6 Informing the Field of Substance Misuse: Progress and Challenges

David A. Deitch, Ph.D.

University of California, San Diego, CA, USA

These three chapters and particularly their sequence offer not only relevant information to a broad array of professionals; medical, treatment practitioners and policy investigators, but also serve as an update to addiction educators. Furthermore, this well-organized and current description of the state of our addiction knowledge reminds us (and for this commentator painfully) of the struggle in our knowledge acquisition regarding the most complex phenomena of how people can get stuck in behaviours that both limit achievement and can result in social disruption that provokes pain and cost to others.

It is clear to me that our field still has within it unending controversy in spite of scientific advancement in understanding the biopsychosocial substrata of addictive behaviour and that for over the last three centuries for every two steps forward there has been one step back. This can be illustrated most aptly in our response to substances in particular; the context of their first appearance, how introduced and by whom, how represented to the public, the degree of class acceptance or stigmatization, the role of politics and the politicization of substance use; the defining of users (relevant to licit or elicit) as deviant, of weak morals, criminals, inebriates, or character disorders, to name just a few, or the description of the addictive process as 'incurable diseases of pleasures and appetites'[*][1] or intemperance.[*][2] Most of these descriptors led to interventions to 'correct the person' through mutual confession and criticism. These attitudes that repeatedly, in spite of our current hard-won advances in the understanding of addictive behaviour still not only exist but remain prevalent. The degree and scope of the current worldwide use, misuse and/or abuse the concomitant cost relevant to health, loss of productivity and social marginalization; the limits of our prevention activities and the mixed outcomes of our treatment interventions clearly demand the promulgation of our latest understanding and information along with a clear picture of

[*] J. Boyle, University of Surrey, UK – Gary Lynch, University of California, Irvine.
[1] Philo Judaeus Alexandria, Egypt 5AD.
[2] Wesley Brothers at Oxford, 1738.

Substance Abuse Disorders: Evidence and Experience, First Edition. Edited by Hamid Ghodse, Helen Herrman, Mario Maj and Norman Sartorius.
© 2011 John Wiley & Sons, Ltd. Published 2011 by John Wiley & Sons, Ltd.

our greatest challenges – these three chapters contribute greatly to that end. In each chapter I will select one point (or more) that, because of my own history and oversight of addiction behaviour teaching and treatment, I feel I can make a contributing comment.

Dr. Mora and her colleagues offer us a quite stunning overview of epidemiology theory and practice as well as a quite comprehensive worldview of incidence and prevalence as well as aspects of production, availability and distribution patterns. In her review we learn yet again some rather 'axiomatic truths', simply put that the greater the availability of any substance, there will be increased use and of this increased use population, there will, of course, follow more people who will get behaviourally stuck in patterns of high risk (be they health or other consequences) chronic and relapsing use. As we review the many resources of data Dr. Mora and her colleagues' cite, as well as other data (World Drug & Crime Report to the UN 2007) we are led to a very high number of illicit drug taking of 222.8 million users (there is, of course, some overlap between the drug categories). Further, for alcohol dependence and problem use an additional 40 million (WHO Report, 2004). If one considers any use of illicit drugs as 'problem use' due to risk for social, if not medical consequences this total then represents a phenomenon that must be attributed to more than availability, but rather the propensity of the human species to desire altered states of consciousness and novelty. Admittedly, for millennia this occurred through dance, song, chanting, prayer and other rituals, but as more Botany and Chemistry have advanced, substances have become the easier and more passive methods to achieve these altered states. Now add to this volatile mix performance-enhancing drugs – be they sexual, physical, attentional and finally cognitive, these numbers will (and have already) climb dramatically. In our world of competitive striving most humans are further vulnerable to not only a drive to alter consciousness, but also to define themselves' by performance, be that athletic, academic, sexual and, of course cognitive. Already in the developed countries physical enhancers for athletic performance are being used in most colleges and high schools. Further, while not reviewed in specific the stimulant attention enhancers Adderall, Ritalin, Concerta and straight Amphetamines are being traded by high-school and college students with each other not for altered state but rather for academic and work performance needs. And as our laboratories work feverishly to develop memory stimulators for Dementia and Alzheimer disease the byproduct use is already known to aid in test taking and recruiting many parts of the brain into tasks (cognitive) that normally only single parts of the brain work on (ampakines[*]). This is the twenty-first century the 'genie' is out of the bottle and I seriously doubt if it can be pushed back!

This then leads to a key problem addressed in 'Drugs: Prevention' by Drs. Vladimir Poznyak, James White and Nicholas Clark. And that is the efficacy of prevention efforts. Poznyak and his colleagues offer us useful dimensions and categories of prevention and also the context of international treaties and conventions as well as worldwide agreements on key strategies to, hopefully, reduce both prevalence of misuse and its multiple levels of cost. This chapter certainly covers in a differentiated way the latest conceptualization of levels of prevention/intervention.

There are two areas in which I would like to comment: media and prevention effectiveness in general. Regarding media what I feel needs to be said is actually media has been and continues to this date delivering far more messages that excite interest in drugs and their use then they help provide prevention messages. Repeatedly in the last sixty years their interest in sensationalizing new drugs; the exotic effects of drugs and the controversies within populations over drug use. They have minimized harm or incredibly exaggerated harm or benefits. They have within film, video and print stimulated interest of most licit misuse and illicit use of drugs. My own interviews of college youths in the late 1960s and early 1970s repeatedly indicated the role of video reports of hallucinogenic drug use on different college campuses as stimulating their interest in consuming, experimenting with these drugs – 'Well if they are dropping acid at Yale this has got to be an exciting experience that we should try here at the University of Chicago'. A useful classroom activity is to ask students to review films at any given time that romanticize or minimize risky use and to further analyse for discussion pro-use messages versus caution messages. The cultural norming that excitement, fun and celebration are deeply associated with intoxication regardless of substance is now worldwide and we have yet to have agreement on a prevention strategy for this norming.

However, for me the sad and reminded truths in this chapter are that thus far 'Conventions' that attempt to control supply (intercontinental) have some but limited success. Further, that targeted interventions that promote protective factors are deeply underfunded and are at constant risk to sacrifice by political economic factors. A case in point is the current economic crises worldwide and California in specific whose first and deepest cuts in financing were aimed at population-specific protective factors. Finally, that both school and nonschool prevention studies after years of funding and improvement in delivery strategies still do not provide us with guidance about what to do but rather what to stop doing.

There are, however, gleams of light that caught my attention: At the secondary level of prevention the use of physician and medical office personnel to screen, assess, provide brief interventions and motivational engagement as well as referral strategies; which have certainly proven their worth in both reducing risk and altering behaviour; the positive impact of pro-health, social skill development and decision-making skill development on decreasing and/or delaying 'hard' drug initiation as well as classroom-centred interventions also achieving a delay.

The failure of any of these interventions to significantly impede marijuana use may indeed be a graphic sign of the times not unlike the use of alcohol that when legally prohibited increased multiple levels of social disruption and did not reduce alcoholism but only shifted populations of vulnerability.

Considering the world political and economic realities as well as the limits of prevention activities we are then led to the absolute necessity of finding appropriate interventions for those who get behaviourally stuck in consuming substances. This leads us to both the content and its necessity in Chapter 3. Drugs: Treatment and Management by Dr. Fabrizio Schifano.

At onset I think it is fair to say there are many treatments and interventions, none of which has emerged as the treatment of choice. None is effective in all cases, but most are effective in some. Further, regardless of which treatment is initiated what appears to matter most is how one sustains and manages their post-acute care recovery. To date this appears best done through peer mutual help provided without bias toward one model or another.

Dr. Schifano certainly has offered a primer for physicians and nursing specialists in agonist, partial agonist and antagonist medication-assisted therapies including dosing safety challenges and mixed-drug overdose risk. He further has provided useful rapid checklist and medication efficacy review for stimulant users as well as management guidelines for hallucinogenic stimulant mixes such as 'ecstasy'-like drugs. He further provides very useful Benzodiazepine crossover preferences and dose equivalencies. Of great interest to me was his urging a simple, but far too often neglected prescribing practice for insomnia-symptom drug abusers, of advice for sleep hygiene .... a singularly most neglected part of Psychiatric/Medical prescribing of sedative effect drugs be they benzodiazepines or anti-anxiety agents, and so on. Dr. Schifano explores some of the psychosocial interventions found useful in adolescents as well as adults. I have been for some time considering the rate of relapse painfully aware of a single greatest need – medications that can reduce and/or ameliorate craving. Admittedly, depending on which locale, age group and culture CBTs (of which there are many, and I wish were more frequently mentioned by name) are being found of use. But the reality of substance-use disorder treatment is that most frequently those who finally show up at our doors are at the intermediate and end stage disease levels. This presents a set of problems that could have been far better addressed earlier if interventions were available in locations that most people frequent, such as their doctor's office and health clinics. The use of screening, brief motivational interviewing and referral to treatment techniques mentioned in the prevention chapter are sorely needed. Our current reality is that many, many people in publicly funded drug management and treatment systems have eroded social, vocational, family and friendship resources, and that regardless of which initial treatment model or method, and regardless of CBT offerings while in treatment are at high risk of relapse in the absence of social recovery capitol. The craving-drive state, which is an inevitable part of recovery, is even more pronounced when there are no alternate sources of reward other than drugs. It is interesting in the face of this reality how effective we have found reinforcement contingency management CBTs in retaining people while in acute care, but how quickly it is extinguished in the face of loneliness, homelessness and the absence of meaningful work. Thus, my plea for the continuing investigation into anti-craving interventions. While not explicitly discussed in these three chapters, the need for public-health parity in the treatment of addictive behaviour and co-occurring illness must be advocated for in as many teaching and policy settings as possible as well as in this commentary to three very useful chapters in offering realistic appraisals of both the problem, its prevention and finally treatment challenges.

Alcohol

section 2

Alcohol

CHAPTER 5

Epidemiology of Alcohol Abuse: Extent and Nature of the Problem

Alcohol Consumption, Alcohol-Use Disorders and Global Burden of Disease

Jayadeep Patra[1,2], PhD; Andriy V. Samokhvalov[1,3], MD, PhD and Jürgen Rehm[1,2,3,4], PhD

[1]*Centre for Addiction and Mental Health, Toronto, Ontario, Canada*
[2]*Dalla Lana School of Public Health, University of Toronto, Ontario, Canada*
[3]*Department of Psychiatry, University of Toronto, Ontario, Canada*
[4]*Clinical Psychology & Psychotherapy, Technische Universität Dresden, Dresden, Germany*

5.1 INTRODUCTION

Alcohol is accountable for high levels of mortality, morbidity and social problems. Results from studies investigating deaths attributable to alcohol vary by country and methodology. Worldwide, alcohol consumption proved to be one of the most important risk factors for global burden of disease, ranking fifth, just behind tobacco (alcohol attributable burden in 2000: 4.0% of global burden compared to 4.1% of tobacco; e.g., [1–4]; for details on alcohol see [5,6]). Only underweight resulting mainly from malnutrition and underfeeding, unsafe sex and high blood pressure had more impact on global burden of disease than these two substances.

This contribution gives a comprehensive background and tries to update the comparative risk assessments and its calculations on alcohol-attributable global burden of disease. It is based on:

Substance Abuse Disorders: Evidence and Experience, First Edition. Edited by Hamid Ghodse, Helen Herrman, Mario Maj and Norman Sartorius.
© 2011 John Wiley & Sons, Ltd. Published 2011 by John Wiley & Sons, Ltd.

- a review of evidence on developments of alcohol exposure in different parts of the world between 2001 and 2003 based on the WHO Global Information System on Alcohol and Health (GISAH; http://www.who.int/globalatlas/default.asp);
- an update of current knowledge on the relationships between consumption of alcohol and disease and injury outcomes;
- new calculations on burden of disease for the year 2004 undertaken by Colin Mathers and his team at the WHO [7].

The contribution of alcohol to global burden of disease is multifaceted and related to effects of acute and chronic alcohol consumption as well as behavioural consequences of drinking [8, 9]. Traditionally, the basic description of alcohol is limited to its effects on central nervous system, whereas alcohol affects multiple organ systems either directly or by changes in their regulation [10]. Therefore it is highly important to understand the whole spectrum of alcohol effects, both acute and chronic, for evaluation of alcohol-attributable burden of disease.

Short-term effects of alcohol consumption vary depending on the amount of alcohol consumed. They include primarily inhibition of the central nervous system and a set of typical changes in other systems. In particular, direct CNS effects of alcohol depend on the alcohol concentration in the blood (BAC). At the level of 50 mg/dL, the drinker becomes euphoric, talkative, feels relaxation and stress relief; at the level of 100 mg/dL signs of CNS depression appear – impairment of motor and sensory functions as well as cognitive impairment are seen; at the level of 300 mg/dL, the drinker becomes stuporous and might lose consciousness. 400 mg/dL level is considered to be critical as at this level one might die due to the inhibition of respiration [11]. Of course, tolerance may lead to much higher BAC levels without fatal outcomes.

Acute alcohol effects on other organs and systems are various and are briefly described below. Due to the toxicity of ethanol and its metabolites severe alcohol intoxication may cause acute hepatitis. Irritation of the sphincter of Oddi together with the increased production of digestive enzymes by the pancreas constitute one of the causes of acute pancreatitis in many binge drinkers [12]. Vomiting is a typical result of alcohol overdose and may lead to several life-threatening conditions like tears of mucosa in the area of the gastroesophageal junction also known as Mallory-Weiss syndrome and loss of electrolytes with the gastric contents [13]. Alcohol is also known to cause cardiac rhythm disorders described as Holiday Heart Syndrome [14]. Besides inhibition of respiratory centres one of the pernicious consequences of acute alcohol intoxication might be acute pneumonia secondary to aspiration of one's own vomit [15].

Alcohol, in particular binge drinking, is also one of the major contributors to hazardous behaviour involving aggression such as bar fights or domestic violence [16, 17]. Also, binge drinking is associated with unsafe sex and the spread of sexually transmitted diseases like HIV, syphilis, gonorrhoea, viral hepatitis B and many others [18–22]. However, the causality of these relations is not clear yet, as there may be personality features which contribute to both heavy drinking and unsafe sex (e.g., risk proneness or sensation seeking).

Also, alcohol affects thermoregulation by peripheral vasodilatation that increases the loss of thermal energy and at the same time gives a fake feeling of warmth, which in turn increases the risk of freezing-related injuries. This is just one example for alcohol-attributable unintentional injuries, which are all linked to acute levels of BAC [23, 24]. More importantly from a public-health point of view are traffic accidents, falls and fires.

Although acute alcohol intoxication significantly contributes to the burden of disease as described above, chronic alcohol consumption leads to a higher burden of disease based on a number of severe complications, most of which are inevitable and irreversible. In fact, chronic alcohol consumption correlates to a wide spectrum of health problems [9]. These health conditions may be divided into two major groups. The first group includes disorders directly related to alcohol consumption such as alcoholic liver cirrhosis, alcoholic encephalopathy, alcoholic polyneuropathy, alcoholic cardiomyopathy and others. Disorders of the second group are those that have alcohol as a risk or predisposing factor for their onset (e.g. ceratin cancer types, tuberculosis, chronic pancreatitis, etc.) [6, 9, 25, 26].

In addition to alcohol-use disorders, alcoholic dementia also known as Wernike–Korsakoff syndrome is one the major psychiatric disorders directly caused by alcohol consumption. It is characterized by a combination of symptoms of Wernike encephalopathy and Korsakoff psychosis, both of which are pathogenically caused by alcohol-related thiamine deficiency. Wernike encephalopathy is clinically presented by ataxia, ophtalmoplegia, nystagmus, confusion and impairment of short-term memory. Korsakoff psychosis is represented with anterograde and retrograde amnesia, confabulations that replace nonexisting memories and amnestic disorientation. These two conditions have poor prognosis when untreated and are highly disabling as they result in irreversible CNS changes [27]. Other CNS impairments related to chronic alcohol consumption include a number of psychiatric manifestations such as cognitive and intellectual deficits, changes of personality, cravings and so on. [27]. Alcoholic polyneuropathy is also related to thiamine deficiency and clinically presents with symmetric loss of sensation, painful paresthesias, decrease of deep tendon reflexes and muscle weakness [27].

Alcoholic liver cirrhosis also known as a last stage of alcoholic liver disease continuum is a result of toxic effects of alcohol and its metabolites and is characterized by necrosis of liver tissue followed by its replacement with fibrous tissue. It results in irreversible liver function decrease and has several major health consequences. Increasing block of portal circulation results in active involvement of porto-caval anastomoses in order to enable the blood shunting from the veins to right atrium. As a consequence, veins that constitute these anastomoses become dilated and may rupture or become a source of thromoemboli. The most prominent clinical signs of portal hypertension are oesophageal varices, haemorrhoids and paraumbilical vein's distension and engorgement also known as 'caput medusae' sign. Another complication of liver cirrhosis is decreased production of albumins resulting in decreased oncotic pressure, which manifests in ascites. Liver also produces clotting factors and patients with liver cirrhosis usually tend to have haemorrhagic complications. Decreased metabolic function of the liver leads to build-up of toxic substances and ultimately – to hepatic encephalopathy. Decreased bile production leads to malabsorption of fats that in turn causes number of nutritional problems including deficiency of lipid-soluble vitamins (A, D, E, K) and subsequent pathological changes [28, 29].

Seizures in chronic alcohol abusers may be related not only to withdrawals but also to alcohol-induced epilepsy that develops due to cerebral atrophy, traumatic and vascular cerebral lesions, 'kindling' effect, chronic ionic imbalance and so on [30].

Chronic pancreatitis in alcoholics usually develops as a result of repetitive acute inflammations of pancreas. Pathogenic mechanism of chronic pancreatitis involves intracellular activation of zymogen granules leading to autodigestion of pancreas and replacement of its parenchyma with connective tissue. Chronic pancreatitis leads to decrease of endocrine and exocrine function of the gland resulting in malabsorption due to the decreased production of pancreatic enzymes and diabetes mellitus due to the death of islet of Langerhans [12].

Alcohol is also known for suppressing the immune system and therefore increasing the risk of multiple infections, especially opportunistic ones. It also worsens the course of pre-existing chronic infections such as tuberculosis [31, 32].

Another negative aspect of chronic alcohol consumption involves toxic effects of ethanol and its metabolites to all cells that they come into contact with. It results in metaplasia and dysplasia in various locations and makes alcohol carcinogenic agent. In fact, alcohol is related to various types of neoplasia in gastrointestinal tract, liver, pancreas, gall bladder, lungs and other organs [26].

As well as acute intoxication chronic consumption of alcohol correlates to injuries, domestic violence, unsafe sex, car accidents and other behavioural components of burden of disease [16, 17, 21, 22, 25].

Foetal alcohol syndrome is the consequence of alcohol ingestion by pregnant woman that affects the child. Children with *in utero* exposure to alcohol represent with a triad of symptoms: mental retardation, retarded physical development and specific coarse facial features. This disorder also contributes to burden of disease estimations [8].

Overall, alcohol consumption has multiple detrimental health effects, both acute and chronic, that contribute to global burden of disease in various ways and estimation of the risks and harm related to alcohol consumption is complex.

5.1.1 Establishing Alcohol as a Risk Factor for Burden of Disease

5.1.1.1 Dimensions of Alcohol Relevant for Burden of Disease and Social Harm

The relationship between alcohol consumption and health and social outcomes is complex and multidimensional, see [9]. Alcohol consumption is linked to health and social consequences through three intermediate outcomes: acute intoxication (F10.0), alcohol-use disorders (F10.0–F10.9), especially alcohol dependence (F10.2) and direct biochemical effects [9]. It should be noted that in a situation where a drunk driver kills somebody and, due to the emotional impact of this event on the drunk driver, he or she loses employment and becomes socially marginalized. In this example, the model would cover the effects of alcohol on the acute consequence (i.e. the driving accident), but does not explicitly cover the subsequent job loss and social marginalization. An example of such direct biochemical effects is the promotion of blood-clot dissolution or direct toxic effects on acinar cells triggering pancreatic damage. Intoxication and dependence are of course also influenced by biochemistry. However, since these two intermediate outcomes are central in shaping the effect of alcohol on many health and social outcomes, they are discussed separately. The other pathways are often specific for one disease or a limited group of diseases. Both intoxication and dependence are defined as health outcomes in ICD-10.

In the following, the three pathways are explained in more detail: direct biochemical effects of alcohol may influence chronic disease either in a beneficial or harmful way. Beneficial effects include the influence of moderate drinking on coronary heart disease via effects on reduction of plaque deposits in arteries, on protection against blood-clot formation and on promotion of blood clot dissolution. Examples of harmful effects include increasing the risk for high blood pressure, direct toxic effects on acinar cells triggering pancreatic damage or hormonal disturbances. The label of direct toxic and beneficial effects is used to summarize all the biochemical effects of alcohol on body tissue and functions, which are independent of intoxication and dependence. In terms of the level of burden, special emphasis should be given to the hepatotoxic properties of some forms of alcohol, such as surrogate alcohol in Russia and other countries in Central and Eastern Europe [33].

Intoxication is a powerful mediator mainly for acute outcomes, such as accidents, or intentional injuries or deaths, domestic conflict and violence, although intoxication episodes can also be implicated in chronic health and social problems. The effects of alcohol on the central nervous system mainly determine the subjective feeling of intoxication. These effects are felt and can be measured even at consumption levels that are light to moderate. A comprehensive review by Eckardt and colleagues [34] concluded that the threshold dose for negative effects on psychomotor tasks is generally found at around 40 to 50 mg% (equivalent to 0.04–0.05%).

Alcohol dependence is a disorder in itself, but is also a powerful mechanism sustaining alcohol consumption and mediating its impact on both chronic and acute physiological and social consequences of alcohol [6].

This chapter is restricted to health consequences only. However, in analysing the burden of disease linked to alcohol one should not overlook that in some regions and countries the social harm related to alcohol is more important or costly than the health consequences.

5.1.1.2   To Which Disease and Injury Conditions is Alcohol Causally Relevant?

As indicated above, two general types of disease and injury conditions causally impacted by alcohol can be distinguished [5]:

- disease and injury conditions that are caused by alcohol by definition (e.g. alcohol dependence, harmful use of alcohol, or alcohol intoxication);
- disease and injury conditions where alcohol was a contributory cause (e.g. ischaemic heart disease or some cancers).

In identifying the latter, that is disease and injury conditions where alcohol is a contributory cause, the usual epidemiological standards were applied. Thus, to establish sufficient evidence of causality: (1) that there had to be consistent evidence of an association (positive or negative) between alcohol consumption and the disease or injury; (2) that chance, confounding variables and other bias could be ruled out with reasonable confidence as factors in this association and (3) that there was evidence of a plausible mediating process [35]. These judgements were made using the usual criteria for establishing causality in epidemiology, with the most weight placed on the following four criteria:

- consistency across studies;
- established experimental biological evidence of mediating processes or at least physiological plausibility (biological mechanisms);
- strength of the association (effect size);
- temporality (i.e. cause before effect).

5.1.1.3   Disease and Injury Conditions Wholly Attributable to Alcohol

With regard to the attribution of alcohol-relatedness, the following conditions are, by definition, wholly attributable to alcohol (100% alcohol attributable: acute intoxication

(F10.0), alcohol-use disorders (F10.0–F10.9), especially alcohol dependence). In other words, in a counterfactual scenario of no presence of alcohol, these disease conditions would not exist. For these conditions, no statistical procedures are necessary to estimate risk relationships. This does not mean that the underlying data are always free of measurement error, that is that all diagnoses of 'alcoholic cirrhosis of liver' are in fact caused by alcohol. However, measurement error may also work in the opposite direction, where alcoholic liver cirrhosis are not identified as such and erroneously classified as other forms of liver cirrhosis.

5.1.1.4   Chronic Disease Conditions and Injuries where Alcohol is a Contributory Cause

Table 5.1 gives an overview of chronic conditions that are not wholly attributable to alcohol, but where alcohol has been identified as causally relevant, based on the above criteria.

Two examples of considerations regarding somewhat controversial outcomes may illustrate this process. For lung cancer, after adjusting for smoking, meta-analyses showed a consistent effect with a relatively large effect sizes. However, since evidence for the possible biological mechanism was not conclusive and residual confounding from smoking could not be excluded, English and colleagues [35] as the first seminal assessment decided to exclude lung cancer from the list of diseases causally influenced by alcohol. A decade later, we still believe this judgement is correct, although some tentative pathways have meanwhile been established.

On the other hand, although English and colleagues [35] concluded there was not sufficient evidence linking alcohol consumption and breast cancer, recent advances both in biological and epidemiological research have changed this evaluation, so that breast cancer was included in the present study as an alcohol-related outcome. Similar scientific advances hold true for colorectal cancer. These two conditions were the only two that had been added to the list in the last decade.

5.2   METHODS

5.2.1   Definition of Regions

The regional classification used in this study was defined by the WHO on the basis of levels of adult and of infant mortality [42]. The regional groups are organized as follows: A stands for very low child and very low adult mortality, B for low child and low adult mortality, C for low child and high adult mortality, D for high child and high adult mortality, and E for high child and very high adult mortality. There were 14 subregions defined in total. The allocation of countries into different subregions can be found in Table 5.2.

5.2.1.1   Exposure Estimates: Key Indicators of Alcohol Consumption at Country and Regional Levels

The following key indicators of exposure are involved in estimating alcohol related burden of disease ([6]; see also detailed description in [43]): adult per capita consumption of

Table 5.1 Relative risks for alcohol-attributable diseases and injuries by consumption stratum (reference group is 'current abstainers').

Disease condition	ICD-10	GBD code	Drinking category I RR	Drinking category II RR	Drinking category III RR	Sources and comments
Conditions arising during the perinatal period: Low birthweight	P05-P07	U050	M/W 1.00	M/W 1.40	M/W 1.40	[36]
Mouth and oropharynx cancers	C00-C14	U061	M/W 1.45	M/W 1.85	M/W 5.39	[36]
Oesophageal cancer	C15	U062	M/W 1.80	M/W 2.38	M/W 4.36	[37]
Colon and rectal cancers	C18-C21	U064	M/W 1.00	M 1.16 / W 1.01	M 1.41 / W 1.41	[36]
Liver cancer	C22	U065	M/W 1.45	M/W 3.03	M/W 3.60	[38]
Breast cancer	C50	U069	<45 yrs W 1.15 / 45+ yrs W 1.14	<45 yrs W 1.41 / 45+ yrs W 1.38	<45 yrs W 1.46 / 45+ yrs W 1.62	[39]
Other neoplasms	D00-D48	U078	M/W 1.10	M/W 1.30	M/W 1.70	[36]
Diabetes mellitus (A regions)	E10-E14	U079	M 0.99 / W 0.92	M 0.57 / W 0.87	M 0.73 / W 1.13	[36]
Diabetes mellitus (Non-A regions)	E10-E14	U079	M/W 1.00	M/W 1.0	M 1.00 / W 1.13	[6]
Alcohol-use disorders	F10	U086	–	–	–	AF 100%
Unipolar depressive disorders[a]	F32-F33	U082				[36]
Epilepsy	G40, G41	U085	M 1.23 / W 1.34	M 7.52 / W 7.22	M 6.83 / W 7.52	[69]
Hypertensive heart disease	I10-I14	U106	M 1.33 / W 1.15	M 2.04 / W 1.53	M 2.91 / W 2.19	[40]
Ischaemic heart disease[a]	I20-I25	U107	M/W 0.82	M/W 0.83	M 1.00 / W 1.12	[6, 41]
Haemorrhagic stroke (A regions)	I60-I62	U108	M 1.12 / W 0.74	M 1.40 / W 1.04	M 1.54 / W 1.94	[41]
Haemorrhagic stroke (Non-A regions)	I60-I62	U108	M 1.12 / W 1.00	M 1.40 / W 1.04	M 1.54 / W 1.94	[41]
Ischaemic stroke (A regions)	I63	U108	M 0.94 / W 0.66	M 1.13 / W 0.84	M 1.19 / W 1.53	[41]

(Continued)

Table 5.1 (Continued)

Disease condition	ICD-10	GBD code	Drinking category I RR	Drinking category II RR	Drinking category III RR	Sources and comments
Ischaemic stroke (Non-A regions)	I63	U108	MW 1.00	M 1.13 / W 1.00	M 1.19 / W 1.53	[6]
Cirrhosis of the liver[a]	K74	U117	MW 1.26	MW 9.54	MW 13.0	[6]
Road-traffic accidents[a]	b	U150	For all injury categories (shaded areas), the approach assuming that consumption strata specific RRs are generalizable across countries was only used as a sensitivity analysis. The main analyses used region-specific alcohol-attributable fractions, based on both the level of consumption and drinking pattern (for derivation see [6]).			[6]
Poisonings[a]	X40-X49	U151				[6]
Falls[a]	W00-W19	U152				[6]
Drownings[a]	W65-W74	U154				[6]
Other unintentional injuries[a]	Rest of V, W20-W64, W75-W99, X10-X39, X50-X59, Y40-Y86, Y88, Y89	U155				[6]
Self-inflicted injuries[a]	X60-X84, Y870	U157				[6]
Violence[a]	X85-Y09, Y871	U158				[6]
Other intentional injuries[a]	Y35	U160				

RR – relative risk.

[a] AAFs are taken from CRA (based on pooled cross-sectional time-series analyses and calibrated to Australia; cf. [6]).

[b] V01-V04, V06, V09-V80, V87, V89, V99. For countries with four-digit ICD-10 data, use: V01.1-V01.9, V02.1-V02.9, V03.1-V03.9, V04.1-V04.9, V06.1-V06.9, V09.2, V09.3, V10.4-V10.9, V11.4-V11.9, V12.3-V12.9, V13.3-V13.9, V14.3-V14.9, V15.4-V15.9, V16.4-V16.9, V17.4-V17.9, V18.4-V18.9, V19.4-V19.6, V20.3-V20.9, V21.3-V21.9, V22.3-V22.9, V23.3-V23.9, V24.3-V24.9, V25.5-V25.9, V26.3-V26.9, V27.3-V27.9, V28.3-V28.9, V29.4-V29.9, V30.4-V30.9, V31.4-V31.9, V32.4-V32.9, V33.4-V33.9, V34.4-V34.9, V35.4-V35.9, V36.4-V36.9, V37.4-V37.9, V38.4-V38.9, V39.4-V39.9, V40.4-V40.9, V41.4-V41.9, V42.4-V42.9, V43.4-V43.9, V44.4-V44.9, V45.4-V45.9, V46.4-V46.9, V47.4-V47.9, V48.4-V48.9, V49.4-V49.9, V50.4-V50.9, V51.4-V51.9, V52.4-V52.9, V53.4-V53.9, V54.4-V54.9, V55.4-V55.9, V56.4-V56.9, V57.4-V57.9, V58.4-V58.9, V59.4-V59.9, V60.4-V60.9, V61.4-V61.9, V62.4-V62.9, V63.4-V63.9, V64.4-V64.9, V65.4-V65.9, V66.4-V66.9, V67.4-V67.9, V68.4-V68.9, V69.4-V69.9, V70.4-V70.9, V71.4-V71.9, V72.4-V72.9, V73.4-V73.9, V74.4-V74.9, V75.4-V75.9, V76.4-V76.9, V77.4-V77.9, V78.4-V78.9, V79.4-V79.9, V80.3-V80.5, V81.1, V82.1, V83.0-V83.3, V84.0-V84.3, V85.0-V85.3, V86.0-V86.3, V87.0-V87.8, V89.2, V89.9, V99, Y850.

Table 5.2   Classification of countries into WHO subregions.

Africa D	Algeria, Angola, Benin, Burkina Faso, Cameroon, Cape Verde, Chad, Comoros, Equatorial Guinea, Gabon, Gambia, Ghana, Guinea, Guinea-Bissau, Liberia, Madagascar, Mali, Mauritania, Mauritius, Niger, Nigeria, Sao Tome and Principe, Senegal, Seychelles, Sierra Leone, Togo
Africa E	Botswana, Burundi, Central African Republic, Congo, Côte d'Ivoire, Democratic Republic of the Congo, Eritrea, Ethiopia, Kenya, Lesotho, Malawi, Mozambique, Namibia, Rwanda, South Africa, Swaziland, Uganda, United Republic of Tanzania, Zambia, Zimbabwe
Americas A	Canada, Cuba, United States of America
Americas B	Antigua and Barbuda, Argentina, Bahamas, Barbados, Belize, Brazil, Chile, Colombia, Costa Rica, Dominica, Dominican Republic, El Salvador, Grenada, Guyana, Honduras, Jamaica, Mexico, Panama, Paraguay, Saint Kitts and Nevis, Saint Lucia, Saint Vincent and the Grenadines, Suriname, Trinidad and Tobago, Uruguay, Venezuela
Americas D	Bolivia, Ecuador, Guatemala, Haiti, Nicaragua, Peru
Eastern Mediterranean B	Bahrain, Iran (Islamic Republic of), Jordan, Kuwait, Lebanon, Libyan Arab Jamahiriya, Oman, Qatar, Saudi Arabia, Syrian Arab Republic, Tunisia, United Arab Emirates
Eastern Mediterranean D	Afghanistan, Djibouti, Egypt, Iraq, Morocco, Pakistan, Somalia, Sudan, Yemen
Europe A	Andorra, Austria, Belgium, Croatia, Cyprus, Czech Republic, Denmark, Finland, France, Germany, Greece, Iceland, Ireland, Israel, Italy, Luxembourg, Malta, Monaco, Netherlands, Norway, Portugal, San Marino, Slovenia, Spain, Sweden, Switzerland, United Kingdom
Europe B	Albania, Armenia, Azerbaijan, Bosnia and Herzegovina, Bulgaria, Georgia, Kyrgyzstan, Poland, Romania, Slovakia, The Former Yugoslav Republic Of Macedonia, Tajikistan, Turkmenistan, Turkey, Uzbekistan, Yugoslavia
Europe C	Belarus, Estonia, Hungary, Kazakhstan, Latvia, Lithuania, Republic of Moldova, Russian Federation, Ukraine
South East Asia B	Indonesia, Sri Lanka, Thailand
South East Asia D	Bangladesh, Bhutan, Democratic People's Republic of Korea, India, Maldives, Myanmar, Nepal
Western Pacific A	Australia, Brunei Darussalam, Japan, New Zealand, Singapore
Western Pacific B	Cambodia, China, Cook Islands, Fiji, Kiribati, Lao People's Democratic Republic, Malaysia, Marshall Islands, Micronesia (Federated States of), Mongolia, Nauru, Niue, Palau, Papua New Guinea, Philippines, Republic of Korea, Samoa, Solomon Islands, Tonga, Tuvalu, Vanuatu, Viet Nam

recorded and unrecorded alcohol; prevalence of abstention by age and sex; prevalence of different categories of average volume of alcohol consumption by age and sex; and score for patterns of drinking.

Exposure data on recorded and unrecorded adult per capita alcohol consumption were taken from the WHO Global Status Report on Alcohol 2004 [44]. Unrecorded alcohol consumption is a proportion that is not reflected in official national records or surveys. Principally, the sources of unrecorded alcohol include: 1) home production (especially spirits); 2) alcohol intended for industrial, technical and medical uses; 3) illegal industrial production or import; 4) beverages with alcohol levels below the legal definition [44]. Per capita consumption records were obtained from the WHO Global Alcohol Database (GAD) [45]. The GAD estimates are based on industry publications on alcohol produced and sold, as well as on data from the Food and Agriculture Organization (FAO) and national sources [46].

Prevalence of abstention was taken from large representative surveys, which were in closest proximity to the year 2002 and adjusted for total adult per capita consumption (i.e. average consumption by everyone aged 15 and above) (see [6]).

Prevalence of different categories of average volume of alcohol consumption by age and sex was also assessed by surveys. The categories of drinking as first defined in study English and colleagues [35] were used and constructed in a way that the risk of many chronic diseases such as alcohol-related cancers were roughly the same for both men and women in the same category, for example [6, 9]. To adjust for underreporting, prevalence estimates were adjusted by adult per capita consumption by sex [43].

Scores that measure patterns of drinking scores have been assessed by a mixed methodology of key expert interviews and surveys. They are part of the GAD, and currently only one score per country has been calculated. For the detailed methodology see [6, 46, 47].

5.2.1.2 Data Indicating Burden of Disease

Both event-based and time-based measures indicating population health status were used in the present analyses. Mortality measured by number of deaths, was the event measure; years of life lost (YLL) due to premature mortality and burden of disease, as measured in disability-adjusted life years (DALYs), constituted the time-based gap measures [6, 48]. The DALY measure combines YLL with years of life lost to living with a disability. Estimates for mortality and DALYs for the year 2002 were directly obtained by WHO Headquarters (Dr. C. Mathers). YLL and DALYs were 3% age-discounted and age-weighted to be comparable with the Global Burden of Disease (GBD) study. Population data were obtained from United Nations (UN) population division (United Nations, 2005). Age groups used were: 0–4 years, 5–14 years, 15–29 years, 30–44 years, 45–59 years, 60–69 years and 70+ years.

5.2.1.3 Relating Alcohol Exposure to Disease and Injury Outcomes

5.2.1.3.1 Defining Alcohol-Attributable Diseases

Alcohol consumption was found to be related to the following GBD categories [6, 8, 9, 49]: conditions arising during the perinatal period: low birthweight; cancers: mouth and oropharynx cancers, oesophageal cancer, colon and rectal cancers, liver cancer, breast cancer and other neoplasms; diabetes mellitus; neuropsychiatric conditions: alcohol-use disorders, epilepsy; cardiovascular diseases: hypertensive heart disease, ischaemic heart disease, cerebrovascular diseases: haemorrhagic stroke, ischaemic stroke; cirrhosis of the liver; unintentional injuries: road-traffic accidents, poisonings, falls, drownings and other unintentional injuries; intentional injuries: self-inflicted injuries, violence and other intentional injuries.

These disease categories are the same as for the CRA 2000 with one exception: colorectal cancer has been added. In other words, all of the major review studies in the 1990s and the early 2000s concluded a causal relationship between alcohol and the respective disease or injury category selected [9], except for colorectal cancer, where some of the evidence is newer [37,50].

5.2.2 Risk Relations

The details on the procedure to quantify the risk of disease attributable to alcohol are described elsewhere [51]. For most chronic disease categories, alcohol-attributable fractions (AAFs) of disease were derived from combining prevalence of exposure and relative risk estimates based on meta-analyses [9,35–38,40] (see Table 5.3). For depression and injuries, AAFs were taken from Comparative Risk Analysis (CRA) study (see [6]), for a detailed description of underlying assumptions and calculations). Protective effects of alcohol consumption on ischaemic heart disease, strokes and diabetes were not estimated in all non-A regions due to the evidence that the pattern of drinking for most alcohol consumption is not protective in these regions (for physiological mechanisms: [52–54] for epidemiological evidence [6,8,55]. Thus, where in A regions (very low child and low adult mortality) a relative risk of less than 1 would represent the protective effect for strokes and diabetes; in

Table 5.3 Characteristics of alcohol consumption in the world in 2003.

WHO Region	Percent of abstainers		Total alcohol consumption	Unrecorded consumption	Pattern value	Recorded beverage most consumed
	M	W				
AFR	57.2	71.2	7.0	3.5	3.0	Other fermented beverages
Africa D	59.3	69.3	7.2	2.2	2.8	Other fermented beverages
Africa E	55.4	73.3	6.9	2.7	3.1	Other fermented beverages and beer
AMR	25.7	45.6	8.6	1.9	2.6	Beer
America A	32.0	52.0	9.4	1.1	2.0	Beer
America B	18.0	39.1	8.4	2.6	3.1	Beer
America D	32.1	51.0	7.4	4.0	3.1	spirits and beer
EMR	89.9	98.1	0.7	0.5	2.6	Beer
Eastern Mediterranean B	86.9	95.0	1.0	0.7	2.6	Spirits
Eastern Mediterranean D	90.8	98.9	0.6	0.4	2.6	Beer
EUR	17.3	32.6	11.9	3.0	2.5	Beer and spirits
Europe A	11.4	23.0	12.1	1.3	1.5	Beer and wine
Europe B	38.6	62.4	7.5	2.8	2.9	Spirits and beer
Europe C	13.0	26.9	14.9	6.1	3.9	Spirits
SEAR	79.0	97.6	2.0	1.5	3.0	Spirits
South East Asia B	77.6	96.9	2.3	0.9	3.0	Spirits
South East Asia D	79.0	98.0	1.9	1.6	3.0	Spirits
WPR	24.9	59.5	6.4	1.2	2.1	Spirits
Western Pacific A	13.0	29.0	9.4	1.7	2.0	Spirits
Western Pacific B	26.3	62.5	6.0	1.1	2.2	Spirits
World	44.8	65.6	6.2	1.7	2.6	spirits (53%)

M = Men, W = Women.
AFR = African region; AMR = American region; EMR = eastern Mediterranean region; EUR = European region; SEAR = southeast Asian region; WPR = western Pacific region.

non-A regions a relative risk of 1 was used. For ischaemic heart disease, the results of a pooled cross-sectional time-series analyses were used [6].

To estimate stroke subtypes (ischaemic stroke and haemorrhagic stroke), we used the region and age-specific proportions of stroke subtypes so that weighted RRs could be applied [56].

For most chronic disease categories, AAFs of disease were derived from combining prevalence of exposure and relative risk estimates based on meta-analyses [9, 35–38, 40]; using the following formula [57, 58]:

$$\text{AAF} = \left[\sum_{i=1}^{k} P_i(\text{RR}_i - 1) \right] \bigg/ \left[\sum_{i=0}^{k} P_i(\text{RR}_i - 1) + 1 \right]$$

where

i: exposure category with baseline exposure or no exposure $i = 0$,

RR(i): relative risk at exposure level i compared to no consumption,

P(i): prevalence of the ith category of exposure,

AAFs, as derived from the formula above can be interpreted as reflecting the proportion of disease that would disappear if there had been no alcohol consumption.

5.3   RESULTS

5.3.1   Global Patterns of Drinking and Burden of Disease

Figure 5.1 gives an overview of adult per capita consumption in different countries.

Overall, there is wide variation around the global average of 6.2 litres of pure alcohol per year (Table 5.3). The countries with highest overall consumption are in Eastern Europe around the Russian Federation, but other areas of Europe also have high overall consumption (Europe region 11.9 litres overall). The Americas are the region with the next highest overall consumption (Americas region 8.6 litres). Except for some individual countries, alcohol consumption is lower in other parts of the world (Eastern Mediterranean being lowest with 0.70 litres). In interpreting these numbers one should keep in mind that the majority of the adult population around the world actually abstains from drinking alcohol (45% of men and 66% of women).

5.3.2   Mortality

Overall, deaths relatively increased in comparison to the CRA analyses for 2000 [5], both for men and women (see Table 5.4). This increase is mainly due to chronic disease deaths.

The net impact of alcohol was relatively larger in younger age groups, again for both sexes. About 3.8% of all deaths were attributable to alcohol for all age groups (6.3% in men; 1.1% in women). Injury deaths, the top contributor to alcohol-attributable mortality occur relatively early in life.

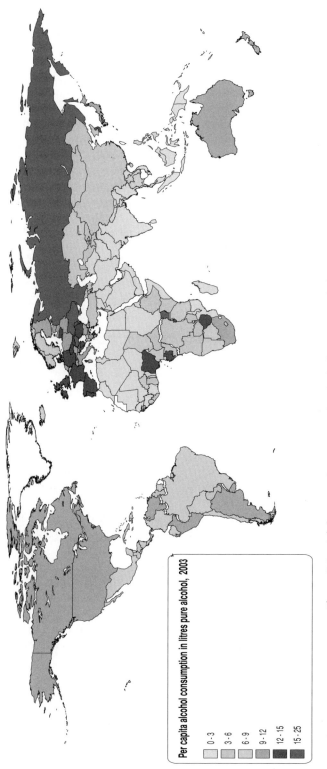

Per capita alcohol consumption in litres pure alcohol, 2003

0 - 3
3 - 6
6 - 9
9 - 12
12 - 15
15 - 25

Figure 5.1   Adult per capita consumption including unrecorded consumption in 2003.

Table 5.4 Deaths[a] attributable to alcohol consumption in the world in 2004.

Disease category	M	W	Total M and W	%M	%W
Maternal and perinatal conditions (low birth weight)	2	1	3	0.1%	0.3%
Cancer	377	111	487	18.5%	25.0%
Diabetes mellitus	0	0	0	0.0%	0.1%
Neuropsychiatric disorders	109	25	135	5.4%	5.7%
Cardiovascular diseases	466	80	545	22.8%	18.0%
Cirrhosis of the liver	297	76	373	14.6%	17.1%
Unintentional injuries	556	110	666	27.3%	24.8%
Intentional injuries	232	40	272	11.4%	9.0%
Total 'detrimental effects' attributable to alcohol	2039	443	2482	100.0%	100.0%
Diabetes mellitus	−8	−4	−12	8.3%	3.2%
Cardiovascular diseases	−88	−128	−215	91.7%	96.8%
Total 'beneficial effects' attributable to alcohol	−96	−132	−227	100.0%	100.0%
All alcohol-attributable net deaths	1944	311	2255		
All deaths	31 063	27 674	58 738		
Percentage of all net deaths attributable to alcohol	6.3%	1.1%	3.8%		

M = Men, W = Women.
[a]Numbers are rounded to the nearest thousand. Zero (0) indicates fewer than 500 alcohol-attributable DALYs in the disease category.

Most of the global death (Table 5.5; details for each region in Table 5.5) was related to acute causes, with 25% due to unintentional injuries and 9% due to intentional injuries. Cancer was the next most important category, accounting for 25%, followed by cardio-vascular disease (18%) and liver cirrhosis (17%) of the overall alcohol-related mortality burden. Globally, about 65% of the mortality due to neuropsychiatric disorders was directly attributable to alcohol-use disorders.

The detrimental effect of alcohol mortality by far outweighed the beneficial effects, which were mainly due to cardiovascular diseases and diabetes mellitus (227 000 prevented deaths versus a net total of 2 255 000 deaths).

More men than women died from alcohol, with a ratio of 6 : 1, due to higher alcohol consumption by men. For men, the estimates range from less than 1% in the Eastern Mediterranean D (represented by Islamic countries) to 15% in Europe C (represented mainly by the countries of the Former Soviet Union). In terms of women, only in one region (Europe A) more deaths were prevented than caused by alcohol (101 000 vs. 56 000 deaths, respectively) (data not shown). In Europe C, alcohol-attributable mortality amongst women was the highest in the world: 6.3% (110,851/1 764 469).

5.3.3 Disability-Adjusted Life Years (DALYs)

Alcohol-attributable DALYs for the year 2004 are summarized in Table 5.6.

Table 5.5 Deaths[a] attributable to alcohol consumption in WHO regions in 2004.

Disease category	AFR			AMR			EMR			EUR			SEAR			WPR		
	M	W	T	M	W	T	M	W	T	M	W	T	M	W	T	M	W	T
Maternal and perinatal conditions (low birth weight)	1	1	1	0	0	1	0	0	0	0	0	1	0	0	1	0	0	0
Cancer	27	12	39	30	20	50	2	1	3	64	40	105	36	2	39	217	36	252
Diabetes mellitus	0	0	0	0	0	0	0	0	0	0	0	0	0	0	0	0	0	0
Neuropsychiatric disorders	17	7	24	23	5	28	3	0	3	28	8	35	18	2	19	21	4	25
Cardiovascular diseases	25	9	34	63	14	77	5	0	5	157	47	204	76	1	77	140	8	148
Cirrhosis of the liver	13	4	17	54	15	69	3	0	3	90	44	134	58	3	61	79	9	88
Unintentional injuries	80	12	93	84	13	97	6	1	7	190	35	225	104	22	126	92	25	117
Intentional injuries	54	8	61	70	6	76	1	0	1	63	11	74	26	5	31	19	9	29
Total 'detrimental effects' attributable to alcohol	216	53	269	324	74	398	20	3	23	592	186	778	319	36	355	569	91	661
Diabetes mellitus	0	0	0	−4	−1	−5	0	0	0	−4	−3	−7	0	0	0	−1	0	−1
Cardiovascular diseases	0	0	0	−25	−21	−46	0	0	0	−54	−98	−152	0	0	0	−9	−8	−17
Total 'beneficial effects' attributable to alcohol	0	0	0	−29	−22	−51	0	0	0	−57	−101	−159	0	0	0	−10	−9	−18
All alcohol-attributable net deaths	216	53	269	296	52	347	20	3	23	534	85	619	319	36	355	560	83	642
All deaths	5787	5475	11262	3286	2920	6206	2396	1910	4306	4847	4646	9493	8103	7176	15 279	6644	5548	12 191
Percentage of all net deaths attributable to alcohol	3.7%	1.0%	2.4%	9.0%	1.8%	5.6%	0.8%	0.1%	0.5%	11.0%	1.8%	6.5%	3.9%	0.5%	2.3%	8.4%	1.5%	5.3%

M = Men, W = Women.

[a]Numbers are rounded to the nearest thousand. Zero (0) indicates fewer than 500 alcohol-attributable deaths in the disease category.

AFR = African region; AMR = American region; EMR = eastern Mediterranean region; EUR = European region; SEAR = southeast Asian region; WPR = western Pacific region.

Table 5.6   Disability-adjusted life-years (DALYs)[a] attributable to alcohol consumption in the world in 2004.

Disease category	M	W	Total M and W	%M	%W
Maternal and perinatal conditions (low birth weight)	64	55	119	0.1%	0.5%
Cancer	4732	1536	6268	7.6%	13.5%
Diabetes mellitus	0	28	28	0.0%	0.3%
Neuropsychiatric disorders	23 265	3417	26 682	37.6%	30.1%
Cardiovascular diseases	5985	939	6924	9.7%	8.3%
Cirrhosis of the liver	5502	1443	6945	8.9%	12.7%
Unintentional injuries	15 694	2910	18 604	25.4%	25.6%
Intentional injuries	6639	1021	7660	10.7%	9.0%
Total 'detrimental effects' attributable to alcohol	61 881	11 349	73 231	100.0%	100.0%
Diabetes mellitus	−238	−101	−340	22.2%	8.1%
Cardiovascular diseases	−837	−1145	−1981	77.8%	91.9%
Total 'beneficial effects' attributable to alcohol	−1075	−1246	−2321	100.0%	100.0%
All alcohol-attributable net DALYs	60 806	10 104	70 910		
All DALYs	799 536	730 631	1 530 168		
Percentage of all net DALYs attributable to alcohol	7.6%	1.4%	4.6%		

M = Men, W = Women.
[a] Numbers are rounded to the nearest thousand. Zero (0) indicates fewer than 500 alcohol-attributable DALYs in the disease category.

Alcohol-attributable DALYs were also slightly higher in 2004 compared to 2000 [5,6]. The notable difference between the impact of disease categories for DALYs compared to mortality was found with respect to neuropsychiatric disorders (38% of alcohol-attributable DALYs versus 5% of alcohol-attributable deaths, respectively). Close to 88% of the neuropsychiatric disease burden was directly attributable to alcohol-use disorders. The second major contributor to alcohol-attributable DALYs were unintentional injuries (26% of alcohol-attributable DALYs, which was similar to mortality). Similar to deaths, men had a far greater alcohol-attributable disease burden than women: about 6 : 1.

The regional differences were also striking and followed a pattern similar to that of mortality. It should be noted that for disease burden there was no region where alcohol had an overall beneficial impact on either gender. The detrimental effect of alcohol on disease burden was many times higher than beneficial (Table 5.7).

5.3.4   The Contribution of Alcohol-Use Disorders to Burden of Disease

Globally, the impact of alcohol-attributable neuropsychiatric disorders first came to light with the first Comparative Risk Analysis Study, particularly in the context of burden of disease [59]. In developed countries, this study shows that this burden continues to be particularly high, but in developing countries, neuropsychiatric disorders continue to levy a serious burden, either due to inadequate care and unmet needs [60] or due to the fact that it may be highly underreported [61].

Table 5.7 Disability-adjusted life-years (DALYs)[a] attributable to alcohol consumption in WHO regions in 2004.

Disease category	AFR			AMR			EMR			EUR			SEAR			WPR		
	M	W	T	M	W	T	M	W	T	M	W	T	M	W	T	M	W	T
Maternal and perinatal conditions (low birth weight)	29	25	55	12	10	22	1	1	1	11	9	20	10	11	21	0	0	0
Cancer	407	192	599	364	277	641	28	10	38	782	516	1298	473	34	506	2679	507	3186
Diabetes mellitus	0	9	9	0	11	11	0	0	0	0	7	7	0	0	0	0	2	2
Neuropsychiatric disorders	1184	337	1521	4457	1233	5691	278	17	294	4573	1018	5591	4061	380	4441	8713	432	9145
Cardiovascular diseases	383	172	554	767	178	945	74	1	75	1927	489	2416	1311	10	1321	1524	89	1612
Cirrhosis of the liver	266	89	355	1017	278	1295	62	5	67	1680	839	2519	1122	68	1189	1356	165	1521
Unintentional injuries	2570	444	3014	2465	343	2808	221	40	262	4725	738	5463	3123	695	3819	2589	651	3239
Intentional injuries	1583	225	1809	2321	179	2499	29	9	37	1549	256	1806	698	142	840	459	210	669
Total 'detrimental effects' attributable to alcohol	6422	1493	7915	11 403	2508	13 911	693	83	776	15 246	3872	19 118	10 798	1339	12 137	17 319	2055	19 374
Diabetes mellitus	0	0	0	−91	−33	−125	0	0	0	−116	−56	−172	0	0	0	−31	−12	−43
Cardiovascular diseases	0	0	0	−250	−208	−458	0	0	0	−488	−832	−1320	0	0	0	−98	−105	−203
Total 'beneficial effects' attributable to alcohol	0	0	0	−342	−241	−583	0	0	0	−604	−889	−1493	0	0	0	−129	−116	−245
All alcohol-attributable net DALYs	6422	1493	7915	11 062	2267	13 328	693	83	776	14 642	2983	17 625	10 798	1339	12137	17 190	1939	19 129
All DALYs	188 525	188 182	376 706	78 015	66 702	144 717	75 467	66 916	142 383	84 476	67 271	151 747	227 531	222 135	449 665	145 524	119 425	264 949
Percentage of all net DALYs attributable to alcohol	3.4%	0.8%	2.1%	14.2%	3.4%	9.2%	0.9%	0.1%	0.5%	17.3%	4.4%	11.6%	4.7%	0.6%	2.7%	11.8%	1.6%	7.2%

M = Men, W = Women.
LBW – low birth weight.
[a] Numbers are rounded to the nearest thousand. Zero (0) indicates fewer than 500 alcohol-attributable DALYs in the disease category

Table 5.8 Cancer related deaths and disease burden (15+ years) attributable to alcohol consumption in the world in 2004.

Malignant neoplasms	Death			DALYs		
	M	W	M and W	M	W	M and W
Mouth and oropharynx cancers	68	10	78	928	134	1063
Oesophagus cancer	132	25	157	1476	307	1783
Colon and rectum cancers	15	3	18	205	42	247
Liver cancer	154	30	185	2026	398	2424
Breast cancer	7	38	38	—	603	603
Other neoplasms	377	4	11	96	52	149
Alcohol-attributable cancers	4106	111	487	4732	1536	6268
All cancers (15+ years)	9.2%	3225	7332	40 191	34 463	74 654
Percentage of cancers attributable to alcohol		3.4%	6.6%	11.8%	4.5%	8.4%

The burden of disease of alcohol-use disorders as a disease category were detailed above (Tables 5.6 and 5.7). They constitute 88% of the burden of alcohol-attributable neuropsychiatric disorders and 38% of the global burden by alcohol. However, as laid out in the conceptual model, alcohol-use disorders also can lead to other disease categories. For instance, a major part of alcoholic liver cirrhosis is probably caused by alcohol-use disorders. There are not many estimates that try estimate this indirect pathway. Patra and colleagues [62] recently attempted a quantification for Canada via heavy drinking occasions, and estimated that about 60% of the mortality and morbidity in Canada were due to alcohol-use disorders. The burden of malignant neoplasms attributable to alcohol, on the other hand, was 8.4% overall (Table 5.8).

Figure 5.2 depicts 1-year prevalence of alcohol-use disorders in people aged 15–64 years by sex and WHO region in 2004 (Figure 5.2).

Average prevalence for both genders worldwide is 3.6% with significantly higher prevalence in men in comparison to women (6.3% versus 0.9%) with the male:female ratio of 7. The same tendency of male prevalence prevailing over female prevalence is seen in all regions with the ratio variation between 2.6 in American region to 28.3 in Western Pacific region. The prevalence of AUD varies also between different regions depending on the levels and patterns of drinking with the highest prevalence in Eastern European region (10.9%) where the alcohol consumption is the highest especially consumption of strong alcohols. The lower prevalence is seen in Eastern Mediterranean region (0.3%), African region (1.1%) and South-East Asian region (2.4%) that is in the regions with lower alcohol consumption per capita and traditional preference of beverages with lower alcohol content. It is also remarkable that in these areas male:female ratios of AUD prevalence are very high.

5.4   DISCUSSION

Before discussing the implications for prevention, we would like to point out some methodological limitations in this study. First, the RRs were derived from the meta-analyses and are assumed to be consistent globally, mainly because they reflect biological mechanisms. This assumption may be challenged for developing countries (Non-A regions), as most

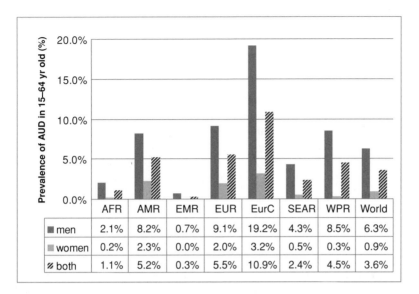

	AFR	AMR	EMR	EUR	EurC	SEAR	WPR	World
▪ men	2.1%	8.2%	0.7%	9.1%	19.2%	4.3%	8.5%	6.3%
▪ women	0.2%	2.3%	0.0%	2.0%	3.2%	0.5%	0.3%	0.9%
▨ both	1.1%	5.2%	0.3%	5.5%	10.9%	2.4%	4.5%	3.6%

AFR=African region. AMR=American region. EMR=eastern Mediterranean region. EUR=European region. EurC=eastern European region with proportionally higher adult mortality than other European parts (most populous country: Russia). SEAR=southeast Asian region. WPR=western Pacific region.

Figure 5.2 1-year prevalence of alcohol-use disorders (AUD) in people aged 15–64 years by sex and WHO region in 2004.

studies included in the meta-analyses are from European or North American countries with similar genetic background and comparable health care systems. Secondly, the AAFs for injury may be more problematic, as the relationship between alcohol and injury has been shown to be quite influenced by culture. Thirdly, the estimates for the age groups 70 years and older are certainly an overestimate, both for beneficial and detrimental effects. RRs have been shown to decrease with age. While there are quantifications of this effect for major tobacco-related risks, no quantification exists for alcohol-attributable disease (see also [63]) for references and further information). Fourth, the procedure for adjustment of the survey data may overestimate consumption in heavy-drinking categories, if the key assumption for this procedure, that is that undercoverage is a result of missing certain heavy-drinking populations such the homeless and the institutionalized, is not valid (see [64]). Despite these limitations, the estimates are the best possible globally and for lack of better estimates, should influence policy.

As was mentioned above, alcohol-use disorders contribute to global burden of disease on several levels including health effects directly related to alcohol intoxication, burden of alcohol-use disorders themselves and health conditions remotely related to alcohol consumption. Prevalence of AUD to a great extent on patterns of drinking, namely, on amounts of alcohol consumed on a daily basis, frequency and quality of alcohol and so on that can be well seen at the distribution of AUD in different world regions – AUD are more prevalent in regions with the higher alcohol consumption and with stronger alcohols consumed traditionally (Eastern European region). At the same time in regions where the alcohol consumption is low and/or beverages with lower alcohol content are consumed traditionally AUD prevalence is significantly lower (African region, Eastern Mediterranean region and South-East Asian region).

Overall, alcohol continues to be one of the most important risk factors for burden of disease. Given the current trends both in exposure and, with expected increases in alcohol consumption in the most populous countries India and China and in outcomes, with an overall relative increase in alcohol-attributable causes of death, the detrimental impact of alcohol is expected in increase in the future if no additional interventions are introduced.

A large part of alcohol-attributable burden is avoidable, however, and some of it in the short term [3]. It was not the aim of this contribution to detail potential interventions to achieve this goal. It suffices to say that such interventions exist (e.g. [65–67]), including for developing countries (e.g. [51]), and that they are cost effective in comparison to other public-health measures [39]. One prerequisite for focused interventions is the establishment of national and regional monitoring and surveillance systems [68]. We hope that the present contribution will help establish such systems.

ACKNOWLEDGEMENTS

The Comparative Risk Assessment (CRA) for Alcohol project was financially supported by the WHO and the Research Institute for Public Health and Addiction in Zurich, a WHO Collaborative Centre. In addition, support to Centre for Addiction and Mental Health (CAMH) for the salary of scientists and infrastructure has been provided by the Ontario Ministry of Health and Long Term Care. The views expressed here do not necessarily reflect those of the Ministry of Health and Long Term Care or of other funders.

REFERENCES

1. Ezzati, M., Lopez, A.D., Rodgers, A.D. *et al.*, Comparative Risk Assessment Collaborating Group (2002) Selected major risk factors and global and regional burden of disease. *Lancet*, **360**, 1347–1360.

2. Ezzati, M., Lopez, A., Rodgers, A. and Murray, C. (2004) *Comparative Quantification of Health Risks. Global and Regional Burden of Disease Attributable to Selected Major Risk Factors*, WHO, Geneva, Switzerland.

3. WHO (2002) *The World Health Report 2002: Reducing Risks, Promoting Healthy Life*, WHO, Geneva, Switzerland.

4. Lopez, A.D., Mathers, C.D., Ezzati, M. *et al.* (2006) *Global Burden of Disease and Risk Factors*, Oxford University Press and the World Bank, New York and Washington.

5. Rehm, J., Room, R., Monteiro, M. *et al.* (2003d) Alcohol as a risk factor for global burden of disease. *Eur Addict Res.*, **9**: 157–164.

6. Rehm, J., Room, R., Monteiro, M. *et al.* (2004) Alcohol use, in *Comparative Quantification of Health Risks: Global and Regional Burden of Disease Attributable to Selected Major Risk Factors*, Vol. **1** (eds. M. Ezzati, A.D. Lopez, A. Rodgers and C.J.L. Murray), WHO, Geneva, pp. 959–1109.

7. WHO (2008) *The Global Burden of Disease: 2004 Update*, WHO, Geneva, Switzerland.

8. Rehm, J., Greenfield, T. and Kerr, W. (2006b) Patterns of drinking and mortality from different diseases – an overview. *Contemp Drug Probl.*, **33**, 205–235.

9. Rehm, J., Room, R., Graham, K., *et al.* (2003c) The relationship of average volume of alcohol consumption and patterns of drinking to burden of disease – an overview. *Addiction.*, **98**, 1209–1228.

10. Spanagel, R. (2009) Alcoholism: A systems approach from molecular physiology to addictive behaviour. *Psychol Rev.*, **89**, 649–705.

11. Pohorecky, L.A. and Brick, J. (1988) Pharmacology of ethanol. *Pharmacol Ther.*, **36**: 335–427.

12. Irving, H.M., Samokhvalov, A. and Rehm, J. (2009) Alcohol as a risk factor for pancreatitis. A systematic review and meta-analysis. *JOP.*, **10**, 387–392.

13. Caroli, A., Follador, R., Gobbi, V., *et al.* (1989) Mallory-Weiss syndrome. Personal experience and review of the literature. *Minerva dietologica e gastroenterologica.*, **35**, 7–12.

14. Balbão, C.E.B., de Paola, A.A.V., Fenelon, G. (2009) Effects of alcohol on atrial fibrillation. *Ther Adv Cardiovasc Dis.*, **3**: 53–63.

15. Szabo, G. and Mandrekar, P. (2009) A recent perspective on alcohol, immunity, and host defense. *Alcohol Clin Exp Res.*, **33**, 220–232.

16. Room, R. (2001) Intoxication and bad behaviour: understanding cultural differences in the link. *Soc Sci Med.*, **53**, 189–198.

17. Rossow, I. (2001) Alcohol and homicide: cross-cultural comparison of the relationship in 14 European countries. *Addiction.*, **96**, 77–92.

18. Rehm, J., Shuper, P.A., Neuman, M. *et al.* (2009b) *Causal Considerations on Alcohol and HIV/AIDS – a Systematic Review*, CAMH, Toronto, ON.

19. Shuper, P.A., Joharchi, N., Irving, H. and Rehm, J. (2009) Alcohol as a correlate of unprotected sexual behavior among people living with HIV/AIDS: review and meta-analysis. *AIDS Behav.* [Epub ahead of print July 18].

20. Fisher, J.C., Bang, H., Kapiga, S.H. (2007) The association between HIV infection and alcohol use: a systematic review and meta-analysis of African studies. *Sex Transm Dis.*, **34**, 856–863.

21. Kalichman, S.C., Simbayi, L.C., Kaufman, M. *et al.* (2007) Alcohol use and sexual risks for HIV/AIDS in sub-Saharan Africa: systematic review of empirical findings. *Prev Sci.*, **8**, 141–151.

22. Baliunas, D., Rehm, J., and Irving, H. (2008) *Alcohol Consumption and Risk of Incident Human Immunodeficiency Virus Infection: a Meta-Analysis*, Centre for Addiction and Mental Health, Toronto, Canada.

23. Gmel, G. and Rehm, J. (2003) Harmful alcohol use. *Alcohol Res Health.*, **27**, 52–62.

24. Rehm, J., Gmel, G., Sempos, C. and Trevisan, M. (2003a) Alcohol-related mortality and morbidity. *Alcohol Res Health.*, **27**, 39–51.

25. Rehm, J., Mathers, C., Popova, S. *et al.* (2009a) Global burden of disease and injury and economic cost attributable to alcohol use and alcohol-use disorders. *Lancet*, **373**, 2223–2233.

26. Baan, R., Straif, K., Grosse, Y. *et al.*, on behalf of the WHO International Agency for Research on Cancer Monograph Working Group (2007) Carcinogenicity of alcoholic beverages. *Lancet Oncol.*, **8**: 292–293.

27. Kaplan, H.I. and Sadock, B.J. (1997) *Kaplan and Sadock's sysnopsis of Psychiatry: Behavioral Sciences, Clinical Psychiatry*, 8th edn, Williams & Wilkins, Baltimore, MD.

28. Lieber, C.S. (1988) Biochemical and molecular basis of alcohol-induced injury to liver and other tissues. *N Engl J Med.*, **319**, 1639–1650.

29. Bautista, A.P. (2005) Liver injury during alcohol use and withdrawal, in *Comprehensive Handbook of Alcohol Related Pathology* (eds. V.R. Preedy and R.R. Watson), Elsevier Academic Press, London, UK, pp. 491–500.

30. Bartolomei, F. (2006) Epilepsy and alcohol. *Epileptic Disord.*, **8**, S72–S78.

31. Parry, C.D.H., Rehm, J.R., Poznyak, V. and Room, R. (2009) Alcohol and infectious diseases: are there causal linkages? *Addiction*, **104**, 331–332.

32. Lönnroth, K., Williams, B., Stadlin, S. *et al.* (2008) Alcohol use as a risk factor for tuberculosis – a systematic review. *BMC Public Health.*, **8**, 289.

33. McKee, M., Suzcs, S., Sarvary, A. *et al.* (2005) The composition of surrogate alcohols consumed in Russia. *Alcohol Clin Exp Res.*, **29**, 1884–1888.

34. Eckardt, M., File, S., Gessa, G. *et al.* (1998) Effects of moderate alcohol consumption on the central nervous system. *Alcohol Clin Exp Res.*, **22**, 998–1040.

35. English, D., Holman, C., Milne, E. *et al.* (1995) *The Quantification of Drug Caused Morbidity and Mortality in Australia 1995*, Commonwealth Department of Human Services and Health, Canberra, Australia.

36. Gutjahr, E., Gmel, G. and Rehm, J. (2001) The relation between average alcohol consumption and disease: an overview. *Eur Addict Res.*, **7**: 117–127.

37. Cho, E., Smith-Warner, S., Ritz, J., *et al.* (2004) Alcohol intake and colorectal cancer: a pooled analysis of 8 cohort studies. *Ann Intern Med.*, **140**, 603–613.

38. Ridolfo, B. and Stevenson, C. (2001) *The Quantification of Drug-Caused Mortality and Morbidity in Australia 1998*, Australian Institute of Health and Welfare, Canberra.

39. Chisholm, D., Rehm, J., van Ommeren, M. and Monteiro, M. (2004) Reducing the global burden of hazardous alcohol use: a comparative cost-effectiveness analysis. *J Stud Alcohol.*, **65**, 782–793.

40. Corrao, G., Rubbiati, L., Bagnardi, V. *et al.* (2000) Alcohol and coronary heart disease: a meta-analysis. *Addiction.*, **95**, 1505–1523.

41. Reynolds, K., Lewis, B., Nolen, J., *et al.* (2003) Alcohol consumption and risk of stroke: a meta-analysis. *JAMA*, **289**, 579–588.

42. WHO (2000b) *World Health Report 2000. Health Systems: Improving Performance*, WHO, Geneva, Switzerland.

43. Rehm, J., Klotsche, J. and Patra, J. (2007) Comparative quantification of alcohol exposure as risk factor for global burden of disease. *Int J Methods Psychiatr Res.*, **16**, 66–76.

44. WHO (2004) *Global Status Report on Alcohol 2004*, WHO, Geneva, Switzerland.

45. WHO (2006) *Global Alcohol Database*, WHO, Geneva, Switzerland.

46. Rehm, J., Rehn, N., Room, R., *et al.* (2003b) The global distribution of average volume of alcohol consumption and patterns of drinking. *Eur Addict Res.*, **9**, 147–156.

47. Gmel, G., Rehm, J. and Frick, U. (2001) Methodological approaches to conducting pooled cross-sectional time series analysis: the example of the association between all-cause mortality and per capita alcohol consumption for men in 15 European states. *Eur Addict Res.*, **7**, 128–137.

48. Murray, C., Salomon, J., Mathers, C. and Lopez, A. (2002) *Summary Measures of Population Health: Concepts, Ethics, Measurement and Applications*, WHO, Geneva, Switzerland.

49. Mathers, C., Vos, A., Lopez, A.D. *et al.* (2001) *National Burden of Disease Studies: a Practical Guide. Global Program on Evidence for Health Policy*, 2nd edn, WHO, Geneva.

50. Boffetta, P., Hashibe, M., La Vecchia, C. *et al.* (2006) The burden of cancer attributable to alcohol drinking. *Int J Cancer.*, **119**, 884–887.

51. Rehm, J., Patra, J., Popova, S. (2006c) Alcohol-attributable mortality and potential years of life lost in Canada 2001: implications for prevention and policy. *Addiction.*, **101**, 373–384.

52. McKee, M. and Britton, A. (1998) The positive relationship between alcohol and heart disease in Eastern Europe: potential physiological mechanisms. *J R Soc Med.*, **91**, 402–407.

53. Puddey, I.B., Rakic, V., Dimmitt, S.B. and Beilin, L.J. (1999) Influence of pattern of drinking on cardiovascular disease and cardiovascular risk factors – a review. *Addiction*, **94**, 649–663.

54. Rehm, J., Sempos, C., Trevisan, M. (2003e) Average volume of alcohol consumption, patterns of drinking and risk of coronary heart disease – a review. *J Cardiovasc Risk.*, **10**, 15–20.

55. Gmel, G., Rehm, J. and Frick, U. (2003) Trinkmuster, Pro-Kopf-Konsum von Alkohol und koronare Mortalitat. *Sucht.*, **49**, 95–104.

56. Clinical Trials Research Unit (2002) *Estimating Stroke Subtypes*, University of Auckland, New Zealand.

57. Walter, S.D. (1976) The estimation and interpretation of attributable risk in health research. *Biometrics.*, **32**, 829–849.

58. Walter, S.D. (1980) Prevention of multifactorial disease. *Am J Epidemiol.*, **112**: 409–416.

59. Murray, C. and Lopez, A. (1997) Global mortality, disability, and the contribution of risk factors: global burden of disease study. *Lancet.*, **349**, 1436–1442.

60. Wang, P., Aguilar-Gaxiola, S., Alonso, J. *et al.* (2007) Use of mental health services for anxiety, mood, and substance disorders in 17 countries in the WHO world mental health surveys. *The Lancet*, **370**, 841–850.

61. Moussavi, S., Chatterji, S., Verdes, E. *et al.* (2007) Depression, chronic diseases, and decrements in health: results from the World Health Surveys. *The Lancet.*, **370**, 851–858.

62. Patra, J., Taylor, B. and Rehm, J. (in press) Deaths associated with high-volume drinking of alcohol among adults in Canada in 2002: a need for primary care intervention? *Contemporary Drug Problems.*

63. Rehm, J., Chisholm, D., Room, R. and Lopez, A. (2006a) Alcohol, in *Disease Control Priorities in Developing Countries* (eds. D.T. Jamison, J.G. Breman, A.R. Measham *et al.*), Oxford University Press and World Bank, Washington, D.C., pp. 887–906.

64. Gmel, G. and Rehm, J. (2004) Measuring alcohol consumption. *Contemp Drug Probl.*, **31**, 467–540.

65. Babor, T., Caetano, R., Casswell, S. *et al.* (2003) *Alcohol: No Ordinary Commodity. Research and Public Policy*, Oxford University Press, Oxford and London.

66. Room, R., Graham, K., Rehm, J. *et al.* (2003) Drinking and its burden in a global perspective: policy considerations and options. *Eur Addict Res.*, **9**, 165–175.

67. Room, R., Babor, T. and Rehm, J. (2005) Alcohol and public health: a review. *Lancet*, **365**, 519–530.

68. WHO (2000a) *International Guide for Monitoring Alcohol Consumption and Related Harm*, WHO, Department of Mental Health and Substance Dependence, Geneva.

69. Corrao, G., Bagnardi, V., Zambon, A. and Arico, S. (1999) Exploring the dose-response relationship between alcohol consumption and the risk of several alcohol-related conditions: a meta-analysis. *Addiction*, **94** (10), 1551–1573.

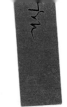

CHAPTER 6

The Prevention of Alcohol Problems

John B. Saunders[1], MD, FRACP, FAFPHM, FAChAM, FRCP and Noeline C. Latt[2], MB, BS, M Phil, MRCP, FAChAM

[1]*Centre for Youth Substance Abuse Research, Faculty of Health Sciences, University of Queensland, Herston and Faculty of Medicine, University of Sydney, NSW, Australia*

[2]*Area Drug and Alcohol Service, Royal North Shore Hospital, St Leonards, Sydney, and Faculty of Medicine, University of Sydney, NSW, Australia*

6.1 INTRODUCTION

Alcohol is a special commodity. It is a source of pleasure to millions when used in moderation but it is also a cause of widespread disease, premature mortality and an array of psychological, social and financial problems. Alcohol is consumed by approximately half the world's adult population. However, there are major differences from region to region in the prevalence of its use, which is influenced by prevailing religious beliefs, cultural mores and social practices.

The prevention of alcohol-related harm is a laudable goal. It might at first sight seem straightforward but in reality it has proven difficult to achieve in the modern world. Alcohol is a source of employment and a source of considerable tax revenue for governments. Furthermore, the producers of alcohol are a politically powerful lobby. Individuals are often conflicted because of the traditional place of alcohol in their own societies and in their personal life. The prevention of alcohol-related harm is an endeavour charged with political and personal emotion.

6.2 THE IMPACT OF ALCOHOL ON HEALTH

6.2.1 Global Burden of Disease, Mortality and Morbidity

Alcohol is the fifth most important cause of the global burden of disease, accounting for an estimated net harm of 4.4%, as measured by disability-adjusted life years (DALYs) [1]. On

Substance Abuse Disorders: Evidence and Experience, First Edition. Edited by Hamid Ghodse, Helen Herrman, Mario Maj and Norman Sartorius.
© 2011 John Wiley & Sons, Ltd. Published 2011 by John Wiley & Sons, Ltd.

a global basis, alcohol-related unintentional injury and neuropsychiatric disorders head the list, while cirrhosis contributes to 10% of the burden of disease [2]. Overall, approximately 4% of deaths worldwide are caused by alcohol. Its impact, in particular as a cause of fatal injuries, is greater in younger age groups – of both sexes. Of all alcohol-related deaths, unintentional injuries (25%), cardiovascular diseases (22%), cancer (20%) are the three biggest categories [1].

Alcohol, therefore, causes an immense burden of harm, which falls on the individual, on the family and the community, and on health services, law-enforcement agencies, the criminal justice system and insurance companies. The total annual cost to the US economy was estimated in 1998 to be $184 billion [3] and in the UK in 2001 it was estimated to be £20 billion [4,5]. In Australia the estimated costs of alcohol-related harm are AU$15 billion each year, when crime ($1.6 billion) health ($1.9 billion), productivity in the workplace ($3.5 billion) and road-traffic accidents ($2.2 billion) are all taken into account [6].

The medical, psychiatric and social harm arising from alcohol consumption is related both to the overall level of intake, but also to the pattern of drinking. Some types of harm occur typically because of 'binge' drinking [7]. Others arise from chronic excessive drinking, itself often reflecting alcohol dependence [8].

6.2.2   Acute Complications of Alcohol

Acute medical, psychiatric and social problems are typically related to episodic binge drinking. The most common of these types of harm are alcohol-related motor-vehicle accidents. These occur as a result of impairment of psychomotor reactions but also from alcohol's effects in increasing the individual's self-confidence in being able to manoeuvre a vehicle. Other common acute harms include alcohol-fuelled violence and trauma (particularly amongst the young), drowning, burns, suicide and homicide and acute illnesses such as acute gastritis and acute pancreatitis [9]. More people die from the acute complications of alcohol than the long-term ones [10].

6.2.3   Long-Term Harms from Alcohol

The chronic complications of alcohol consumption are innumerable, as alcohol's toxic effects can involve nearly every organ system in the body [11]. The commonest cause of morbidity and mortality amongst the chronic physical diseases is cirrhosis of the liver (accounting for 10% of DALYs worldwide). In the UK a fourfold increase in deaths from cirrhosis was recorded between 1970 and 2000, mainly in those aged 35–44 years and principally from alcohol [5].

Much of the long-term harm occurs in the alcohol-dependent population. Alcohol dependence causes an additional direct burden of disease due to the withdrawal syndrome. As an example, delirium tremens, comprising confusion, hallucinations and paranoia ideation, has a mortality of 30% if not adequately treated [12].

6.2.4   Alcohol Dependence

Alcohol is a dependence-inducing (addictive) substance. Alcohol dependence is a psychobiological syndrome which is the manifestation of a 'driving force' that constitutes the addictive process. The latter develops in meso-cortico-limbic systems in response to repeated exposure of these systems to alcohol [13–15]. The mechanisms involved include (i) a resetting of the reward and salience-incentive pathways subserved by dopamine and endogenous opioids, (ii) recruitment of the brain stress systems mediated by glutamate and corticotrophin-releasing factor (CRF) and (iii) impairment of inhibitory control pathways coursing from the frontal lobes to the reward and stress pathways. As its severity increases, alcohol dependence becomes an increasingly fixed entity. In several Western societies alcohol dependence has a (12-month) period prevalence of 4–10% [16–17].

6.3 ALCOHOL CONSUMPTION IN THE COMMUNITY

6.3.1 The Distribution of Alcohol Consumption

An important reason that alcohol is a special commodity is that it is socially infectious. An individual's consumption is influenced considerably by the level of use in society as a whole. In the early 1950s the French mathematician and demographer, Ledermann, proposed a 'single distribution' theory of alcohol consumption in society. He provided empirical support for this theory by analysing alcohol consumption and related harms [18]. Essentially, the single distribution model states that alcohol consumption is distributed unimodally and conforms to a logarithmic normal distribution.

The implications of this theory are:

(1) there is no group of people within a population whose alcohol consumption is entirely separate from that of the general population (if this were the case the distribution would be bimodal);
(2) if alcohol consumption overall increases in a society, the number of people drinking the highest amounts also increases and the increase, because of the log-normal curve, is proportionately greater than the average increase in the number of drinkers; and
(3) factors that influence the level of alcohol consumption overall in society will therefore increase the number of the heaviest drinkers.

The Ledermann model has been an extremely influential one and has underpinned alcohol control measures that seek to reduce the overall consumption of alcohol in society. Several criticisms have been made of the single distribution theory and in particular the assumption of log-normality [19]. However, the essential implication of the model, namely that when alcohol consumption changes overall in society, so does the proportion of people who are drinking in a harmful way, remains valid. This has resulted in a groundswell of opinion that the primary approach to the prevention of alcohol-related harm should be to reduce the overall level of use through various forms of restrictive legislation [17].

Skog, a leading researcher on distribution theory, developed the notion of 'social contagion'. This states that a person's drinking has a societal impact and *vice versa*. In Skog's words 'If a person increases his alcohol consumption, the likelihood that he will offer his friends alcohol will increase. Their consumption increases and it is more likely that they will also offer their friends alcohol. And so it continues, with the semblance of a passing wave' [19].

6.3.2   Influences

Alcohol is a market commodity. Its use therefore conforms to market forces. When its price is low, consumption is higher than when the price is high [1, 17, 20, 21]. There is a considerable literature that demonstrates that the cost of alcohol (in relation to disposable income) is a key influence on the level of alcohol consumption in society, as usually expressed by *per capita* intake [1, 17].

The impact of a high alcohol intake in society is very evident. As an example, France had the highest *per capita* alcohol consumption in the world for most of the twentieth century. This has been attributed to the very low cost of alcohol, its protected agrarian economy, the prominence of wine production and the free allocation of wine for soldiers after the First World War [18]. *Per capita* alcohol intake remained high by world standards through to the early 1990s. Not surprisingly France has had exceptionally high rates of alcohol-related disorders, such as cirrhosis of the liver [8]. Other countries in Europe, such as Portugal and Luxembourg, have now overtaken it, and *per capita* intake is now rapidly increasing in the UK and some Nordic countries, with attendant increases in cirrhosis deaths [22].

Because of the close relationship between the cost of alcoholic drinks and intake, several countries have employed taxation as a means of reducing alcohol-related harm. In particular, the Nordic countries have a long tradition of imposing high taxes on alcoholic drinks, such that they are regarded as luxury commodities. In recent years this traditional approach has been challenged by cross-European legislation, consequent on the formation of the European Union and the dominance of the single European market. This has resulted in deregulation of markets in those counties joining the EU, through so-called 'harmonization' of legislation. In Finland, alcohol sales have increased threefold since that country joined the European Union and was therefore subjected to EU legislation [22]. In the period from 2001 to 2006 alcohol-related injuries in Finland increased three-fold, and the prevalence of cirrhosis of the liver increased by 70%.

In contrast to the increase in *per capita* alcohol intake in many Northern European counties, alcohol intake overall has declined in some Mediterranean countries, notably France and Italy, and alcohol-related deaths have fallen. In its European Alcohol Action Plan, the WHO Regional Office for Europe set a target for all member countries to reduce *per capita* alcohol consumption by 25% by 2001 [23]. This occurred in France and Italy, and was achieved in Italy within the timeframe of the Action Plan. The extent to which this was a response to policy initiatives is uncertain. Many consider the decreases to be due to urbanization, shifts to factory and service work, to changes in family structure and 'destructuring' of meals, supported in more recent years by increased health consciousness and alcohol policies [24].

6.3.3   Universal Versus Targeted Interventions

A constant theme in the debate about effective measures of reducing alcohol-related harm is whether it is better to concentrate on universal population measures to reduce *per capita* consumption and thereby alcohol-related harm, or to target subgroups of the population at particular risk of harm. This debate is fuelled not only by the scientific evidence but also by the cultural and political views of those participating. To what extent should individual behaviour – in this case alcohol consumption – be controlled by the (presumably benevolent) state?

The arguments in favour of universal measures are scientifically compelling. As indicated, above, there is a wealth of data gathered over more than 100 years – and historical data dating over several centuries – that demonstrates that control measures affecting consumption of the whole population significantly reduce indices of alcohol use, alcohol misuse, alcohol-related harm, medical morbidity and mortality [17, 18, 20, 25].

Although controlling *per capita* alcohol intake reduces consumption in the heaviest drinkers, alcohol-related harm is prevalent amongst those with lower consumption. The 'preventive paradox', a term originally coined by Kreitman [26] indeed states that the majority of alcohol-related harm occurs not in the heaviest drinkers in society but in those whose consumption is at lesser levels. The reason for the supposed paradox is that there are many more people with lower-level alcohol consumption. Even though harm is less frequent in them, their greater number means they account for a substantial proportion of harm. Reducing the consumption of the entire population will lessen alcohol-related harm in the community to a greater extent than measures that target only those with alcohol dependence and others with peak consumption levels.

Recent analyses have caused a reinterpretation of the preventive paradox. Stockwell and colleagues have shown the need to analyse particular patterns of alcohol consumption with regard to the consequences [7]. Episodic high-level drinking is strongly associated with accidents, trauma, aggressive behaviour and domestic violence. The overall alcohol consumption of this particular group may not be especially high – because of the episodic nature of their drinking. When expressed, therefore, as average daily alcohol intake, their consumption might be in the middle range. In reality, this pattern of drinking is not moderate but high risk and only considered middle-range by the somewhat artificial measure of average daily intake. Nonetheless, reducing overall alcohol intake in society would have beneficial effects by reducing consumption across the range of patterns and levels of consumption.

Targeted interventions are logical in focusing on the consumption patterns of particular subgroups or individuals. For example, an important target group would be drivers operating motor vehicles. Random breath testing has been shown to reduce drink-driving and alcohol-related motor-vehicle deaths [27]. Other target groups could be (i) workers using industrial machinery, (ii) young people gathering in particular drinking environments and (iii) patients attending doctors or in a range of health-care settings. This has led to the development of approaches for screening for hazardous or harmful drinking patterns [28] and individualized intervention of those identified with such alcohol use [29]. There is considerable evidence for the benefit of brief structured interventions aimed to reduce alcohol intake in people with hazardous and harmful consumption. The key issue that has emerged in recent years is whether these individualized interventions can be delivered systematically through health care and other providers so that the promise of reduced alcohol-related harm in the community becomes a reality [30, 31].

6.4   APPROACHES TO PREVENTION

6.4.1   The Evidence Base

Several systematic reviews are available to guide the development of preventive approaches. These have been undertaken under the auspices of the World Health Organization [1, 23, 32–34], by several national and regional governments [4, 35, 36], and by academic and research institutions and groups over 40 years and more. Despite its varied provenance, there is consistency in the evidence on prevention and its interpretation. The first such review was written by an expert group headed by Kettil Bruun who had worked extensively for WHO [37]. A similarly constituted group headed by Griffith Edwards undertook a subsequent review of the literature and published 'Alcohol Policy and the Public Good' [38]. Later this group (with a modified membership) produced 'Alcohol: No Ordinary Commodity' [17]. At the global level, WHO published a 'Global Status Report: Alcohol Policy' in 2004 [32] and the WHO Regional Office for Europe published a review of preventative strategies in 2005 [39] and a WHO expert committee reported in 2007 [40].

In its review of 32 preventive strategies, the WHO European Office [34, 39] summarized the most effective approaches to reduce alcohol-related harm at a population level as:

(1) alcohol-control policies, including increasing price through taxation policies;
(2) drink-driving countermeasures, and
(3) brief intervention for hazardous and harmful drinking.

The review concluded that positive effects were difficult to find with measures commonly advocated such as (1) education in schools, (2) media campaigns and announcements and (3) voluntary regulation by the alcohol industry.

The Global WHO report [1, 40] drew the following conclusions:

• Reductions in per capita consumption result in decreased alcohol problems.
• As the price of alcohol beverages increases demand declines and *vice versa*.
• Heavy drinkers are affected by policy measures including price, availability and alcohol regulations as much as lighter drinker.
• Limiting access and discouraging drinking under the legal purchasing age are likely to reduce harm linked to specific drinking patterns.
• Individual approaches to prevention for example school-based prevention programs have a much smaller effect on drinking patterns and problems than population-based approaches that affect drinking environment and availability of alcohol beverages.
• Legislative interventions to reduce permitted blood alcohol levels for drivers, raising the legal driving age and controlling outlet density are effective in lowering alcohol-related problems [1, 40].

Because of the evidence supporting the relationship between total consumption and alcohol-related harm and the effectiveness of alcohol-control policies, the European Office of WHO set a target of 25% reduction in overall consumption by 2001 [23].

In the United Kingdom a review of the evidence was published in 2004 by the Academy of Medical Sciences. Their report, 'Calling Time' emphasized the primary importance of controlling alcohol-related harm by reducing the average level of alcohol consumption in the population [41]. Consistent with the conclusions of WHO, they noted that there was a strong correlation between average consumption in the community and the prevalence of heavy alcohol consumption and between the latter and alcohol-related harm. Its primary recommendations were that:

• the price of alcohol be raised; and
• alcohol availability is limited through appropriate legislation.

They relegated education about alcohol, voluntary codes of conduct by the alcohol industry and treatment to more minor roles [41].

In Australia, the National Preventative Health Task Force identified 39 interventions (see Table 6.1) and examined them for their effectiveness, cost, breadth of evidence and cross-cultural applicability [42]. Approximately half are universal interventions and half targeted interventions. Controlling consumption through (i) legislation, for example on minimum drinking age and hours of operation of alcohol outlets, (ii) taxation and pricing policy and (iii) targeting drink-driving were again judged to be the most effective approaches.

In the United States, the focus has been on influencing drinking behaviour through means such as responsible beverage service (RBS) programs for alcohol servers and establishment managers. The effectiveness of these programs depend, though, on strong legislative provisions and enforcement [43].

6.4.2 Government Responses

Reports emanating from governments tend to have a very different emphasis – even when government is informed by scientific bodies that have conducted systematic reviews. A salient example is an official UK Government report produced by the Prime Minister's Strategy Unit [44], 'Alcohol Harm Reduction Strategy for England'. Some months before, an interim report 'Alcohol Project: Interim Analytical Report' was made available and commentators noted curious differences between the interim and final versions [45].

The report from the Prime Minister's strategy unit as finally published emphasized four elements:

(1) education and communication;
(2) identification and treatment of alcohol problems;
(3) dealing with alcohol-related crime and disorder; and
(4) supply and industry responsibility.

The interim report stated clearly that there is poor evidence for the effectiveness of education and communication and that this should not be a major arm of policy [45].

In the final report, the sections for dealing with crime and cooperation with the alcohol industry place much emphasis on voluntary codes of conduct [44]. As Plant has commented, 'voluntary agreements have a tendency to result in token or minimal compliance' [46]. Room [47] has further noted that none of the policies identified by the WHO or the Academy of Medical Sciences that are rated as having high impact form part of the UK government official strategy. Increasing taxation and therefore the price of alcohol drinks is rejected in the final report as having 'unwanted side effects and ... not a viable option' [45].

6.4.3 The Reality of Prevention Policy

Crombie and colleagues [48] surveyed public health policies to reduce alcohol-related harm in 12 developed countries, Australia, Canada, Denmark, England, Ireland, Japan, New Zealand, Northern Ireland, Scotland, Sweden, USA and Wales. Australia, Canada,

Table 6.1

Strategy area	Intervention	Effectiveness	Cost to implement
Regulating Physical Availability (Population based approach to reduce overall per capita alcohol consumption – Restrict availability; Supply reduction – Primary prevention of alcohol related problems)	Total ban on sales	***	High
	Minimum legal purchase age	***	Low
	Hours and days of sale restrictions	**	Low
	Restrictions on density of outlets	**	Low
	Staggered closing times for bars and clubs		–
	Server liability	***	Low
	Different availability by alcohol strength	**	Low
	Control availability at public events where alcohol related harm is likely to occur for example sporting events.		
Taxation and Pricing (Increasing taxation and increasing prices of alcohol-Population based approach to reduce overall alcohol consumption – Restrict availability; Supply reduction) – Demand Reduction – Primary prevention of alcohol-related problems	Alcohol taxes	***	Low
	Hypothecated tax to pay for treatment/prevention		
	Setting floor prices/banning discounting.		
Drink-driving countermeasures/ (Legislation/high-visibility law enforcement; reducing blood alcohol concentrations – Targeting vulnerable populations/ high-risk problem drinkers) Primary prevention of alcohol-related problems	Sobriety checkpoints	**	Moderate
	Random breath testing	***	Moderate
	Lowered BAC limits	***	Low
	Administrative license suspension	**	Moderate
	Low BAC for young drivers	***	Low
	Graduated licensing for novice drivers	**	Low
	Designated drivers and ride services	o – no studies	Moderate
	Ignition interlocks.		
Treatment and intervention (Brief/Early Intervention; Targeting vulnerable populations/ high risk drinkers and problem drinkers – Secondary intervention Treatment of alcohol related problems including alcohol dependence	Brief Intervention in Primary Health Settings	**	Moderate
	Alcohol problems treatment		
	Thiamine supplementation	*	High
	Workplace interventions	*	Low
	Mutual help/self-help	*	Moderate
	Mandatory treatment for repeat drink drivers		

Altering the drinking context (targeting vulnerable populations, managing drinking venues to reduce violence in places where alcohol is drunk for example sports and music events)	Bans on serving intoxicated persons	*	Moderate
	Training staff to prevent intoxication/aggression	*	Moderate
	Voluntary codes of bar practice	—	
	Enforcement of on-premises regulations and laws	o – no studies	Low
	Promoting alcohol-free events	**	Low
	Community mobilization		High
	Plastic or tempered-glass serving containers	o – no studies	High
	Food service	**	High
Regulating promotion and alcohol advertising-Primary prevention of alcohol-related problems? Targeting whole populations)	Advertising bans	no evidence available	Low
	Advertising content controls	no evidence available	Low
Education / Encouragement of responsible drinking (Culture change and training-Primary prevention of alcohol-related problems – targeting whole populations?)	Alcohol education in schools	o – no studies	High
	College-student education	o – no studies	High
	Parent education	no evidence available	Moderate
	Public service messages/mass-media campaigns	Warrants further research	Moderate
	Warning labels/National drinking guidelines	Nil – no studies	Low

Adapted from National Preventative Health Taskforce Technical Report no. No3 Preventing alcohol related harm in Australia: a window of opportunity Commonwealth of Australia 2008.

o – Lack of effectiveness/no studies undertaken/limited investigations.
* – Limited effectiveness.
** – Moderate effectiveness.
*** – High degree of effectiveness.

New Zealand, Sweden, the UK and USA had substantial alcohol policies. Denmark and Japan had shorter sections within an overall public-health and health-promotion agenda. Of these countries, only Ireland, Sweden and the USA explicitly state the goal of reducing overall alcohol consumption. In the Australian reports there has been a shift from average consumption to particular patterns of drinking, especially binge drinking. The English report states (to the amazement of the authors of this chapter) that 'there is no direct relationship between the amounts or patterns of consumption and types or level of harms caused' [45].

Taxation policy varies widely with Ireland and New Zealand stating the need for taxes on alcohol to be as high as possible. In striking contrast, the Prime Minister's strategy report, covering England, makes a clear commitment not to increase price as a means to reduce alcohol-related harm.

6.5   PRACTICAL COMPONENTS OF PREVENTION

In the next section of this review, we shall outline what we consider, on the basis of the evidence, to be the six most important approaches to reducing alcohol-related harm.

1. Determining the Legal Status of Alcohol

Although in the aftermath of the prohibition experience in the United States (1919–1932), most Western societies rejected the notion that alcohol be classified as an illicit substance, world-wide this remains an important approach. This is most evident in many Islamic countries where there is prohibition of any consumption of alcohol. Religious principle also influences alcohol consumption in countries such as Turkey, which are constitutionally secular states but where Islam is the dominant religion. For example, Turkey has a *per capita* alcohol intake of under 1 litre per adult per annum (compared with 6–20 in Western societies), and alcohol-related harm is correspondingly low. In India, the Federal Constitution entreaties its citizens to abstain from consuming alcohol and to promote abstinence as the national ethos; 6% of adult Indians consume alcohol. In the Western world there is no serious move to alter the general legal status of alcohol. Any moves by a political party towards prohibition would likely cause such an outcry that none would contemplate it.

Legislation to ban consumption of alcohol by young people is, however, a key legislative plank to minimize alcohol consumption and related harm. Legislation may cover the consumption of alcohol by young people, purchase of alcohol in a pub or licensed shop, and provision of alcohol to young people. For many countries the minimum age for purchasing alcohol is 18 years and in several that is also the minimum age for consuming it. Notably, the minimum age in the United States is 21 years [49]. Comparisons of alcohol use and related problems show that these are fewer in US samples of 18–20 year-olds than in countries where the minimum purchase age is 18 years [50]. Furthermore, when the minimum purchase age is decreased, there is a corresponding increase in alcohol-related harm in the 18–20 year age group [51]. In the US, a lower minimum legal age of drinking than the current 21 years was found to be associated with higher rates of motor-vehicle accidents [49]. This resulted in restricting sales of alcohol and zero-tolerance laws for those under the age of 21 years. Raising the minimum legal drinking age from 18 to 21 years of age showed significant beneficial effects with fewer traffic crashes, injuries and fatalities [52].

The scientific argument for raising the minimum purchase (or consumption) age becomes more compelling with increasing evidence for the deleterious effect of alcohol consumption on brain development and the fact that brain development continues until the mid-20s [53].

Legislating a minimum purchase age should therefore be a major part of a national strategy to reduce alcohol-related harm. Proposals to increase the minimum purchase age have in recent years been few in number and have been generally unpopular. A proposal to increase the age to 20 years in New Zealand did not gain the support of any major political party. One may conclude therefore that there would have to be considerably more community concern about the effects of alcohol in young people for raising the minimum purchase age to be a realistic possibility. This is where campaigns to raise public awareness of the toll of youth drinking have an important role.

2. Regulating Physical Availability

Regulating physical availability has been a more usual approach. Such legislation includes (1) restrictions on the number of alcohol sales outlets, typically requiring authorization of licensing authorities; (2) restrictions on the hours of opening of outlets and therefore sales of alcohol; (3) restriction of alcohol sales to particular types of premises; (4) operation of a state monopoly for sale of alcohol and (5) restriction of sales at sports and social events.

Regulating the number and location of alcohol sales outlets is another evidence-based strategy. The prevalence of alcohol-related harm (for example, assaults and alcohol-related motor accidents) is correlated with the density of sales outlets in the local community [17, 54–56]. The argument to restrict these outlets by licensing approaches is strong. The Nordic countries have long adopted restrictions on the physical availability of alcohol, especially through restricting the numbers and nature of sales outlets. There is similar evidence for the effectiveness of restricting the hours of operation of alcohol sales outlets [57, 58]. In addition to such measures, Sweden and Finland operated state alcohol monopolies for many years. There is also evidence that restriction of sales of alcohol at social and sports events by legislation and law enforcement reduces assaults and injuries [17, 48].

These approaches, which are of considerable public-health benefit, often succumb to commercial considerations. These partly reflect pressure from local producers and owners of sales outlets, but also pressures within a free market economy. These include the principle of open competition, the desire for harmonization of laws within economic communities and the influence of multinational alcohol producers. Nonetheless, where there is community concern, restrictions on sales outlets by the relevant licensing authorities (number of outlets and opening hours) remain an important means of modifying consumption and reducing alcohol-related harm.

3. Taxation and Pricing

The most consistently effective approach to reducing harm from alcohol involves changes to the cost of alcohol, typically through taxation policy. When the price of alcohol decreases (in relation to disposable income), alcohol-related harm increases. When alcohol prices increase, alcohol-related harm decreases [17, 20, 42].

The extent to which alcohol consumption can be modified through taxation depends on the degree to which sales of alcohol are affected by changes in price. This is known as price elasticity and is a general phenomenon that influences sales of all consumer goods. The elasticity of alcoholic drinks varies according to the type of drink – beer, wine or spirits. In turn, this reflects the extent to which particular drinks are part of the social fabric of that society. In the United Kingdom, for example, beer is relatively price inelastic, whereas wine and spirits have higher values for elasticity; their purchase is influenced to a great extent by price [17, 38].

Increasing taxation, whether on alcoholic drinks overall or on specific types of drink, is therefore an effective control measure available for governments. Increasing taxation on alcohol also holds the attraction to governments of greater revenue. In many periods governments have adopted taxation policy as a primary tool to reduce alcohol consumption and related harm. Historical examples include the tax imposed on gin in eighteenth-century England. In Norway in the late nineteenth century, taxation was increased and likewise in Sweden in the early twentieth century. Following introduction of this legislation consumption in these countries declined substantially and alcohol-related harm remained relatively low for several decades [17].

Raising taxation on alcoholic drinks is straightforward in principle to enact and there are established systems in developed countries to channel the increased tax levies into the public purse. The economic interests of alcohol producers typically result in an orchestrated campaign to prevent such tax increases. This can include mass-media campaigns invoking the right of people to drink at a 'fair' price, the rights of people to self-determine their consumption, the generation of suspicion and ulterior motives for governments to increase the price of alcohol and in short, a series of tactics designed to dissuade governments to take such action, based on the arguments that it would cause major electoral unpopularity and they will be voted out of office.

Alternative taxation-based approaches have been developed in recent years. These include volumetric taxation that is based on the principle of taxing alcoholic drinks according to their alcohol content. Although this might seem an obvious approach, taxation policy in individual countries has tended to develop as an amalgam of different individual pieces of tax legislation rather than through a concerted and considered tax policy based on clear strategic goals (at least until the era of harmonization laws). The introduction of volumetric taxation would for many countries require a significant legislative process involving revoking multiple laws and taxation schedules and their replacement with uniform legislation. What appears to be straightforward in principle does require a considerable commitment on the part of any government and its ability to secure, in a democratic society, majority support from the electorate. A related approach is setting a minimum purchase price for alcohol. Other interventions include increasing the cost of drinks that appeal to the young and banning price promotions [59].

The real issue is the willingness of governments to legislate for such tax increases. The refusal of the UK government to legislate in response to recommendations of the advisory bodies is an example, and is testimony to the difficulties in enacting evidence-based policy [45].

4. Countering Drink-Driving

In many countries the single commonest cause of death and disability from alcohol consumption is motor-vehicle accidents where the driver is impaired because of recent drinking. Many countries set limits for the blood alcohol concentration above which it is illegal to drive. The limits may vary according to the age and experience of the driver. However, an important principle is that criminal conviction is based on the blood alcohol concentration *per se*, rather than on a measure of impairment of driving performance, although the latter may lead to additional charges.

Drink-driving countermeasures include random breath testing, sobriety check points, imposing and reducing limits for blood alcohol concentration for driving, the differential blood alcohol concentration limits for subgroups of drivers (e.g. those under the age of 21 and those learning to drive), ignition interlocks and designated drivers (drivers who agree to abstain from alcohol and will be responsible for taking home those who are drinking).

Evidence suggests that drink-driving countermeasures consistently produce long-term problem reductions of between 5 and 30% [17, 58]. Random breath testing has been shown to be effective in several countries in reducing road crashes, injuries and fatalities [58].

Lowering limits of BAC for younger drivers and suspension of licence if caught driving with BAC above legal limits has been found to be very effective in reducing road crashes, injuries and fatalities [42, 58].

Court diversion of drink drivers and educative treatment programs and ignition interlock devices that prevent a vehicle from being started until the driver passes a breath test are also effective [17].

5. Early and Brief Interventions

Early and brief intervention is a good example of a targeted approach to reducing alcohol-related harm. It entails identifying people who have hazardous and harmful alcohol consumption and providing brief therapy before they develop a more serious alcohol problem [28, 29, 60]. Screening and brief intervention is therefore analogous to screening for asymptomatic hypertension or hyperlipidaemia. It is predicated on the basis that early detection and treatment of a disorder in its developmental stage has advantages over treatment of the established disorder in terms of (i) reduced morbidity, (ii) better and more guaranteed response to treatment, (iii) avoidance of the costs of treating the advanced disorder, and (iv) prevention of premature mortality.

Screening and brief intervention has its origins in the work of a WHO expert committee in the late 1970s [61]. In the report of its findings the committee recommended 'the development of methods for identifying potentially harmful patterns of alcohol consumption before dependence developed and disease was entrenched'. This resulted in a program of work by WHO on the development of techniques for screening and early identification of hazardous and harmful alcohol consumption [28, 62]. Parallel work in the area was also being undertaken by pioneers such as Kristenson [63] and Heather [64]. A major effort went into the development of screening instruments, a good example being the Alcohol Use Disorders Identification Test (AUDIT) [28] to complement the development of brief structured therapies designed to be used when hazardous alcohol use is identified.

Since that time compelling evidence has been generated to support screening and brief intervention as an effective approach to reduce alcohol-related harm in this population. Brief interventions have been shown to reduce alcohol consumption in men, although the effect amongst women has not been as consistent [29]. Brief interventions have been shown to be effective in a variety of settings, for example in primary care settings, emergency departments, hospital outpatient clinics and trauma centres. There is mixed evidence for the effectiveness of brief intervention in hospital wards.

The overall reduction in alcohol consumption between those receiving brief intervention and control groups receiving no advice or standard care is moderate and amounts to approximately 10 g of alcohol per day. There is a greater effect on hazardous drinking and an even greater effect on alcohol-related injuries, with a relative risk of 0.68 (95% CI 0.57–0.81) for hazardous alcohol consumption at one year [29] and 0.59 (95% CI 0.42–0.84) for alcohol-related injury [65]. Brief intervention reduces mortality over a ten-year follow up, with a relative risk of 0.47 (95% CI 0.25–0.89) [66, 67]. The number needed to treat (NNT) is 58.8 to achieve mortality reduction. Brief counselling also shows beneficial effects on nonfatal injury outcomes such as falls, motor vehicle crashes and suicide attempts. [68]. Other outcome measures following brief intervention have been examined but not yet subject to systematic review. In the brief intervention trial of Fleming and colleagues, hospitalizations were significantly reduced in a four-year follow-up period in those who received brief intervention compared to the control group [69].

Brief interventions are the most consistently effective and potent interventions directed at individuals and considerable effort is being made to incorporate them into the health-care system. This is proving to be more difficult than originally anticipated. Very often screening and brief intervention can be established as a brief project but it tends not to be continued in any systematic way when external support and interest ceases [30]. The efficiency of screening brief intervention will vary according to the prevalence of hazardous alcohol consumption. In general practice where 10–15% of patients in many Western countries would likely be hazardous drinkers, approximately 8 people will need to be screened for each hazardous drinker to be identified. Combining that with the NNT of 5–6 for reducing alcohol consumption leads to the result that on average 45 patients in primary care will need to be screened for each person with hazardous alcohol consumption to become a low-risk drinker. This indicates the degree of effort required to provide brief intervention in practice although information on alcohol consumption is relevant to much of health care when other issues such as the potential for interactions with medications and advice needed for pregnant women and people with a range of chronic medical disorders are taken into consideration.

Opportunities for early detection and brief intervention for alcohol-use disorders exist in many settings. These include general medical/family medical practice, other primary care settings (nurse, psychologist, social worker-delivered), emergency departments and acute-care clinics, student health services [70], work-place health programs and also certain public arenas such as shopping centres. In addition to these primary care or community contact settings, brief interventions can be offered in hospital wards (general and psychiatric) and in a range of specialist services such as diabetes, hypertension and liver clinics. These settings are of course quite diverse and the extent to which a person can be engaged in any alcohol intervention will vary according to the primary task of a particular setting. Still, given that few people specifically request treatment and assistance in an alcohol-use disorder, any attempt to identify these and to place them on the health care agenda is to be welcomed.

6. Treatment

There are numerous controlled trials of various treatments and therapies for alcohol-use disorders. They encompass psychological therapies, medications, support groups and they have been the subject of many systematic reviews and meta-analyses. As these are described in a companion chapter on the treatment of alcohol-use disorders, only brief comment will be made here. In general, the psychological therapies are based on sociocognitive theory. The many versions of cognitive-behaviour therapy, typically as applied to relapse prevention, have consistently been shown to be effective in reducing alcohol consumption and alcohol-related harm. Meta-analyses of the pharmacotherapies have likewise shown reduction in overall alcohol consumption and higher rates of abstention from alcohol in those receiving medication compared to those assigned to a placebo preparation. The cost benefit is comparable to many other forms of treatment but, overall, treatment is a more resource-intensive approach than the broader population-level strategies described above.

Thus, there is considerable debate about the place of treatment as a component of an overall population-level preventive strategy. Some of the considerations are:

- Is there evidence that the provision of treatment reduces in a quantifiable, population-level way, alcohol-related harm including morbidity and mortality from disease, accidents and injuries and social problems?
- To what extent should treatment effectiveness be gauged by its capacity to reduce such harm in the community at large?
- Should treatment be judged only by its capacity to improve the health, well being and life expectancy of individuals?
- Even if there is no evidence that treatment reduces population-level harm or benefits to the community as a whole, is it a right that citizens have – similar to the treatment of diabetes, heart disease and infectious diseases?

These considerations are not simple ones. In terms of the demonstrable effects on population-level harm, the evidence is somewhat limited.

One of the few attempts to identify this was by Smart and Mann [71] who analysed Canadian and US data sets. In analyses of the availability of treatment for alcohol problems, these authors found that clinic numbers could not be linked with subsequent falls in population-level morbidity and mortality. Smart and colleagues did identify a relationship between the availability of AA meetings (focused on abstinence from alcohol for people with alcohol dependence) and a reduction of alcohol-related harm in the community [71]. Studies of health-service utilization by people with alcohol-use disorders have shown considerable declines following treatment, in hospitalization and overall health-care costs, presumably reflecting substantially reduced alcohol-related disease [72].

6.6   OTHER POTENTIAL APPROACHES

1. Altering the Drinking Context

This set of approaches seeks to modify the environment in which alcohol consumption takes place in an effort to make it safer for patrons, and therefore prevent the occurrence of

harm in and around the venue and at, or around, the time of drinking. In Australia, an estimated 60% of alcohol-related assaults were found to have occurred near licensed premises
[73]. Modifying the drinking context, which should avert problems such as drink-driving
and violence to others, needs to be backed up by credible enforcement [40]. Such interventions include codes of responsible bar practice, server training, bans on serving intoxicated
persons, using plastic (rather than glass) containers and promotion of alcohol-free events.
There is also a move to introduce voluntary codes of practice in pubs, bars and liquor outlets. A difficulty with these approaches is that there has been a major shift in the drinking
environment from the licensed and controlled environment to drinking in people's homes
and other nonregulated settings.

Studies of the efficacy of the following have shown mixed results [42, 58]:

- bans on selling or serving intoxicated persons;
- not serving underage drinkers;
- server liability if legal requirements are not met (enforcement);
- support and training sessions for owner and management of alcohol establishments which
  is necessary for enforcement of on-premises regulations and laws, training staff on how
  to prevent intoxication and manage aggression;
- promotion of low-strength or nonalcohol beverages;
- plastic or tempered-glass serving containers to reduce violence in licensed venues; and
- nutritious food service with alcohol.

These are useful complementary approaches but the evidence does not support them as
being the main plank of preventive policy.

2. Promotion, Advertising and Marketing

Advertising of alcohol is variably controlled by legislation and voluntary codes of practice.
Although it would seem logical that advertising would increase overall consumption as
well as influence brand preference, there is only limited evidence on this point. Alcohol
advertising and marketing have been shown to influence the age of onset and amount
of alcohol consumed by adolescents [74, 75]. Much promotion occurs outside formal
advertising, for example the linking of alcohol with sports events and similar popular
activities. While restrictions of advertising have not achieved a major reduction in drinking
and related harms in the short term, countries with greater restrictions on advertising have
less drinking and fewer alcohol-related problems [17].

3. Information and Warning Labels

Mandatory labels on alcohol bottles/casks that reflect the national guidelines on safe levels
of drinking by men and women have been introduced in some jurisdictions, sometimes
accompanied by warnings on harmful effects of alcohol if safe levels are exceeded [58].
The labels may also include the number of units or grams of alcohol or ml of alcohol in a
given drink. Warnings regarding the risk of fetal alcohol spectrum disorder if women drink
during pregnancy are often included.

4. Community Education and Advice

A major emphasis in alcohol prevention has been to include education messages directed at school students in an effort to delay the uptake of alcohol and to deter interest in drinking. Unfortunately, there is no consistent evidence that this works [17, 58]. Certain recent approaches such as harm reduction rather than nondrinking approaches have been shown in some trials to be effective but this is not broadly accepted [76].

The evidence for mass-media campaigns is also controversial. Such campaigns certainly increase the awareness of the community of alcohol as a problem in society. However, it has not been demonstrated that they reduce overall alcohol consumption or any measures of alcohol-related harm [17].

5. Insurance Limitations

In some states in the US the insurer is not liable for any loss sustained or contracted in consequence of the insured being intoxicated or under the influence of alcohol or drugs.

6. Harm-Reduction Strategies

There is evidence for the effectiveness of thiamine fortification of flour (bread) in reducing alcohol-related brain damage at a population level [77]. This is a valuable approach but clearly it is an intervention directed to those with entrenched heavy alcohol consumption (and likely alcohol dependence). Prevention and early intervention, as outlined above, offers scope for reducing the broad range of alcohol-related harm in the community.

REFERENCES

1. World Health Organization (2007) *Evidence-based Strategies and Interventions to Reduce Alcohol Related Harm – Global Assessment of Public Health Problems Caused by Harmful Use of Alcohol. World Health Organization, Geneva.*

2. Anderson, P. (2006) Global use of alcohol, drugs and tobacco. *Drug and Alcohol Review*, **25**, 489–502.

3. Harwood, H. (1998) *Updating Estimates of the Economic Costs of Alcohol Abuse in the United States: Estimates, Update Methods and Data*, National Institute on Alcohol Abuse and Alcoholism, Bethesda.

4. Cabinet Office Strategy Unit (2003) *Alcohol Misuse: How Much does it Cost?* Cabinet Office Strategy Unit, London.

5. Appleby, E. (2005) Alcohol use: consumption and costs, in *ABC of Alcohol*, 4th edn (eds. A. Paton and R. Touquet), BMJ Books, Blackwell Publishing Ltd, Oxford.

6. Collins, D.J. and Lapsley, H.M. (2008) *The Cost of Tobacco, Alcohol and Illicit Drug Abuse to Australian Society in 2004–05. National Drug Strategy Monograph Series no. 64.* Department of Health and Ageing, Canberra.

7. Stockwell, T., Hawks, D., Lang, E. and Rydon, P. (1996) Unravelling the preventive paradox for acute alcohol problems. *Drug and Alcohol Review*, **15**, 7–15.

8. Péquignot, G., Tuyns, A.J. and Berta, J.L. (1978) Ascitic cirrhosis in relation to alcohol consumption. *International Journal of Epidemiology*, **7**, 113–120.

9. Rehm, J., Mathers, C., Popova, S. *et al.* (2009) Global burden of disease and injury and economic cost attributable to alcohol use and alcohol-use disorders. *Lancet*, **373**, 2223–2233.

10. National Health and Medical Research Council (2009) *Australian Guidelines to Reduce Health Risks from Drinking Alcohol*, Commonwealth of Australia, Canberra.

11. Latt, N., Conigrave, K., Saunders, J.B., Marshall, E.J. and Nutt, D. (2009) *Addiction Medicine*, Oxford University Press, Oxford.

12. Saunders, J.B. and Janca, A. (2000) Delirium tremens: its aetiology, natural history and treatment. *Current Opinion in Psychiatry*, **13**, 629–633.

13. Koob, G.F. and Le Moal, M. (2001) Drug addiction, dysregulation of reward, and allostasis. *Neuropsychopharmacology*, **24**, 97–129.

14. Koob, G.F. and Le Moal, M. (2005). Plasticity of reward neurocircuitry and the dark side of drug addiction. *Nature Rev: Neurosci*, **8**, 1442–1444.

15. Koob, G.F. (2006) The neurobiology of addiction: a neuroadaptational view relevant for diagnosis. *Addiction*, **101** s1, 24–31.

16. Grant, B., Dawson, D., Stinson, F. *et al.* (2004) The 12-month prevalence and trends in DSM-IV alcohol abuse and dependence: United States, 1991–1992 and 2001–2002. *Drug and Alcohol Dependence*, **74**, 223–234.

17. Babor, T., Caetano, R., Casswell, S. *et al.* (2003) *Alcohol: No Ordinary Commodity*, Oxford University Press, Oxford.

18. Ledermann, S. (1960) *Alcool, Alcoolism, Alcoolisation: Données Scientifiques de Caractère Physiologique, Économique et Social*, Presses Universitaires de France, Institut National d'Etudes Demographiques, Paris.

19. Skog, O.J. (1985) The collectivity of drinking cultures; a theory of the distribution of alcohol consumption. *British Journal of Addiction*, **80**, 83–99.

20. Seeley, J.R. (1960) Death by liver cirrhosis and the price of beverage alcohol. *Canadian Medical Association Journal*, **83**, 1361–1366.

21. Anderson, P. (2009) Global alcohol policy and the alcohol industry. *Current Opinion in Psychiatry*, **22**, 253–257.

22. Herttua, K., Makela, P. and Martikainen, P. (2008) Changes in alcohol related mortality and its socioeconomic differences after a large reduction in prices. *American Journal of Epidemiology*, **168**, 1110–1118.

23. World Health Organization (1992). *European Alcohol Action Plan (Ref: EUR/RC42/8)*. World Health Organization, Copenhagen.

24. Allamani, P. and Prina, F. (2007) Why the decrease in consumption of alcohol beverages in Italy between the 1970s and 2000s? Shedding light on the Italian mystery. *Contemporary Drug Problem*, **34**, 187–189.

25. Thorsen, T. (1990) *Hundred Ears Alkoholmiskrug (One Hundred Years of Alcohol Misuse)*, Alkohol-og Narkotikaradet, Copenhagen.

26. Krietman, N. (1986) Alcohol consumption and the preventive paradox. *British Journal of Addiction*, **81**, 353–363.

27. Henstridge, J., Homel, R. and Mackay, P. (1997). *The Long-term Effects of Random Breath Testing in Four Australian States: a Time Series Analysis*. Australian Federal Office of Road Safety, Canberra.

28. Saunders J.B., Aasland O.G., Babor T.F., de la Fuente J.R. and Grant M. (1993) Development of the Alcohol Use Disorders Identification Test (AUDIT): WHO Collaborative Project on Early Detection of Persons with Harmful Alcohol Consumption II. *Addiction*, **88**, 791–804.

29. Kaner, E.F.S., Dickenson, H.O., Beyer, F. *et al.* (2009). The effectiveness of brief interventions in primary care settings: a systematic review. *Drug and Alcohol Review*, **28**, 301–323.

30. Gomel, M. K., Wutzke, S. E., Hardcastle, D. M., Lapsley, H. and Reznik, R. B. (1998) Cost-effectiveness of strategies to market and train primary health care physicians in brief intervention techniques for hazardous alcohol use, *Social Science and Medicine*, **47**, 203–211.

31. Funk, M., Wutzke, S., Kaner, E., Anderson P., Pas, L., McCormick, R., Gual, A., Barfod, S. and Saunders, J.B. (2005) A multi-country controlled trial of strategies to promote dissemination and implementation of brief alcohol intervention in primary health care: findings of a World Health Organization Collaborative Study. *Journal of Studies on Alcohol*, **66**, 379–388.

32. World Health Organization (2004) Global Status Report 2004: Alcohol Policy World Health Organization, Geneva.

33. World Health Organization (2000) *European Alcohol Action Plan 2000–2005*, WHO regional office for Europe 1999, Copenhagen. Available from URL http://www.who.dk/adt/; http://www.euro.who.int/documents/E67946.pdf.

34. World Health Organization (2006) *Framework for Alcohol Policy in the WHO European Region*, World Health Organization, Copenhagen, Denmark.

35. U S Department of Health and Human Services (2007) *The Surgeon General's Call to Action to Prevent and Reduce Underage Drinking*, US Department of Health and Human Services, Washington, DC.

36. *National Health and Medical Research Council, Australian Guidelines to Reduce Health Risks from Drinking Alcohol*, Commonwealth of Australia, 2009.

37. Brunn, K., Edwards, G., Lumina, M. *et al.* (1973) *Alcohol Control Policies in Public Health Perspective,* Finnish Foundation for Alcohol Studies, Helsinki.

38. Edwards, G. *et al.* (1994) *Alcohol Policy and the Public Good*, Oxford University Press, Oxford.

39. World Health Organization (2005) *Alcohol Policy in the WHO European Region: Current Status and the Way Forward*. World Health Organization, Copenhagen.

40. World Health Organization (2007) WHO Expert Committee on Problems Related to Alcohol Consumption, Second Report, WHO Technical Report Series no. 944 World Health Organization, Geneva.

41. Academy of Medical Sciences (2004) *Calling Time: The Nation's Drinking as a Major Health Issue*, Academy of Medical Sciences, London.

42. National Preventative Health Taskforce (2008) *Preventing Alcohol Related Harm in Australia: a Window of Opportunity*. Commonwealth of Australia, Canbera World Health Organization.

43. Mosher, J.F., Toomey, T., Good, C. *et al.* (2002) State laws mandating or promoting training programs for alcohol servers and establishment managers: An assessment of statutory and administrative procedures. *Journal of Public Health Policy*, **23**, 90–106.

44. Cabinet Office Strategy Unit (2004) *Alcohol Harm Reduction Strategy for England*, Cabinet Office Strategy Unit, London.

45. Marmot, M.J. (2004) Evidence based policy or policy based evidence. *British Medical Journal*, **328**, 906–907.

46. Plant, M. (2004) The alcohol harm reduction strategy for England. *British Medical Journal*, **328**, 905–906.

47. Room, R. (2004) Disabling the public interest: Alcohol strategies and policies for England. Addiction.

48. Crombie, I.K., Irvine, L., Elliott, L. and Wallace, H. (2007) How do public health policies tackle alcohol related harm: A review of 12 developed countries. *Alcohol and Alcoholism*, **42**, 492–499.

49. Wagenaar, A.C. (1993) Minimum drinking age and alcohol availability to youth: issues and research needs, in (eds. M.E. Hilton and G. Bloss), Alcohol and Health monograph.

50. Toumbourou, J., Hemphill, S., McMorris, J., Catalano, F. and Patton, G. (2009) Alcohol use and related harms in school students in the USA and Australia. *Health Promotion International*, **24**, 373–382.

51. Kypri, K., Voas, R.B., Langley, J.D. *et al.* (2006). Minimum purchasing age for alcohol and traffic crash injuries among 15-to 19-year-olds in New Zealand. *American Journal of Public Health*, 96, 126–131.

52. Wagenaar, A.C. and Toomey, T.L. (2002) Effects of minimum drinking laws age: review and analysis of the literature from 1960–2000.

53. Tapert, S.F., Brown, G.G., Kindermann, S.S. *et al.* (2001) fMRI measurement of brain dysfunction in alcohol dependent young women. *Alcohol CLin Exp Res*, **25**, 236–245.

54. Chikritzhs, T. and Stockwell (2006) The impact of later trading hours for hotels on levels of impaired driver road crashes and driver breath alcohol levels. *Addiction*, **101**, 1254–1264.

55. Britt, H., Carlin, B.P., Toomey, T.L. and Wagenaar, A.C. (2005) Neighborhood-level spatial analysis of the relationship between alcohol outlet density and criminal violence. *Environmental and Ecological Statistics*, **12**, 411–426.

56. Gruenewald, P.J., Freisthler, B., Remer, L., *et al.* (2006) Ecological models of alcohol outlets and violent assaults: crime potentials and geospatial analysis. *Addiction*, **101**, 666–677.

57. Gruenewald, P.J., Millar, A., Treno, A.J. *et al.* (1996) The geography of availability and driving after drinking. *Addiction*, **91**, 967–983.

58. Loxley, W., Toumbourou, J.W., Stockwell, T. *et al.* (2004) *The Prevention of Substance Use Risk and Harm in Australia: a Review of the Evidence*, Commonwealth of Australia, Canberra.

59. Chikritzhs, T.N., Dietze, P.M., Allsop, S.J., Daube, M.M., Hall, W.D. and Kypros, K. (2009) The 'alcopops' tax: heading in the right direction, *Medical Journal of Australia*, **190**, 294–295.

60. Saunders J.B. and Lee N.K. Hazardous alcohol use: its delineation as a subthreshold disorder, and approaches to its diagnosis and management. *Comprehensive Psychiatry*, **41**, 95–103.

61. World Health Organization (1980) *Problems Related to Alcohol Consumption, Technical Report Series no. 650*. World Health Organization, Geneva.

62. Babor T. F., Acuda A., Campillo C., Del Boca F. K., Grant M., Hodgson R., Rollnick S., Ivanets N., Lukomskaya M., Machona M., Saunders J. B., Skutle A. and the WHO Brief Intervention Study Group. (1996) A cross-national trial of brief interventions with heavy drinkers. *American Journal of Public Health* **86**, 948–955.

63. Kristenson, H., Ohlin, H., Hulter-Nosslin, M. *et al.* (1983) Identification and intervention of heavy drinkers in middle-aged men: results and follow up at 24-60 months of long term study with randomised controls. *Alcoholism: Clinical and Experimental Research*, **7**, 203–209.

64. Heather, N., Campion, P.D., Neville, R.G. and MacCabe, D. (1987) Evaluation of a controlled drinking minimal intervention for problem drinkers in general practice (the DRAMS scheme) *Journal of the Royal College of General Practitioners*, **37**, 358–63.

65. Havard, A. Shakeshaft, A. and Sanson-Fisher, R. *et al.* (2008) Systematic review and meta-analysis of strategies targeting alcohol problems in emergency departments: interventions reduce alcohol related injuries. *Addiction*, **103**, 368–376.

66. Wutzke S.E., Conigrave, K.M., Saunders, J.B. and Hall, W.D. (2002). The long term effectiveness of brief interventions for unsafe alcohol consumption: a ten year follow up. *Addiction*, **97**, 665–675.

67. Cuijpers, P., Riper, H. and Lenners, L. (2004). The effects on mortality on brief interventions for problem drinking: a meta analysis. *Addiction*, **99**, 939–945.

68. Dinh-Zarr T.B., Goss, C.W., Heitman, E. *et al.* (2009) Interventions for preventing injuries in problem drinkers: The Cochrane Database of Systematic Reviews, 2 *The Cochrane Library*.

69. Fleming M.F., Mundt, M.P., French, M.T., Manwell, L.B., Stauffacher, E.A. and Barry, K.L. (2002) Brief physician advice for problem drinkers: long-term efficacy and benefit-cost analysis. *Alcoholism: Clinical and Experimental Research*, **26**, 36–43.

70. Kypri, K., Langley, J.D., Saunders, J.B., Cashell-Smith, M.L. and Herbison, P. (2008) Randomized controlled trial of web-based alcohol screening and brief intervention in primary care. *Archives of Internal Medicine*, **168**, 530–536.

71. Smart, R. and Mann, R.E. (1990) An increase in treatment levels and Alcoholics Anonymous membership large enough to reduce liver cirrhosis rates. *British Journal of Addiction*, **85**, 1291–1298.

72. Holder, H. and Blose, J. (1992) The reduction of health care costs associated with alcoholism treatment: a 14-year longitudinal study. *Journal Studies on Alcohol*, **53**, 293–302.

73. Briscoe, S. and Donnelly N. (2001) Temporal and regional aspects of alcohol related violence and disorder in NSW: National Drug Research Institute and NSW Bureau of Crime Statistics and Research Report.

74. British Medical Association (2009) *Under the Influence – the Damaging Effect of Alcohol Marketing on Young People*, BMA, London.

75. Anderson, P., de Bruijn, A., Angus, K. *et al.* (2009) Impact of alcohol advertising and media exposure on adolescent alcohol use: a systematic review of longitudinal studies. *Alcohol*, **44**, 229–243.

76. McBride, N., Farrington, F., Midford, R. *et al.* (2004) Harm minimisation in school drug education: final results of the School Health and Alcohol Harm Reduction Program (SHAHRP). *Addiction*, **99**, 278–291.

77. Harper, C.G., Sheedy, D.L., Lara, A.I. and Garrick, T.M. (1998) Prevalence of Wernicke-Korsakoff syndrome in Australia: has thiamine fortification made a difference? *Medical Journal of Australia* **168**, 542–545.

CHAPTER 7

Alcohol-Use Disorders – Treatment and Management

**Filippo Passetti[1], MD, PhD, MRCPsych and
Colin Drummond[2], MBChB, MD, FRCPsych**

[1]*Division of Mental Health, St George's University of London, London, UK*
[2]*National Addiction Centre, Institute of Psychiatry, King's College London, UK*

7.1 INTRODUCTION

Alcohol-use disorders exist along a continuum of severity, from hazardous drinkers, that is individuals whose drinking puts them at risk of experiencing alcohol-related problems; through harmful drinkers, who are already experiencing problems related to drinking; to a range of severities of alcohol dependence, characterized by symptoms including tolerance, withdrawal, craving, impaired control and continued use despite adverse consequences [1]. To meet the needs of such a wide spectrum of disorders, treatment should be tailored to levels of severity, contexts and individual needs. In this chapter we first outline the principles of treatment and management, with particular reference to the issue of matching treatment to severity of drinking problems; then we review interventions for hazardous and harmful drinkers across a range of settings; and discuss the management of alcohol dependence in specialist settings, including pharmacological, psychological and psychosocial interventions. We conclude with a discussion of service organizations, including a brief review of research on cost-effectiveness and the treatment of special groups, such as ethnic minorities and women, who may find access to services more difficult.

7.2 PRINCIPLES OF TREATMENT AND MANAGEMENT

The first principle of management of alcohol problems has already been enunciated and refers to the notion of a spectrum of severity needing a range of treatment approaches (Figure 7.1, top part of the triangle). Until as recently as the 1980s the concept of alcoholism focused attention on a small group of drinkers with very severe problems, and on intensive specialist treatment aimed at lifelong abstinence from alcohol. It became apparent that much larger proportions of the general population were vulnerable to developing

Substance Abuse Disorders: Evidence and Experience, First Edition. Edited by Hamid Ghodse, Helen Herrman, Mario Maj and Norman Sartorius.
© 2011 John Wiley & Sons, Ltd. Published 2011 by John Wiley & Sons, Ltd.

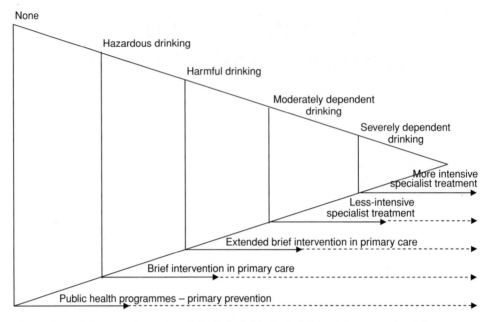

Figure 7.1   The range of severity of alcohol problems and their treatment approaches (adapted from Raistrick *et al.* [2] Review of effectiveness of treatment for alcohol problems).

alcohol-related problems, though less severe and that these individuals could benefit from some form of treatment, though generally of a lesser intensity and in nonspecialist settings [3]. It was even suggested that such opportunistic early interventions may achieve greater health gains, overall, than the more expensive treatment used to target the much smaller group of individuals with severe alcohol dependence: a suggestion that was described as 'the preventive paradox'. This concept led to an expansion of the range of individuals offered alcohol treatment, as well as of the range and locations of interventions. Treatment is no longer delivered solely in specialist services, but also in a variety of other settings and by nonspecialist staff, as we will discuss in the next section.

A second principle of the management of alcohol-use disorders is that, in order to match the spectrum of problem severity, treatment must also diversify to achieve a spectrum of intensities of interventions (Figure 7.1, lower part of the triangle). This principle is supported not only by evidence of effectiveness of brief interventions in patients at the less severe end of the spectrum (e.g. [4]), but also by studies showing that even amongst alcohol-dependent individuals there are many who do not require the most intensive specialist treatments (e.g. [5]). The most intensive treatments should be reserved for the more severely dependent drinkers [6] and the least intensive treatment, such as brief interventions, to the less severe alcohol disorders [7].

Figure 7.2 illustrates a third principle of the management of alcohol-use disorders. Stepped care refers to the pragmatic approach of offering first the least intensive (and least expensive) treatment that is likely to be beneficial to an individual, to then move to more intensive interventions if this is unsuccessful. This approach, which has been supported by research conducted in primary-care settings [8,9], is increasingly applied to the management

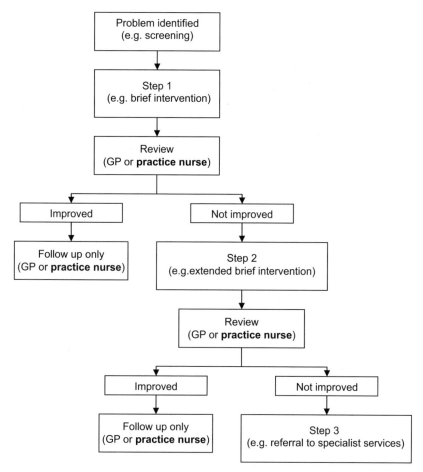

Figure 7.2 Example of stepped care for alcohol-use disorders in nonspecialist health services.

of alcohol-use disorders across the spectrum of severities. Thus, in nonspecialist settings such as primary care, Step 1 may be a brief intervention, delivered by a GP or a practice nurse, Step 2 an extended brief intervention delivered by a counsellor and, for those who do not respond, Step 3 referral to specialist alcohol services. In a specialist setting (e.g. a community alcohol team), Step 4 may be a care plan comprising alcohol detoxification followed by four sessions of Motivational Enhancement Therapy [10], while further steps will involve increasingly more intensive interventions, such as an intensive day programme or a residential rehabilitation programme.

Stepped care is not the only principle guiding the choice of the most appropriate treatment for each individual with an alcohol-use disorder. The importance of negotiating the goals of treatment with each drinker is intuitively obvious and cannot be understated ([11], cf. [12]). As for all interventions aimed at engendering behaviour change, the most effective approach is one that emphasizes personal responsibility and informed choice (these aspects are captured by the acronym FRAMES used to summarize the crucial elements of effective brief interventions, see below). In addition, the principle of minimizing harm may be applied to the alcohol, as well as to the drug-treatment field. In alcohol treatment, these principles are supported by evidence that individuals choosing a moderation goal, as opposed to abstinence, may benefit significantly from treatment providing they are not severely alcohol dependent [13].

7.3   THE TREATMENT OF HAZARDOUS/HARMFUL DRINKERS

This section deals with the treatment of that large proportion of the population, 23% in the UK [14], who drink to hazardous or harmful levels, without satisfying the criteria for alcohol dependence [15]. By definition, these interventions are a form of secondary prevention, as they are aimed at reducing the likelihood that these drinkers will develop the severe alcohol-related problems that characterize alcohol dependence. The first step is of course to identify these individuals. To this aim, screening programmes have been developed, which use well established research tools such as the Alcohol Use Disorders Identification Test (AUDIT, [16]) in a variety of settings, including primary care, accident and emergency departments, and the general hospital. The next step is, in keeping with stepped care, to offer the least intensive intervention that is likely to prove beneficial. Brief interventions can be delivered by nonspecialist staff in a variety of settings and are therefore particularly well suited to follow directly from screening, involving whenever possible the same staff.

7.3.1   Brief Interventions

These are the most well-supported intervention for alcohol problems. A recent large systematic review of studies of alcohol treatment found over 30 well-conducted studies on 'brief intervention' [17]. Brief interventions can be defined as advice and/or counselling directed at reducing alcohol consumption. Simple brief interventions consist of a single session, lasting between 5 and 60 minutes, while extended brief interventions include 2–3 sessions of short duration. Focus of the intervention is information and advice on the effects of alcohol across a range of personal domains and on ways to reduce consumption.

   Particularly in primary-care settings there is now very strong evidence that brief interventions are effective at reducing alcohol consumption in hazardous and harmful drinkers [4]. In contrast, alcohol-dependent individuals seeking treatment in specialist settings do not seem to benefit from brief interventions [7]. There is no clear evidence to indicate who should be offered simple and who should be offered extended brief intervention as a first treatment step (see [2]). Some have suggested using a cut-off on the AUDIT questionnaire used for screening [18], but in practice this may be a decision that is more pragmatic than evidence-based.

   In addition to a specific duration and focus, brief interventions are associated with a specific counselling style, which is modelled on the concepts of motivational interviewing developed by Miller and Rollnick [19]. The six aspects of counselling, which are more strongly associated with effective brief interventions can be summarized using the acronym FRAMES [20]:

(1) providing individualized **F**eedback on the risks of continuing to drink at current levels;
(2) emphasizing personal **R**esponsibility for implementing behavioural changes;
(3) offering specific **A**dvice on treatment goals, be these to cut down or to become abstinent;

(4) suggesting a **M**enu of options, rather than few cut and dry solutions;

(5) using an **E**mpathic interviewing style and also one that;

(6) enhances **S**elf-efficacy.

It is important to emphasize that the features of brief interventions can be incorporated into the interviewing style of nonspecialist staff without a need for extensive training. This makes them suitable for being delivered in a variety of nonspecialist settings.

7.3.2 Primary Care

Primary care is where the bulk of research supporting the effectiveness of brief interventions has been accrued [4, 21–23]. There are several reasons why this might be the ideal setting for brief interventions. Primary care is often the first point of presentation for patients with any complaint. For example, in the UK 64% of all adults consult their general physician (GP) every year and this figure is higher in excessive drinkers [14]. In addition, primary-care health settings may be seen as less stigmatizing than specialist alcohol services. Thus, primary care may be ideally placed for picking up alcohol-use disorders at an early stage, using a screening tool such as the AUDIT (or shorter variants such as AUDIT-C, FAST or Single Item Screening Questionnaire). Individuals scoring above a cut-off may then be offered a 5–30 minute brief intervention by a nonspecialist member of staff (e.g. GP, practice nurse, counsellor).

7.3.3 General Hospital

Accident and emergency (A&E) departments are the other health-care setting where patients present as first port of call, with hazardous and harmful users being over-represented amongst all attenders [24]. Brief interventions in A&E departments can reduce both the alcohol consumption of harmful and hazardous drinkers and also the frequency of their attendance following accidents and other alcohol-related problems [24, 25]. In the UK, it is becoming more common to include an alcohol health worker in the staff of A&E departments, to ensure that patients with alcohol-use disorders can be swiftly referred for formal screening and, if appropriate, treatment. In general hospital wards, the effectiveness of brief interventions is less well researched. A systematic review found inconclusive evidence to endorse their routine introduction [26], but studies conducted since are beginning to provide more substantial support [27].

7.3.4 Mental-Health Settings

Given the high prevalence of alcohol-use disorders in psychiatric populations, mental-health services may be another important setting for a programme of screening and treatment for alcohol-use disorders. For example, in a study of psychiatric inpatients conducted in the UK 49% were found to be drinking in the hazardous/harmful range [28]. There are reciprocal interactions between psychiatric and alcohol-use disorders. This means that interventions aimed at reducing drinking may be particularly helpful in this group as they may improve the outcome of psychiatric treatment. It also means that compared to the general population lower levels of drinking may carry significant health consequences and that more extended interventions might be required [29]. The crucial issue is not the duration or type of intervention, as this can be easily incorporated into the general psychiatric treatment, but, rather, how to ensure that alcohol-use disorders are identified by psychiatric staff [30].

7.3.5 Other Settings

A range of nonhealth-related settings could also lend themselves to screening and brief intervention for alcohol-use disorders. The criminal justice system (e.g. prison, probation, police custody) and educational establishments are two obvious ones to consider: the first because of the link between alcohol and crime; and the second because of the opportunity to reach vulnerable individuals at an early stage of their drinking career. Other possible locations may include social services, the workplace, youth programmes and sports centres. These contexts are relatively underresearched as potential settings for screening and brief interventions, but they are appealing, because they may provide an opportunity to screen individuals who, compared to the general population, may less readily access their general physicians.

7.3.6 Summary

Screening and brief interventions are an effective way to reduce alcohol consumption in hazardous and harmful drinkers. There is good evidence for short- and longer-term reduction of alcohol use [4, 29, 31] and also some evidence suggesting a reduced use of health-care services [24, 25], as a result of these interventions. Other benefits of such programmes for health, for example reduced mortality and for society, for example reduced crime, are likely, but have been less firmly established. Although screening and brief intervention programmes are comparatively inexpensive, their implementation poses substantial organizational challenges, as it requires the coordination of a range of organizations that are not primarily focused on alcohol treatment, and in some cases not even on health (e.g. the criminal justice system).

7.4 THE TREATMENT OF ALCOHOL DEPENDENCE

The treatment of alcohol dependence is, compared with the treatment of harmful/hazardous drinkers, much more firmly within the realm of specialist services. This is because it generally requires the formulation of a more comprehensive package of care, aimed at addressing the range of physical, psychological and psychosocial antecedents and consequences of dependent drinking. It commonly also involves pharmacological intervention, be this to facilitate progression through withdrawal states, to address co-morbidity, or to enhance relapse prevention. For different drinkers the pathway to recovery may follow a variety of different routes, but for clarity the treatment of alcohol dependence can be described as consisting of three stages of unequal durations: i) management of alcohol withdrawal (1–2 weeks); ii) relapse prevention (3–6 months); iii) aftercare (years). In this section we look at each of these aspects of treatment in turn. Since the location and intensity of specialist treatment has been the subject of intense research and debate, we begin by considering these first.

7.4.1 Treatment Settings and Models

In an influential study Edwards *et al.* [5] randomized alcohol-dependent individuals to two intensities of treatment, specialist inpatient care versus assessment and advice, and found no difference in outcome between the two groups at 1 year. The findings of several subsequent UK and US studies were generally consistent with those results [32–34]. Similarly, studies that looked specifically at the management of alcohol withdrawal, found no substantial difference in outcome between inpatient and outpatient detoxification [35]. The problem with these studies (particularly those looking at detoxification, as we will discuss below) is that they have tended to exclude patients with particularly poor prognosis, such as those with severe psychiatric or physical co-morbidity. This means that if a higher intensity of treatment (or treatment in inpatient setting) were only relevant for these groups of patients, the studies would not be suited to pick up any differential effects of the treatments under investigation. In keeping with this notion, some later studies did find an interaction of severity of dependence (or complexity of alcohol-related problems) and intensity of treatment ([36–38]; see also [39, 40]). Bringing together findings spanning 30 years, a currently prevalent view is that while the majority of alcohol-dependent individuals can be treated in the community, those with more complex problems may be more likely to benefit from more intensive treatment in a residential setting [2].

The move of treatment from inpatient to community settings for the majority of alcohol-dependent cases has advantages beyond reducing costs. It enables a treatment that is less stigmatizing and minimizes any interference with other aspects of a patient's life, such as family and work, thus supporting sustained recovery. These are good reasons to support a move of services away from hospital settings and alcohol treatment is now primarily community-based in many Western countries ([41]; Drummond, 2009). A consequence of this shift from hospital-based to decentralized treatment is that the organization of specialist services have had to change, both in terms of their *modus operandi* and, as we shall see in the final section of this chapter, in the planning and coordination of local treatment systems.

In a community-based system, a variety of professional roles may become responsible for the delivery of distinct aspects of treatment and specialist services may be required to take a more coordinating rather than a direct care role. The Community Alcohol Team model of treatment delivery that has become established in the UK over the past 30 years [42] encapsulates these principles. A typical Community Alcohol Team, comprising members of a range of disciplines (medicine/ psychiatry, nursing, social work and psychology), is primarily engaged in advising and training in the management of alcohol-use disorders staff in primary care, hospital, general psychiatry, social work and criminal justice settings. In this capacity, the Community Alcohol Team may coordinate interventions such as admission to day or residential care (for detoxification or rehabilitation), most often managed by other agencies. The team may also take a more direct involvement in the management of the more complex cases, but always in a time-limited manner. This model of treatment delivery has received support from research comparing the outcome of treatment in 'shared care' versus treatment fully based within a specialist service [43]. The model has variants that incorporate a longer-term community psychiatric nurse follow up [44], a more assertive approach for difficult-to-engage patients [45], or provision for the implementation of a 'community reinforcement approach', discussed in more detail below. In addition, the Specialist Alcohol Treatment centre is a compromise between a Community Alcohol Team and a hospital-based centre. It is centred on a multidisciplinary alcohol team, which also coordinates and supports other treatment providers, but is based at a facility that hosts an outpatient clinic, and/or a day centre, and/or an inpatient unit.

It is important to realize that someone with an alcohol-use disorder may receive treatment through a combination of the different agencies that provide treatment for alcohol dependence. For example, after screening in a general hospital, a man with alcohol dependence may be referred by a physician to a Community Alcohol Team, which facilitates inpatient detoxification followed by residential rehabilitation. Towards the end of detoxification and during treatment at a residential rehabilitation facility, the man may be encouraged to attend Alcoholics Anonymous (AA) meetings and may be referred to homeless persons' services for rehousing into an environment that will support sustained recovery. This example highlights the importance of the coordinating role of a Community Alcohol Team (or a Specialist Alcohol Treatment team) is underscored by the wide range of services that may be involved in the individual's care pathway [47]. Importantly, the services that may become involved may have different philosophy, remits and funding priorities. For example, in the case of residential rehabilitation, there are themes that are common to all or most organizations: treatment takes place in a nonmedical setting, tends to be based on a therapeutic community approach [48] and is aimed at gradually redressing the balance of incentives for alcohol- and nonalcohol-related activities. However, within this description any number of variations are possible. Many are based on the 12-step model, some are based on a religious philosophy and yet others are based on a variety of eclectic therapeutic models.

7.4.2 Achieving Abstinence – Treatment of Withdrawal States

Folk wisdom has known and talked about withdrawal states well before the scientific era. 'If I don't have a drain o' rum, Jim, I'll have the horrors' says the seaman to Jim Hawkins in Stevenson's *Treasure Island*, knowing what would happen if he were to stay without for long, after years of continuous heavy drinking ([49]; p. 19). A scientific demonstration of the consequences of a rapid fall of blood alcohol level in dependent drinkers is reported by Isbell *et al.* [50]. They kept ten experimental subjects (who were detoxified opioid dependent prisoners) continuously intoxicated with alcohol for periods of between 6 and 12 weeks, then withdrew the alcohol abruptly. All subjects developed a syndrome that included tremors, weakness, nausea, vomiting, hyperreflexia and fever, with the severity of these features being related to the severity and duration of prior drinking. Two had seizures and three developed delirium tremens.

The treatment of alcohol withdrawal includes pharmacological and psychosocial interventions and its aim is twofold. First, it is aimed at removing a barrier hindering engagement in structured psychological interventions. Secondly, it aims to prevent the most dangerous consequences of the abrupt discontinuation of drinking, in particular seizures and delirium tremens. The timing and location of assisted withdrawal are therefore crucial aspects of this part of treatment. Assisted alcohol withdrawal is more likely to lead to long-term abstinence when it is immediately followed by some form of relapse prevention [51]. Thus, alcohol withdrawal and its treatment should be, whenever possible, planned, and tied in with a post-detoxification care plan, aimed at consolidating lifestyle changes associated with long-term abstinence (see below, *Preventing Relapse*). The importance of carefully considering the timing of detoxification is underscored by evidence that multiple detoxifications tend to be associated with poorer outcome [52] and possibly cognitive impairment [53].

In terms of the location of treatment, the majority of assisted alcohol withdrawal is carried out in the community and we discussed in the previous section the evidence supporting this. A decision to carry out detoxification in a residential setting may be triggered by: i) a history of delirium tremens or seizures, particularly if these occurred during medically assisted withdrawal; ii) a history of medical conditions that may make it unsafe to manage alcohol withdrawal in a community setting (e.g. recent myocardial infarction, poorly controlled high blood pressure or diabetes, chronic obstructive pulmonary disease, cirrhosis) or a history of mental illness that suggests that more close monitoring may be required than is possible to provide in a community setting (e.g. a depressive illness associated with significant suicide risk); iii) a home environment that is unsuitable for community withdrawal from alcohol, for example with no one to provide monitoring and support; iv) alcohol intake that is too great for withdrawal to be managed safely and comfortably in the community (e.g. above 40 Units per day, with 1 Unit = 8 g alcohol); v) in keeping with stepped care, inpatient detoxification may also be chosen if a previous attempt at community detoxification has been unsuccessful.

When detoxification takes place in the community, in keeping with the model described by Stockwell and colleagues [54], treatment involves daily contact with a psychiatric nurse, either at the patient's home or at a community alcohol team clinic. With this arrangement it is possible to monitor closely for complications, adjust the medication regime as required and avoid the potential dangers of dispensing large amounts of medication at once. Daily contact also enables the consolidation of a resolve to maintain abstinence, and the reinforcement of strategies to cope with craving and to avoid alcohol. Whether detoxification takes place in the community or in hospital, rating scales are useful to assess the severity of withdrawal to titrate medication and detect complications early. The psychological interventions administered alongside medication during assisted withdrawal have not been extensively researched. Aside from a greater emphasis on self-monitoring and the here-and-now, they tend to run along similar themes as those described below in the section on *Preventing Relapse – Psychological Interventions*.

In terms of the medication to be used, a large body of evidence supports the effectiveness of benzodiazepines in mitigating the severity of alcohol withdrawal and preventing the development of delirium tremens and alcohol-related seizures [55–57]. Different long-acting benzodiazepines are comparable in their effectiveness, although longer-acting benzodiazepines (e.g. chlordiazepoxide, diazepam) are easier to titrate, to manage withdrawal. Other benzodiazepines may suit specific situations better than chlordiazepoxide. For example, in view of its shorter metabolism and half-life, lorazepam may be preferable in patients with liver failure.

The initial dose of medication is decided based on a combination of a structured assessment of current withdrawal and on the severity of past drinking and dependence. For example, when using chlordiazepoxide, the revised Clinical Institute Withdrawal Assessment for Alcohol (CIWA-Ar; [58]) or the Severity of Alcohol Dependence Questionnaire (SADQ, [59]) can be used to guide prescription of the initial dose (see [60]). The dose is then gradually reduced over the course of 7–10 days. Ideally, a symptom triggered-approach would be preferable to a fixed regime, as it avoids prescribing unnecessarily high doses [61], but this is only suitable for inpatient detoxification and with appropriate staffing levels and training. An alternative technique for reducing the total amount of medication required involves a front-loading dose prior to a decreasing regime [62].

Of the alternatives to benzodiazepines, chlormethiazole, although effective [56] is no longer recommended, as it has no advantage over chlordiazepoxide and has a higher abuse and overdose potential [63]. Carbamazepine has been shown to be as effective as some benzodiazepines [55, 56, 64], making this a reasonable alternative to chlordiazepoxide or lorazepam in patients with liver failure. Since carbamazepine is primarily an anti-epileptic medication it may also seem intuitively appropriate to add it to a benzodiazepine decreasing regime when treating patients with a history of alcohol-related seizures. However, although both carbamazepine and benzodiazepines are effective in preventing alcohol-related seizures, there appears to be no advantage in using them together [65].

In severe alcohol dependence thiamine deficiency may lead to Wernicke's encephalopathy, a preventable condition that can lead to Korsakoff syndrome. Since many cases are undiagnosed, as suggested by post-mortem studies [66], it is appropriate to prescribe thiamine supplementation alongside benzodiazepine medication, as a preventative measure, to all patients who have had a heavy alcohol intake. In the case of low-risk individuals, that is drinkers of only moderate severity, not malnourished and showing no signs of neurological complications, oral thiamine doses of 300 mg daily for the duration of withdrawal will be sufficient. For heavier, malnourished drinkers parenteral doses (250 mg daily as Pabrinex IM or IV) will be required, as in these individuals absorption is likely to be impaired as a result of the chronic damage caused by alcohol to the intestinal mucosa [67]. Higher parenteral doses (500 mg daily as Pabrinex IM or IV) will be required to treat confirmed or strongly suspected Wernicke's encephalopathy [65].

7.5   PREVENTING RELAPSE – PSYCHOLOGICAL INTERVENTIONS

The majority of individuals who undertake assisted alcohol withdrawal in a specialist setting successfully achieve abstinence, but rates of relapse following detoxification are substantial (around 70% at one year). Over the one hundred years or so of history of modern treatment for alcohol-use disorders, a large number of programmes and interventions have been proposed, tested and championed [68]. In trying to make sense of this vast literature, it is useful to emphasize at the outset that many of these interventions share common elements, such as an interviewing stile consistent with the FRAMES paradigm (see above), an emphasis on developing new coping skills or the involvement of a patient's social network. This is probably one of the reasons why in clinical trials it appears to be difficult to demonstrate the superiority of one approach over another [2]. In addition, it should be made explicit that in contrast with the treatment of withdrawal states, which has relatively narrow and focused goals, relapse prevention has much broader scope. First, the drinking goal may be abstinence, moderation, or a reduction of alcohol-related problems. Secondly, since in alcohol dependence drinking can have many different maintaining factors, treatment must address in each individual case as many as possible of those factors. It is not surprising, therefore that there should be so many alternative approaches to choose from.

In 2002 the Scottish Advisory Committee on Alcohol Misuse commissioned a review of available evidence relevant to the issue of which psychological treatment, to be instigated after alcohol detoxification, is most likely to produce a positive clinical outcome and to do so cost effectively. The review highlighted four treatment options: i) Motivational Enhancement Therapy, ii) Behavioural Self-Control Training, iii) Coping and Social Skills Training and iv) Marital and Family Therapies [69]. The results of three other systematic reviews [2, 57, 70] and two large clinical trials [10, 71] are consistent with these findings, adding a fifth treatment to the list of effective approach, 12-Step Facilitation Therapy. In the rest of this section we review these treatments and discuss in more detail the findings of Project MATCH, which are relevant to the issues of intensity of treatment and treatment matching.

Motivational Enhancement Therapy is a psychological treatment approach that capitalizes on concepts derived from the social psychology of persuasion [19]. A central tenet of Motivational Enhancement Therapy is that behavioural change is more likely to be sustained if it is perceived to be internally driven, rather than externally imposed. Thus, a confrontational or didactic style is avoided in Motivational Enhancement Therapy, in favour of a more Socratic approach that makes much use of reflective listening and summarizing of the patient's statements. Motivation is enhanced primarily by engendering a perception of a discrepancy between behaviour and attitudes (cognitive dissonance). For example, the therapist may draw a distinction between a patient's view of themselves as a 'social drinker' and the harm they are experiencing with their drinking. The therapist aims to elicit self-motivational statements from the patient, for example 'I feel I need to cut down on my drinking'. Once a self-motivational statement has been made, the therapist may draw attention to a discrepancy between current behaviour and stated goals. Subsequently, other psychological techniques may be used to shift a patient's position along a continuum of motivation. Motivational Enhancement Therapy is a relatively low-intensity treatment (for example, the manualized version used in Project MATCH consisted of 4 sessions over a 12-week period) and thus is also cost effective and well suited for outpatient settings.

Twelve-Step Facilitation Therapy is an individual psychotherapy derived from the programme of Alcoholics Anonymous (AA). It incorporates the AA philosophy of alcoholism as a disease that can be arrested, but not cured; its action plan, outlined by the twelve steps; and its emphasis on the spiritual aspects of the process of recovery. It also includes encouragement to attend AA meetings outside treatment sessions. The importance of AA to the treatment of alcohol problems cannot be understated. It is estimated that AA has a membership of over 2 million around the world, and more residential programmes are based on this than on any other treatment model in the UK or the US (where it is commonly known as the 'Minnesota Model'). In terms of its effectiveness, Project MATCH found the 12-Step Facilitation version as effective as Motivational Enhancement Therapy or Cognitive Behavioural Coping Skills Therapy [10]. However, large systematic reviews have been less consistent in finding evidence to support its effectiveness. For example, Berglund et al. [57] supported it, but in Miller et al.'s 'Mesa Grande' effectiveness review [70] 12-Step Facilitation and AA only rank 37th and 38th, respectively.

Behavioural Self-Control Training and Coping and Social Skills Training are special developments of cognitive behavioural therapy (CBT), as are Marlatt and Gordon's Relapse Prevention Therapy [72], Cue Exposure Therapy [73] and the Community Reinforcement Approach (see below *Preventing Relapse – Psychosocial interventions*). In all these models, drinking is considered a maladaptive pattern of behaviour, which needs to be unlearned. A crucial step of this process is the development of more appropriate patterns of behaviour. For example, Social Skills Training focuses on assertiveness and communication skills and is aimed at those drinkers who lack confidence (or self-efficacy) in resisting alcohol in 'high-risk' situations. Patients are helped to develop new ways to deal with these situations, using role play, desensitization and other CBT techniques. Similarly, Relapse Prevention Therapy and Behavioural Self-Control Training, which is particularly suited for individuals who have a goal of moderation, rather than abstinence, focus on triggers to drinking and on strategies that may be developed to avoid relapse. Cue Exposure Therapy looks specifically at the capacity of conditioned stimuli, such as the sight and smell of a favourite drink, to trigger craving and drive relapse behaviour. As in CBT, these therapies usually make use of diaries and self-monitoring tools, which are reviewed during therapy sessions, to challenge unhelpful assumptions relating to alcohol and drinking. In terms of effectiveness, several treatments based on CBT models and techniques have been supported by clinical trials [10,57,69,70,73]. Often these treatments are incorporated into a more comprehensive treatment package [14] and their real-life efficacy depends on the skills with which they have been selected and tailored to the individual patient. Behavioural Self-Control Training and Social Skills Training both ranked highly in Miller *et al.*'s systematic review [70].

The relationship between alcohol problems and the family are complex and reciprocal. The inclusion of a patient's closest relative or friend in treatment is but a general principle of good practice in the management of alcohol-use disorders [74]. Marital and Family Therapies make this principle integral to the delivery of treatment, by both focusing on resolving problems and capitalizing on the asset of a stable relationship to address drinking behaviour. For example, behavioural contracts may be negotiated with the patient's spouse and included in the care plan. Marital and Family Therapies have been developed within a variety of psychotherapeutic models (including CBT). Considered as a whole, these therapies have been shown to improve drinking outcomes [75] and rank highly in the 'Mesa Grande' review [70].

With so many treatment approaches, some with quite different theoretical underpinnings, the notion of matching patient to the treatment most likely to be beneficial is intuitively appealing. Project MATCH, a large clinical trial that included over 1700 patients, was designed to test specific matching hypotheses. Patients were randomized, across two arms (outpatient and post-detoxification), to three treatments: 12-Step Facilitation, Motivational Enhancement and CBT Coping Skills Therapy. The three treatments did not differ significantly in efficacy, but some matching hypotheses were supported, albeit with matching providing only small incremental benefits (10% or less, see [76,77]). Only one such match was supported in the post-detoxification care arm and should be mentioned here as it is relevant to the topic of diversifying treatment according to problem severity, which has been a running theme of the present discussion. Patients classified as having low dependence had better outcome if they were offered the CBT-based treatment, while patients classified as having severe dependence had better outcome if they were offered 12-Step Facilitation.

Project MATCH has been widely regarded as disproving the usefulness of matching treatment to patient. This is only true of the systematic matching investigated by Project MATCH. In real-world clinical practice the pragmatic selection of the most appropriate treatment based on a careful assessment of needs and previous treatment history remains a uniquely important aspect of the management of alcohol dependence. This is different from tailoring of treatment to individual patient needs, which incorporates the variety of domains that are relevant to outcome, including the medical, psychiatric, financial, forensic and familial. The other important implication of the findings arising from Project MATCH relates the issue of intensity of treatment. Motivational Enhancement Therapy was found to be as effective as two treatments of greater intensity (12-Step and Behavioural Coping Skills). We already mentioned that the presence of common ingredients across different interventions is one possible reason why statistically significant outcome differences are rarely found in alcohol treatment and others are discussed elsewhere ([2], p. 31–32). These considerations are important, but the finding of similar effectiveness of two treatment approaches of different cost and intensity must have implications for treatment planning. In the UK, reflecting the importance of these results, aspects of Motivational Enhancement Therapy are increasingly being incorporated into the 'basic work of treatment' of alcohol specialists across the National Health Service.

7.5.1   Preventing Relapse – Psychosocial Interventions

The assessment interview is not only the vehicle for the information gathering that is necessary for diagnosis, it is also a crucial opportunity for the therapist to set the tone of the relationship that will evolve from it and to begin the work of enhancing commitment and clarifying goals. In alcohol treatment, assessment is the beginning of treatment also in a more practical sense. In alcohol dependence both the antecedents and the consequences of drinking problems tend to span several domains. A key task, for the assessor, is to identify all the potentially modifiable maintaining factors of the patient's problems, so that interventions aimed at ameliorating as many as possible of these can be built into the management plan. Thus, the care plan of an individual with moderate to severe alcohol dependence commonly includes a variety of psychosocial interventions, aimed for example at supporting the patient with accommodation, employment, financial difficulties or legal problems.

Besides these psychosocial interventions, which are aspects of case management, a range of therapeutic interventions can be described as psychosocial in that they specifically focus on the social context, capitalizing on the availability of social reinforcers to bring about behavioural change. Elements of this theme are integral part of the Marital Therapies and the AA programme, which have already been mentioned. In the AA programme, for example, powerful social reinforcers are at play both during the meetings and outside, as the new member is offered access to a completely new social circle, with which to replace their old drinking network. The Community Reinforcement Approach and Social Behaviour and Network Therapy are two treatment approaches that are explicitly built on the capacity of social networks to modify behaviour.

The Community Reinforcement Approach was originally developed for use in inpatient settings and elements of this approach survive in many residential treatment programmes based on the therapeutic community model. The approach consists of a variety of inter-ventions aimed at organizing contingencies in the drinker's environment in such a way that behaviours consistent with a nondrinking lifestyle are rewarded; intoxication and other alcohol-related behaviours are deliberately not rewarded. The treating team may enlist the drinker's family and friends, social clubs and employment support agencies, to secure as many salient social rewards as possible [78]. The approach is eclectic and may include such varied components as marital therapies, communication skills training and the prescription of sensitizing medication (disulfiram, see below). As a treatment option, the Community

Reinforcement Approach has fared very well in most trials, both in its inpatient [79, 80] and outpatient variety ([81]; see also [70, 78]). Evidence suggests that the community reinforcement approach does particularly well with the difficult-to-engage patients, such as the homeless [82]. Surprisingly, the Community Reinforcement Approach has not yet become very widely adopted in clinical practice, perhaps because of concerns about the amount of coordination it requires and the potentially high associated costs [2]. However, in the UK contingency management, which builds on the Community Reinforcement Approach, is on the way to becoming an important part of drug treatment [84].

A variant of Community Reinforcement Approach was developed for the UK Alcohol Treatment Trial (UKATT) in Social Behaviour and Network Therapy [85]. The UKATT was set up specifically to assess whether the findings of MATCH could be extrapolated to the UK context. UKATT set out to compare Motivational Enhancement Therapy with Social Behaviour and Network Therapy in a large multisite trial. The findings were broadly consistent with the results of Project MATCH. Both treatments resulted in significant therapeutic gains, spanning the domains of drinking, alcohol-related problems and health [71]. There were no significant differences between the two treatment approaches, despite Motivational Enhancement Therapy being less intensive than Social Behaviour and Network Therapy, making Motivational Enhancement Therapy more cost effective (but see [86]).

7.5.2 Preventing Relapse – Pharmacological Interventions

A number of pharmacological interventions have been proposed to facilitate the maintenance of abstinence or attenuation of drinking behaviour, but in practice there are three medications to consider. These are a sensitizing agent, disulfiram, and two other medication, acamprosate and naltrexone, whose precise mechanisms are unknown. Of these, disulfiram appears to be useful in specific circumstances; and for the other two, much of the evidence for their effectiveness comes from studies in which they were used as adjunct to some form of psychological treatment (with few, notable exceptions, e.g. [87]). When used under these circumstances, the effect of naltrexone and acamprosate on measurable aspects of clinical outcome are relatively small but consistent [2].

The effect of disulfiram depends on its ability to interfere with the metabolism of alcohol. When someone taking disulfiram drinks alcohol, the accumulation of an alcohol metabolite, acetaldehyde, leads to an unpleasant reaction, including nausea, vomiting, palpitation and flushing. Thus, disulfiram may act as a deterrent and may be helpful for individuals who have some control over their drinking, but may need extra restraint at times when their motivation is faltering. Lapses into drinking can, however, be planned and so disulfiram seems to be only effective when its administration is supervised, part of a contract with a family member, or imposed by the courts [57, 88, 89]. The reaction triggered by alcohol in the presence of disulfiram, which is at least partly dose dependent, may include tachycardia and hypertension and thus disulfiram is contraindicated in congestive heart failure, hypertension and coronary heart disease, as it is in pregnancy.

Naltrexone is a mu-opioid receptor antagonist that is used in the treatment of opiate addiction. The mu receptor is involved in processes mediating the rewarding properties of alcohol both in animals [90] and in humans [91]. Trials on the effectiveness of naltrexone as an adjunct to psychological treatment for alcohol dependence have begun since the early 1990s. The majority found good statistical evidence of its utility, but with fairly high numbers needed to treat (NNT). For example, Slattery *et al.* [69] calculate the NNT to be around 11, meaning that 11 alcohol-dependent individuals need to be prescribed this drug for one to benefit from it. It is possible that optimization of the timing of prescription [92], dose [93] and compliance (e.g. by using once-monthly prescription of a sustained release, injectable formulation, see [94]) may lead to clearer evidence of efficacy. Naltrexone is licensed as a treatment for alcohol dependence in the US and several other countries, but not, as yet, in the UK.

Acamprosate, a structural analogue of the amino acid taurine, has negative modulatory effects at the NMDA glutamate receptor [95]. Since glutamatergic mechanisms are increased during alcohol withdrawal, it is hypothesized that acamprosate may attenuate the severity of the withdrawal syndrome [96]. Considerations similar to those made about naltrexone apply to acamprosate. Acamprosate has a NNT of 11 [69] and there are uncertainties about the timing at which prescription should begin after detoxification [97]. Identification of predictors of response to either naloxone or acamprosate, based on genetic and neurocognitive analyses, could clarify which patients are more likely to benefit in clinical practice [98–100].

Other pharmacotherapies have been proposed to be useful for the treatment of alcohol dependence. These include older sensitizing agents, such as citrated calcium carbimide, which are no longer in use, nonbenzodiazepine anti-convulsants (e.g. valproic acid, gabapentin, pregabalin, vigabatrin and topiramate), a GABA-B receptor antagonist (baclofen; [101]) and a range of psychotropic medications, including anti-psychotic and anti-depressant drugs, which have been suggested to reduce craving as well as their main target effects on drinking behaviour. While co-morbid anxiety and depression are common antecedents or consequences in alcohol dependence, anti-psychotic and anti-depressant medications do not appear to have intrinsic anti–craving potential and are thus only useful in the presence of co-morbid psychological disorders [57, 102]. Of the other pharmacotherapies, topiramate has generated special interest, as it appears to decrease both symptoms of withdrawal and craving, raising the possibility of a pharmacotherapy that may be useful both during assisted withdrawal and for relapse prevention [103].

7.5.3   Aftercare

For many people alcohol dependence is a chronic relapsing disorder, similar to severe and enduring mental illness or diabetes [104–106] and should therefore be managed whenever possible with long-term recovery in mind. When the active part of treatment is finished, it is important to plan for interventions that will ensure therapeutic gains are maintained over time. This is a relatively recent acquisition. For a long time, services for the treatment of alcohol dependence have been focused on the management of acute problems [107]. Once the acute phase is over, patients may be left in a relative vacuum. There is good evidence that low-key interventions aimed at keeping people well after the end of active treatment may be beneficial [75, 108] and, as we shall discuss further in the final section of this chapter, also cost effective [109].

A successful aftercare programme must be capable of monitoring and strengthening progress in the process of recovery. Crucially, it must also be able to detect a relapse early and facilitate additional treatment to stop problems escalating back to pretreatment levels. Case management is an accepted aspect of the treatment of severe and enduring mental illness that is aimed at achieving these very goals [110]. This model requires an assertive approach and has not been widely employed in the alcohol field, where treatment typically tends to emphasize personal choice and motivation more than assertive engagement. In the UK, where residential treatment is mostly funded through social services, outcome monitoring is a standard part of social work, but the aims of this are generally limited both in scope and duration. The only widely available form of aftercare is the AA fellowship, which offers life-long support to members. However, AA is not acceptable to all alcohol-dependent individuals.

Case management can be labour intensive and costly. However, in keeping with the numerous pieces of evidence discussed in preceding sections of this chapter, showing beneficial effects of interventions of limited duration and intensity, the provision of a successful aftercare programme needs not to be. Capitalizing on experience from research in treatment of tobacco addiction [111], Stout and colleagues [107] proposed an aftercare programme that is based on the delivery of low-key interventions such as counselling telephone contacts of the patient and their closest relatives. In this approach, which they call Extended Case Monitoring, contacts are tailed down over a period of 2 years and, if the patient relapses, may be intensified or lead to a re-entry into active treatment. A pilot study of this approach showed significant beneficial effects, as evidenced by longer times to first drink and a lower percentage of heavy-drinking days, compared to controls [109]. A recent British study capitalized on this and on the experience of assertive outreach treatment increasingly established in general psychiatric services, to improve engagement of 'revolving-door' alcohol-dependent patients [45], and a Medical Research Council trial based on this pilot study is currently under way.

7.5.4 Summary

The treatment of alcohol dependence has changed considerably over the last three decades. The most obvious change has been the shift towards community-based services, which has meant that treatment is now more flexible and inclusive, eliminating some of the barriers (e.g. stigma) to seeking help. It is important to emphasize, however, that for the safe management of severely dependent individuals with complex problems inpatient treatment is still required. The other important change is that treatment is becoming much more evidence based than it used to be [119]. There have been several comprehensive reviews of alcohol treatment [2, 65, 69, 70], as well as three large and well-designed studies (Project MATCH, Project UKATT, Project COMBINE) setting benchmarks for quality of evidence on effectiveness of alcohol treatment. The reviews highlight the availability of a menu of effective treatments for alcohol dependence, including pharmacotherapies, structured psychological interventions and psychosocial interventions aimed at consolidating behaviour change. They also emphasize the fallacy of the notion of a direct relationship between treatment intensity and clinical outcome. This may mean that new innovative research methods are needed, in order to capture the complexities of alcohol treatment and its key 'active ingredients' [112]. Practically, a novel concept of the treatment of alcohol dependence is beginning to emerge, which emphasizes the 'extensity', rather than intensity of treatment, which is more suitable to the management of a chronic relapsing disorder and that may be particularly appropriate for the management of difficult-to-engage, revolving door alcohol-dependent individuals [45, 107].

7.6   SERVICE ORGANIZATION

As we have seen, the treatment of alcohol-use disorders should involve a range of services and professional roles. In this final section, we take a public-health perspective. This is appropriate given the high societal costs of alcohol misuse and the relevance of alcohol treatment to the health of a nation and its public spending. A systems perspective is important for the success of interventions that, as is often the case for alcohol treatment, require the coordination of large numbers of organizations and professionals. We consider the costing arguments, the integration of services and the assessment of needs, including those of special groups that tend to be underrepresented in alcohol treatment.

7.6.1   Cost Effectiveness

From a public-health perspective, the value of an intervention depends as much on evidence of its capacity to improve the symptoms and signs of a disorder, as on its potential impact on society. In general, there is some evidence of beneficial effects of alcohol treatment at a population level. For example, several North American studies showed that a direct relationship exists between increases in the availability or uptake of alcohol treatment services and deaths from cirrhosis [113, 114]. However, in order to drive investment, beneficial effects of alcohol treatment must be quantified and translated into an assessment of potential costs and cost savings. This includes not only the costs of the intervention, but also the potential savings in terms of health care, social services and criminal justice costs that could be generated, and of the potential increase in patients' and carers' productivity that could be achieved, as a result of each intervention. In addition, the effects of an intervention on a patient's quality of life must also be quantified, so that each discrete increment in quality of life that could be achieved as a result of the intervention can be offset directly against its cost. The most commonly used measure of quality of life is the Quality of Life Adjusted Years (QALY), which is derived from a catalogue of statements provided by the general public about how much they value different aspects of one's quality of life. Using this measure, it is possible to express the effectiveness of an intervention in terms of the cost per QALY achieved and to set criteria for cost effectiveness. For example, in the UK a health intervention is considered to be sufficiently cost effective to be implemented in the National Health Service if it is expected to achieve at least one QALY per £20 000 (www.nice.org.uk).

Alcohol-related problems constitute a huge burden for western societies [115, 116]. In addition, the quality of life of individuals who misuse alcohol is poor, leaving ample margin for improvement as a result of treatment. Thus, even when limiting the analysis to whether treatment costs are offset by future health-care savings (i.e. omitting assessments of other costs and of individual benefits), alcohol treatment has been consistently found to be at least cost neutral [117, 118, 120, 121]. Separating this into treatment for hazardous/ harmful drinkers versus treatment for alcohol dependence, the evidence suggests that alcohol dependence is more costly [122] and that although its treatment is also more costly, long term it leads to greater health-care savings ([2], p. 163). A recent large UK study that compared a large range of costs associated with alcohol dependence, including health care, social care and criminal justice costs, in the six months before and after treatment, found a return of £5 for every £1 spent in treatment [86].

In economic evaluations, interventions can be compared with no intervention or with other interventions. When treatments of similar intensities in an inpatient versus outpatient setting were compared with each other, the former were found to be more cost effective [123]. This is not surprising, given the evidence of comparable effectiveness reviewed above (as discussed, these studies tended to exclude the more complex cases). Perhaps more surprising is the evidence, emerged from the UKATT study, that in an analysis that includes the widest range of public-sector costs, the more costly intervention, Social Behaviour and Network Therapy, yields greater savings than the less costly Motivational Enhancement Therapy [86]. The evidence on the cost effectiveness of pharmacotherapies as adjunct to psychological interventions is less detailed than that available for psychotherapies. However, using as a measure of cost per death averted and offsetting for healthcare cost savings, Slattery et al. [69] estimated acamprosate to be cost saving, and naltrexone and disulfiram to be cost effective, at £2076 and £5536 per death averted, respectively.

7.6.2   Planning and Integration

Besides hospital-based teams, the community alcohol team and primary care, alcohol treatment can be based in a variety of other settings, as we have seen, including: residential rehabilitation facilities, self-help groups, services for special groups, such as homeless people or drinkers with child-care responsibilities, and the criminal justice system. With such a wide range of settings the argument for an overall perspective on service provision is strong [124]. In the UK, the last 10 years have seen a significant drive for the development of a centralized strategy for alcohol treatment, which is primarily implemented through the setting of parameters for purchasing decisions [47]. Similarly, 'Managed Care' has been developed to influence purchasing decisions for alcohol treatment in the USA (National Advisory Council on Alcohol Abuse and Alcoholism). In future years, the challenge for these approaches to the planning and integration of services will be to facilitate the establishment of a purchasing system that implements evidence-based aspects of care, such as brief interventions, while retaining the more intensive services required for the more complex cases, which, as we have seen, are also cost effective when economic evaluations are conducted from the broadest perspectives.

The starting point for the planning of alcohol services must be an assessment of needs. Nationwide needs assessment exercises conducted in the USA and in the UK found large regional variations in the provision of alcohol treatment ([3, 14, 83]). In addition, there was limited association between the extent of public-funds investment in alcohol treatment and indices of alcohol related harm. These findings highlight the importance of local needs assessments in order to plan investment into alcohol-treatment services efficiently, including provisions for special groups.

7.6.3   Special Groups

There are specific groups of services users, which deserve special attention in the planning of alcohol services. The reasons for this include the apparent difficulty of these groups to access services, their special needs, or the lack of clarity as to which services would be most appropriate for them (e.g. individuals with psychiatric co-morbidity).

Although women have historically been underrepresented in alcohol treatment beyond the differences in prevalence of alcohol-use disorders a recent UK survey found no evidence of this [14]. Thom and Green [125] reviewed the possible reasons why women may be more reluctant to enter treatment and it is interesting to note that one of them, a fear to have one's children taken away, may actually encourage women to accept help in countries, like the UK, that have placed increased emphasis on the role of substance-misuse services in the minimization of harm to children [126]. There are other arguments to suggest careful consideration of the needs of women when planning services. Women have different alcohol using 'careers' [127]. When in treatment, they tend to do well [128], but not when treatment involves mixed-sex group therapy [129].

Homeless people have high prevalence of substance-use disorders [130]. This is a group for which it makes sense to consider treatment in a residential setting. There will be many in this group, for whom the incentives for not drinking are few and for these abstinence may not be a realistic goal. In addition, a community reinforcement approach may be particularly helpful [82]. In the UK, where health care is strongly primary-care centred, specialist primary care for homeless people services are increasingly common, as are 'wet' hostels, residential facilities where drinking is allowed, but in an environment designed to minimize alcohol-related harm.

Young people and people from ethnic minority groups have also been considered to require special services. The argument for young people is that they are over-represented in alcohol-related accidents and accidental deaths. In the UK, services for young people will in the future be commissioned separately from those of adults. The issue of ethnic minorities is more complex. Some ethnic minorities are over- and some underrepresented in surveys of alcohol-related problems and treatment uptake [131–134]. In general, religious and cultural differences may affect both the pattern of drinking and help-seeking behaviour in these groups, and thus it is appropriate to consider ways to make services ethno-culturally sensitive [2].

The relationship between substance misuse and psychiatric disorders is complex, including problems of diagnosis [135, 136], management [137] and the organization of services [138]. There are three possible service organization models: serial, integrated and shared care. Arguments for the integrated treatment of individuals with dual diagnosis include the intertwining psychopathology [138] and a realization of the risk that patients may 'fall through the net' with that less than perfect handover between distinct teams [139]. However, alcohol misuse is very common amongst individuals with severe mental illness [30, 140] and thus it is difficult to see how patients would be divided between the general psychiatric services and the dual diagnosis integrated service. A shared care model deals with this problems by assigning individuals with dual diagnosis to either mental health or addiction services depending on the relative severity of mental-health and substance-misuse problems [46], and leaving the other agency to take an advisory role. There are advocators of either of the integrated and the shared-care models of service delivery and perhaps there are arguments to suggest that each is best suited to a particular health care system [141, 142]. A recent review concluded that there is currently insufficient empirical evidence to prefer either [143].

7.6.4   Summary

Overall, the evidence base for cost effectiveness of alcohol treatment is strong. However, the planning and commissioning of alcohol services remains, in any country, a difficult balancing act. The pressure to contain costs must be balanced against the long-term effects of planning decisions and against the need to protect the interests of the small number of individuals with the most complex problems, whose care is particularly costly. Historically, research has struggled to keep up with the need to provide the evidence on which such decisions should be based. For example, the large number of studies that have found similar outcome of treatments of differing intensity and setting has at times led to decisions about service organization and planning, which ultimately translated into loss of funding for individuals with complex needs. In addition, specific aspects of service organization, such as integrated care pathways and shared care, have been implemented without systematic research into their effectiveness. In the future, it is hoped that as the quality of treatment research continues to improve and tackle the key issues that are relevant to service planning, its findings will inform the organization of services that provides cost-effective treatment, while remaining inclusive and able to meet the needs of the broadest section of the population.

REFERENCES

1. Edwards, G. and Gross, M. (1976) Alcohol dependence: Provisional description of a clinical syndrome. *British Medical Journal*, **281**, 1058–1061.
2. Raistrick, D., Heather, N. and Godfrey, C. (2006) *Review of the Effectiveness of Treatment for Alcohol Problems*, National Treatment Agency for Substance Misuse.
3. Institute of Medicine (1990) *Broadening the Base of Treatment for Alcohol Problems*, National Academy Press, Washington DC.
4. Kaner, E.F.S., Dickinson, H.O., Beyer, F.R. *et al.* (2007) Effectiveness of brief alcohol interventions in primary care populations. *Cochrane Database of Systematic Reviews* (2), CD004148.
5. Edwards, G., Orford, J., Egert, S. *et al.* (1977) Alcoholism: A controlled trial of treatment and advice. *Journal of Studies on Alcohol*, **38**, 1004–1031.
6. Orford, J., Oppenheimer, E. and Edwards, G. (1976) Abstinence or control: the outcome for excessive drinkers two years after consultation. *Behaviour Research and Therapy*, **14**, 409–418.
7. Moyer, A., Finney, J., Swearingen, C. and Vergun, P. (2002) Brief Interventions for alcohol problems: A meta-analytic review of controlled investigations in treatment-seeking and non-treatment seeking populations. *Addiction*, **97**, 279–292.
8. Drummond, C., Coulton, S., James, D. *et al.* (2009) Effectiveness and cost effectiveness of stepped care intervention for alcohol use disorders in primary care: a pilot study. *British Journal of Psychiatry*, **195**, 448–456.
9. Bischof, G., Grothues, J.M., Reinhardt, S. *et al.* (2008) Evaluation of a telephone-based stepped care intervention for alcohol-related disorders: a randomized controlled trial. *Drug and Alcohol Dependence*, **93** (3), 244–251.
10. Project MATCH Research Group (1997) Matching alcoholism treatment to client heterogeneity: Project MATCH post treatment drinking outcomes. *Journal of Studies on Alcohol*, **58**, 7–29.
11. Booth, P.G., Dale, B., Slade, P.D. and Dewey, M.E. (1992) A follow-up study of problem drinkers offered a goal choice option. *Journal of Studies on Alcohol*, **53**, 594–600.
12. Adamson, S.J. and Sellman, J.D. (2001) Drinking goal selection and treatment outcome in out-patients with mild-moderate alcohol dependence. *Drug and Alcohol Review*, **20**, 351–359.
13. Sobell, L.C. and Sobell, M.B. (1995) Alcohol consumption measures, in *Assessing Alcohol Problems: A Guide for Clinicians and Researchers. NIAAA Treatment Handbook, (Series 4)*

(eds. J.P. Allen and M. Columbus), National Institute on Alcohol Abuse and Alcoholism, Washington DC, pp. 55–74.

14. Drummond, C., Oyefeso, A., Phillips, T. *et al.* (2005) *Alcohol Needs Assessment Research Project (ANARP)*. Department of Health.

15. World Health Organization (1992) *The ICD-10: Classification of Mental and Behavioural Disorders: Clinical descriptions and diagnostic guidelines.* World Health Organization, Geneva.

16. Saunders, J.B., Aasland, O.G., Babor, T.F. *et al.* (1993) Development of the alcohol-use disorders identification test (AUDIT): WHO collaborative project on early detection of persons with harmful alcohol consumption-II. *Addiction*, **88**, 791–804.

17. Miller, W.R. and Wilbourne, P.L. (2002) Mesa Grande: a methodological analysis of clinical trials of treatments for alcohol-use disorders. *Addiction*, **97**, 265–277.

18. Room, R., Babor, T. and Rehm, J. (2005) Alcohol and public health. *Lancet*, **365** (9458), 519–530.

19. Miller, W.R. and Rollnick, S. (1991) *Motivational Interviewing: Preparing People to Change Addictive Behavior*, Guilford Press, New York.

20. Bien, T.H., Miller, W.R. and Tonigan, J.S. (1993) Brief interventions for alcohol problems: a review. *Addiction*, **88**, 315–335.

21. Kahan, M., Wilson, L. and Becker, L. (1995) Effectiveness of physician-based interventions with problem drinkers: a review. *Canadian Medical Association Journal*, **152**, 851–859.

22. Ballesteros, J., Duffy, J.C., Querejeta, I. *et al.* (2004) Efficacy of brief interventions for hazardous drinkers in primary care: systematic review and meta-analyses. *Alcoholism, Clinical and Experimental Research*, **28**, 608–618.

23. Bertholet, N., Daeppen, J.B., Wietlisbach, V. *et al.* (2005) Reduction of alcohol consumption by brief alcohol intervention in primary care: systematic review and meta-analysis. *Archives of Internal Medicine*, **165**, 986–995.

24. Crawford, M.J., Patton, R., Touquet, R. *et al.* (2004) Screening and referral for brief intervention of alcohol-misusing patients in an emergency department: a pragmatic randomised controlled trial. *Lancet*, **364**, 1334–1339.

25. Barrett, B., Byford, S., Crawford, M.J. *et al.* (2006) Cost-effectiveness of screening and referral to an alcohol health worker in alcohol misusing patients attending an accident and emergency department: a decision-making approach. *Drug and Alcohol Dependence*, **81**, 47–54.

26. Emmen, M.J., Schippers, G.M., Bleijenberg, G. *et al.* (2004) Effectiveness of opportunistic brief interventions for problem drinking in a general hospital setting: systematic review. *British Medical Journal*, **328**, 318.

27. Holloway, A.S., Watson, H.E., Arthur, A.J. *et al.* (2007) The effect of brief interventions on alcohol consumption among heavy drinkers in a general hospital setting. *Addiction* **102** (11), 1762–1770.

28. McCloud, A., Barnaby, B., Omu, N. *et al.* (2004) Relationship between alcohol-use disorders and suicidality in a psychiatric population: in-patient prevalence study. *British Journal of Psychiatry*, **184**, 439–445.

29. Hulse, G.K. and Tait, R.J. (2002) Six-month outcomes associated with a brief alcohol intervention for adult in-patients with psychiatric disorders. *Drug and Alcohol Review*, **21**, 105–112.

30. Barnaby, B., Drummond, C., McCloud, A. *et al.* (2003) Substance misuse in psychiatric inpatients: comparison of a screening questionnaire survey with case notes. *BMJ*, **327**, 783–784.

31. Fleming, M.F., Mundt, M.P., French, M.T. *et al.* (2002) Brief physician advice for problem drinkers: long-term efficacy and benefit-cost analysis. *Alcoholism, Clinical and Experimental Research*, **26**, 36–43.

32. Chick, J., Ritson, B., Connaughton, J. *et al.* (1988) Advice versus extended treatment for alcoholism: a controlled study. *British Journal of Addiction*, **83**, 159–170.

33. Walsh, D.C., Hingson, R.W., Merrigan, D.M. *et al.* (1991) A randomised trial of treatment options for alcohol-abusing workers. *The New England Journal of Medicine*, **325**, 775–782.

34. Long, C.G., Williams, M. and Hollin, C.R. (1998) Treating alcohol problems: a study of programme effectiveness according to length and delivery of treatment. *Addiction*, **93**, 561–571.

35. Hayashida, M., Alterman, A.I., McLellan, A.T. *et al.* (1989) Comparative effectiveness and costs of inpatient and outpatient detoxification of patients with mild-to-moderate alcohol withdrawal syndrome. *The New England Journal of Medicine*, **320**, 358–365.

36. Guydish, J., Sorensen, J.L., Werdegar, D. *et al.* (1999) A randomized trial comparing day and residential drug abuse treatment: 18 month outcomes. *Journal of Consulting and Clinical Psychology*, **67**, 428–434.

37. Greenwood, G., Woods, W., Guydish, J. and Bien, E. (2001) Relapse outcomes in a randomised trial of residential and day drug abuse treatment. *Journal of Substance Abuse Treatment*, **20**, 15–23.

38. Rychtarik, R., Connors, G., Whitney, R. *et al.* (2000) Treatment settings for persons with alcoholism: evidence for matching clients to inpatient versus outpatient care. *Journal of Consulting and Clinical Psychology*, **68**, 277–289.

39. Finney, J.W., Hahn, A.C. and Moos, R.H. (1996) The effectiveness of inpatient and outpatient treatment for alcohol abuse: The need to focus on mediators and moderators of setting effects. *Addiction*, **91**, 1773–1796.

40. Brown, J.M. (2003) The effectiveness of treatment, in *Essential Handbook of Treatment and Prevention of Alcohol Problems* (eds. Heather, N. and Stockwell, T.), John Wiley & Sons, Ltd, Chichester, pp. 9–20.

41. Fuller, R.K. and Hiller-Sturmhofel, S. (1999) Alcoholism treatment in the US. *Alcohol Research and Health*, **23**, 69–77.

42. Shaw, S.J., Cartwright, A.K.J., Spratley, T.A. and Harwin, J. (1978) *Responding to Drinking Problems*, Croom Helm, London.

43. Drummond, D.C., Thom, B., Brown, C. *et al.* (1990) Specialist versus general practitioner treatment of problem drinkers. *Lancet*, **336**, 915–918.

44. Patterson, D.G., MacPherson, J., and Brady, N.M. (1997) Community psychiatric nurse aftercare for alcoholics: a five-year follow-up. *Addiction*, **92**, 459–468.

45. Passetti, F., Jones, G.M., Chawla, K. *et al.* (2008) Assertive community treatment methods in alcohol dependence. *Alcohol and Alcoholism* **43** (4), 451–455.

46. Department of Health (2002) Mental Health Policy Guide: Dual Diagnosis Good Practice Guide. Department of Health, London.

47. Department of Health & National Treatment Agency for Substance Misuse (2006) *Models of Care for Alcohol Misusers (MoCAM)*, Department of Health.

48. Kennard, D. (1983) *An Introduction to Therapeutic Communities*, Routledge and Kegan Paul, London.

49. Stevenson, R.L. (1883) *Treasure Island*, Parragon, Glasgow.

50. Isbell, H., Fraser, H., Wikler, A. *et al.* (1955) An experimental study of the etiology of 'rum fits' and delirium tremens. *Q J Stud Alcohol*, **16**, 1–33.

51. Imber, S., Schultz, E., Funderburk, F. *et al.* (1976) The fate of the untreated alcoholic. Toward a natural history of the disorder. *J Nerv Ment Dis*, **162** (4), 238–247.

52. Malcolm, R., Roberts, J., Wang, W. *et al.* (2000) Multiple previous detoxifications are associated with less responsive treatment and heavier drinking during an index outpatient detoxification. *Alcohol*, **22**, 159–164.

53. Duka, T., Townshend, J.M., Collier, K. and Stephens, D.N. (2003) Impairment in cognitive functions after multiple detoxifications in alcoholic inpatients. *Alcohol Clin Exp Res*, **27** (10), 1563–1572.

54. Stockwell, T., Bolt, L., Milner, I. *et al.* (1990) Home detoxification for problem drinkers: Acceptability to clients, relatives, general practitioners and outcome after 60 days. *British Journal of Addiction*, **85**, 61–70.

55. Mayo-Smith, M. (1997) Pharmacological management of alcohol withdrawal. *JAMA*, **278**, 144–151

56. Williams, D. and McBride, A.J. (1998) The drug treatment of alcohol withdrawal symptoms: A systematic review. *Alcohol and Alcoholism*, **33**, 103–115.

57. Berglund, M., Thelander, S. and Jonsson, E. (eds) (2003) *Treating Alcohol and Drug Abuse: An Evidence-Based Review*, Wiley-VCH Verlag GmbH, Weinheim, Germany.

58. Sullivan, J.T., Sykora, K., Schneiderman, J., Naranjo, C.A. and Sellers, E.M. (1989) Assessment of alcohol withdrawal: the revised clinical institute withdrawal assessment for alcohol scale (CIWA-Ar). *Br J Addict.*, **84** (11), 1353–1357.

59. Stockwell, T.R., Hodgson, R.J., Edwards, G. *et al.* (1979) The development of a questionnaire to measure severity of alcohol dependence. *British Journal of Addiction*, **74**, 79–87.

60. Taylor, D., Paton, C. and Kerwin, R. (2007) *The Maudsley Prescribing Guidelines*, Informa Healthcare, London.

61. Saitz, R., Mayo-Smith M.F., Roberts M.S. *et al.* (1994) Individualized treatment for alcohol withdrawal. A randomized double-blind controlled trial. *JAMA*, **272**, 519–523

62. Day, E., Patel, J. and Georgiou, G. (2004) Evaluation of a symptom-triggered front-loading detoxification technique for alcohol dependence: A pilot study. *Psychiatric Bulletin*, **28**, 407–410.

63. Duncan, D. and Taylor, D. (1996) Chlormethiazole or chlordiazepoxide in alcohol detoxification. *Psychiatric Bulletin*, **20**, 599–601.

64. Malcolm, R., Myrick, H., Roberts, J. *et al.* (2002) The effects of carbamazepine and lorazepam on single versus multiple previous alcohol withdrawals in an outpatient randomized trial. *J Gen Intern Med*, **17** (5), 349–355.

65. Lingford-Hughes, A., Welch, S. and Nutt, D. (2004) Evidence based guidelines for the pharmacological management of substance misuse, addiction, and co-morbidity: Recommendations from the British Association for Psychopharmacology. *Journal of Psychopharmacology*, **18**, 293–335.

66. Cook, C.C.H., Hallwood, P.M. and Thomson, A.D. (1998) B vitamin deficiency and neuropsychiatric syndromes in alcohol misuse. *Alcohol and Alcoholism*, **33**, 317–336.

67. Thomson, A.D. (2000) Mechanisms of vitamin deficiency in chronic alcohol misusers and the development of the Wernicke-Korsakoff syndrome. *Alcohol Alcohol Suppl*, **35** (Suppl 1), 2–7.

68. Edwards, G., Marshall, E.J. and Cook. C.C.H. (2003) *The Treatment of Drinking Problems: A Guide for the Helping Professions*, 4th edn, Cambridge University Press, Cambridge.

69. Slattery, J., Chick, J., Cochrane, M. *et al.* (2003) Prevention of Relapse in Alcohol Dependence. Health Technology Assessment Report 3. Health Technology Board for Scotland, Glasgow.

70. Miller, W.R., Wilbourne, P.D. and Hetema, J.E. (2003) What works? a summary of alcohol treatment outcome research, in *Handbook of Alcoholism Treatment Approaches: Effective Alternatives*, 3rd edn (eds. R.K. Hester and W.R. Miller), Allyn and Bacon, Boston, MA, pp. 13–63.

71. UKATT Research Team (2005a) Effectiveness of treatment for alcohol problems: findings of the randomized UK Alcohol Treatment Trial (UKATT). *British Medical Journal*, **311**, 541–544.

72. Marlatt, G.A. and Gordon, J.R. (1985) *Relapse Prevention: Maintenance Strategies in the Treatment of Addictive Behaviors*, Guilford Press, New York.

73. Drummond, D.C., Tiffany, S.T., Glautier, S. and Remington, B. (eds.) (1995) *Addictive Behaviour: Cue Exposure Theory and Practice*, John Wiley & Sons, Ltd, Chichester.

74. Copello, A. and Orford, J. (2002) Addiction and the family: Is it time for services to take notice of the evidence? *Addiction*, **97**, 1361–1363.

75. O'Farrell, T.J., Choquette K.A., Cutter, H.S.G. *et al.* (1993) Behavioural marital therapy with and without additional couples relapse prevention sessions for alcoholics and their wives. *Journal of Studies on Alcohol*, **54**, 652–666.

76. Stout, R.L., Del Boca, F., Coronary, J. *et al.* (2003) Primary treatment outcomes and matching effects: Outpatient arm, in *Treatment Matching in Alcoholism* (eds. T. Babor and F.K. del Boca), Cambridge University Press, Cambridge, pp. 150–165.

77. Randall, C., Del Boca, F.K., Mattson, M.E. *et al.* (2003) Primary treatment outcomes and matching effects: Aftercare arm, in *Treatment Matching in Alcoholism. IRMA Monograph Series No. 4* (eds. T.F. Babor and F.K. del Boca), Cambridge University Press, Cambridge, pp. 135–149.

78. Myers, R.J. and Miller, W.R. (eds) (2001) *A Community Reinforcement Approach to Addiction Treatment. International Research Monographs in the Addictions*, Cambridge University Press, Cambridge.

79. Hunt, G.M. and Azrin, N.H. (1973) A community reinforcement approach to alcoholism. *Behaviour Research and Therapy*, **11**, 91–104.

80. Azrin, N.H. (1976) Improvements in the community reinforcement approach to alcoholism. *Behavior Research and Therapy*, **14**, 339–348.

81. Sisson, R.W. and Azrin, N. (1986) Family-member involvement to initiate and promote treatment of problem drinkers. *Journal of Behaviour Therapy and Experimental Psychiatry*, **17**, 15–21.

82. Smith, J.E. and Delaney, H.D. (2001) CRA with the homeless, in *A Community Reinforcement Approach to Addiction Treatment* (eds. R.J. Meyers and W.R. Miller), Cambridge University Press, Cambridge, pp. 104–122.

83. National Audit Office (2008) *Reducing Alcohol Harm: Health Services in England for Alcohol Misuse*. National Audit Office, London.

84. National Institute of Clinical Excellence (2007) *Drug Misuse: Psychosocial Interventions*. NICE clinical guideline 51, NICE: London.

85. Copello, A., Orford, J., Hodgson, R. *et al.*, on behalf of the UKATT Research Team (2002) Social behaviour and network therapy: Basic principles and early experiences. *Addictive Behaviors*, **27**, 354–366.

86. UKATT Research Team (2005b) Cost-effectiveness of treatment for alcohol problems: Findings of the UK Alcohol Treatment Trial. *British Medical Journal*, **331**, 544–547.

87. De Wildt, W.A.J.M., Schippers, G.M., Van Den Brink, W. *et al.* (2002) Does psychosocial treatment enhance the efficacy of acamprosate in patients with alcohol problems? *Alcohol and Alcoholism*, **37**, 375–382.

88. Azrin, N.H., Sisson, R.W., Meyers, R. and Godley, M. (1982) Alcoholism treatment by disulfiram and community reinforcement therapy. *Journal of Behavior Therapy and Experimental Psychiatry*, **13**, 105–112.

89. Martin, B., Clapp, L., Bialkowski, D. *et al.* (2003) Compliance to supervised disulfiram therapy: A comparison of voluntary and court-ordered patients. *The American Journal of Addictions*, **12**, 137–143.

90. Froelich, J.C., Harts, J., Lumeng, L. and Li, T.K. (1990) Naloxone attenuates voluntary ethanol intake in rats selectively bred for high ethanol preference. *Pharmacol Biochem Behav*, **35**, 385–390.

91. Swift, R.M., Whelihan, W., Kuznetsov, O. *et al.* (1994) Naltrexone-induced alterations in human ethanol intoxication. *Am J Psychiatry*, **151**, 1463–1467.

92. Krystal, J.H., Cramer, J.A., Kroll, W. *et al.*, Veterans Affairs Naltrexone Cooperative Study 425 Group (2001) Naltrexone in the treatment of alcohol dependence. *New England Journal of Medicine*, **345**, 1734–1739.

93. Combine Study Group (2003) Testing combined pharmacotherapies and behavioral interventions for alcohol dependence (the COMBINE Study): a pilot feasibility study. *Alcohol Clin Exp Res.*, **27**, 1123–1131.

94. Garbutt, J.C., Kranzler, H.R., O'Malley, S.S. *et al.* (2005) Efficacy and tolerability of long-acting injectable naltrexone for alcohol dependence: a randomized controlled trial. *Journal of the American Medical Association*, **293** (13), 1617–1625.

95. Littleton, J. and Little, H. (1994) Current concepts of ethanol dependence. *Addiction*, **89**, 1397–1412.

96. Littleton J (1995) Acamprosate in alcohol dependence: how does it work? *Addiction* **90**, 1179–1188.

97. Anton, R.F., O'Malley, S.S. *et al.*, for the Combine Study Group (2006) Combined pharmacotherapies and behavioral interventions for alcohol dependence. The COMBINE study: a randomized controlled trial. *Journal of the American Medical Association*, **295**, 2003–2017.

98. Oslin, D.W., Berrettini, W., Kranzler, H.R. *et al.* (2003) A functional polymorphism of the mu-opioid receptor gene is associated with naltrexone response in alcohol-dependent patients. *Neuropsychopharmaclolgy*, **28**, 1546–1552.

99. Ooteman, W., Naassila, M., Koeter, M.W. *et al.* (2009) Predicting the effect of naltrexone and acamprosate in alcohol-dependent patients using genetic indicators. *Addiction Biology*, **14** (3), 328–337.

100. Kim, S.G., Kim, C.M., Choi, S.W. *et al.* (2009) A micro opioid receptor gene polymorphism (A118G) and naltrexone treatment response in adherent Korean alcohol-dependent patients. *Psychopharmacol (Berl)*, **201** (4), 601–618.

101. Addolorato, G., Leggio, L., Agabio, R. *et al.* (2006) Baclofen: a new drug for the treatment of alcohol dependence. *International Journal of Clinical Practice*, **60** (8), 1003–1008.

102. Garbutt, J.C., West, S.L., Carey, T.S. *et al.* (1999) Pharmacological treatment of alcohol dependence: A review of the evidence. *Journal of the American Medical Association*, **281**, 1318–1325.

103. Kenna, G.A., Lomastro, T.L., Schiesl, A. *et al.* (2009) Review of topiramate: an antiepileptic for the treatment of alcohol abuse. *Current Drug Abuse Review*, **2** (2), 135–142.

104. Fillmore, K.M. (1988) *Alcohol Use Across the Life Course: Review of Seventy Years of International Longitudinal Research*, Addiction Research Foundation, Toronto.

105. McLellan, A.T. (2002) Have we evaluated addiction treatment correctly? Implications from a chronic care perspective. *Addiction*, 97, 249–252.

106. Vaillant, G.E. (2003) A 60-year follow-up of alcoholic men. *Addiction*, **98**, 1043–1051.

107. Stout, R.L., Rubin, A., Zwick, W., Zywiak, W. and Bellino, L. (1999) Optimizing the cost-effectiveness of treatment for alcohol problems: A rationale for extended case monitoring. *Addictive Behaviors*, **24**, 17–35.

108. Ahles, T.A., Schlundt, D.G., Prue, D.M. and Rychtarik, R.G. (1983) Impact of aftercare arrangements on the maintenance of treatment success in abusive drinkers. *Addictive Behaviors*, **8**, 53–58.

109. Hilton, M.E., Maisto, S.A., Conigliaro, J. *et al.* (2001) Improving alcoholism treatment services across a spectrum of services. *Alcoholism: Clinical and Experimental Research*, **25**, 128–135.

110. Korr, W.S. and Cloninger, L. (1991) Assessing models of case management: An empirical approach. *Journal of Social Service Research*, **14**, 129–146.

111. Orleans C.T., Schoenbach, V.J., Wagner, E.H. *et al.* (1991) Self-help quit smoking interventions: Effects of self-help materials, social support instructions, and telephone counseling. *Journal of Consulting and Clinical Psychology*, **59**, 439–448.

112. Curran, H.V. and Drummond D.C. (2006) Psychological treatments for substance misuse and dependence. In Nutt, D.J., Robbins, T.W., Stimson, G.V., Ince, M., Jackson, A. (Eds.) *Drugs and the Future: Brain Science, Addiction and Society*. Academic Press, London.

113. Mann, R.E., Smart, R., Anglin, L. and Rush, B. (1988) Are decreases in liver cirrhosis rates a result of increased treatment for alcoholism? *British Journal of Addiction*, **83**, 683–688.

114. Mann, R.E., Smart, R., Anglin, L. and Adlaf, E. (1991) Reductions in cirrhosis deaths in the United States: associations with per capita consumption and AA membership. *Journal of Studies on Alcohol*, **52**, 361–365.

115. Harwood, H. (2000) Updating estimates of the economic costs of alcohol abuse in the United States: estimates, update methods, and data.

116. Prime Minister's Strategy Unit (2004) *Alcohol Harm Reduction Strategy for England*, Cabinet Office, London.

117. Potaminos, G., North, W., Meade, T. *et al.* (1986) Randomised trial of community-based centre versus conventional hospital management in treatment of alcoholism. *The Lancet*, **8510**, 797–799.

118. Holder, H.D. (1987) Alcoholism treatment and potential health care cost saving. *Medical Care*, **25**, 52–71.

119. Holder, H., Longabaugh, R., Miller, W., *et al.* (1991) The cost effectiveness of treatment for alcoholism: A first approximation. *Journal of Studies on Alcohol*, **52**, 517–540.

120. Luckey, J.W. (1987) Justifying alcohol treatment on the basis of cost savings: The "offset" literature. *Alcohol Health & Research World*, **12**, 8–15.

121. Parthasarathy, S., Weisner, C., Hu, T-W. and Moore, C. (2001) Association of outpatient alcohol and drug treatment with health care utilization and cost: Revisiting the offset hypothesis. *Journal of Studies on Alcohol*, **62**, 89–97.

122. McKenna, M., Chick, J., Buxton, M. *et al.* (1996) The SECCAT Survey 1. The costs and consequences of alcoholism. *Alcohol and Alcoholism*, **31**, 565–576.

123. Godfrey, C. (1994) Assessing the cost-effectiveness of alcohol services. *Journal of Mental Health*, **3**, 3–21.

124. Edwards, G., Anderson, P., Babor, T. *et al.* (1994) *Alcohol Policy and the Public Good*, Oxford University Press, Oxford.

125. Thom, B. and Green, A. (1996) Services for women with alcohol problems: the way forward, in *Alcohol Problems in the Community* (ed. L. Harrison), Routledge, London, pp. 200–222.

126. Home Office (2003) *Hidden harm. Responding to the needs of children of problem drug users.* http://drugs.homeoffice.gov.uk (Accessed 31 August 2010).

127. Davis, T.M., Carpenter, K.M., Malte, C.A. *et al.* (2002) Women in addictions treatment: comparing VA and community samples. *Journal of Substance Abuse Treatment*, **23**, 41–48.

128. Timko, C., Moos, R.H., Finney, J.W. and Connell, E.G. (2002) Gender differences in help-utilization and the 8-year course of alcohol abuse. *Addiction*, **97**, 877–889.

129. Jarvis, T.J. (1992) Implications of gender for alcohol treatment research: A quantitative and qualitative review. *British Journal of Addiction*, **87**, 1249–1261.

130. Farrell, M., Howes, S., Taylor, C. *et al.* (1998) Substance misuse and psychiatric co-morbidity: An overview of the OPCS National Psychiatric Morbidity Survey. *Addictive Behaviors*, **23**, 909–918.

131. Harrison, L., Harrison, M. and Adebowale, V. (1997) Drinking problems among black communities, in *Alcohol Problems in the Community* (ed. L. Harrison), Routledge, London, pp. 223–40.

132. Karlsen, S., Rogers, A. and McCarthy, M. (1998) Social environment and substance misuse: A study of ethnic variations among inner London adolescents. *Ethnicity and Health*, **3**, 265–273.

133. Aharonovich, E., Hasin, D., Rahav, G. *et al.* (2001) Differences in drinking patterns among Ashkenazic and Sephardic Israeli adults. *Journal of Studies on Alcohol*, **62**, 301–305.

134. Orford, J., Johnson, M. and Purser, B. (2004) Drinking in second generation black and Asian communities in the English midlands. *Addiction Research and Theory*, **12** (1), 11–30.

135. Trull, T.J., Sher, K.J., Minks-Brown, C. *et al.* (2000) Borderline personality disorder and substance use disorders: a review and integration. *Clin. Psychol. Rev.*, **20** (2), 235–253.

136. Crawford, V. and Crome, I. (2001) *Coexisting Problem of Mental Health and Substance Misuse*, Royal College of Psychiatrists, London.

137. Johns, A. (1997) Substance misuse: A primary risk and a major problem of co-morbidity. *International Review of Psychiatry*, **9**, 233–241.

138. Graham, H.L., Copello, A., Birchwood, M.J. *et al.* (2003) Cognitive behavioural integrated treatment approach for psychosis and problem substance use, in *Substance Misuse in Psychosis. Approaches to Treatment and Service Delivery* (eds. H.L. Graham, A. Copello, M.J. Birchwood and K.T. Meuser), John Wiley & Sons, Ltd, Chichester.

139. Todd, J., Green, G., Harrison, M. *et al.* (2004) Social exclusion in clients with co-morbid mental health and substance misuse problems. *Social Psychiatry and Psychiatric Epidemiology*, **39**, 581–587.

140. Regier, D.A., Farmer, M.E., Rae, D.S. *et al.* (1990) Comorbidity of mental disorders with alcohol and other drug abuse. *Journal of the American Medical Association*, **264**, 2511–2518.

141. Drake, R., Mercer-McFadden, C., Mueser, K. *et al.* (1998) Review of integrated mental health and substance abuse treatment for patients with dual disorders. *Schizophrenia Bulletin*, **24**, 589–608.

142. Weaver, T., Stimson, G., Tyrer, P. *et al.* (2004) What are the implications for clinical management and service development of prevalent co-morbidity in UK mental health and substance misuse treatment populations? *Drugs: Education, Prevention and Policy*, **11**, 329–348.

143. Cleary, M., Hunt, G.E., Matheson, S.L., Siegfried, N. and Walter, G. (2008) Psychosocial interventions for people with both severe mental illness and substance misuse. Cochrane Database of Systematic Reviews, Issue 1. Art. No.: CD001088. DOI: 10.1002/14651858.CD001088.pub2.

8.1 Perverse Interpretation of Evidence in Alcohol Policy

Steve Allsop, PhD

National Drug Research Institute, Curtin University of Technology, Perth, Australia

An unadorned summary of these three chapters would conclude that while alcohol makes a significant contribution to many countries' burden of disease, and there are other substantial economic and social costs, there is an increasing body of evidence that can guide preventive effort and effective clinical interventions. Over the past two centuries, and especially the last two or three decades, a vast body of evidence has been amassed on 'drunkenness and its effects on the human body' [1], prevention strategies [2, 3] and treatment options [4, 5]. We have also identified evidential gaps that limit our ability to accurately attribute alcohol's contribution to some physical and mental health problems and adverse social outcomes, particularly the secondary impact of alcohol (e.g. adverse impacts on families, bystanders and the broader community). There appears to be an inverse relationship between the evidence and political and community willingness to adopt prevention strategies – those interventions with the strongest evidence base are not always popular, while those that are accepted do not always have the best research support. Finally, while the challenges of treating severe alcohol dependence are well known, we have had limited success in ensuring the widespread adoption of interventions directed at the large proportion of at-risk drinkers who do not enter our specialist treatment services.

As illustrated by all authors in this section, the research evidence about effective interventions has not uniquely influenced policy and clinical decisions about responses to alcohol-related problems. In shaping policy, research evidence competes with: vested interests, such as those of the alcohol manufacturers and retailers; the divergent views of government departments such as treasury, employment, industry and health; and, community and clinician perceptions about the nature and extent of alcohol-related harm. Community views are influenced by individuals' perceived proximity to adverse outcomes of alcohol consumption, and popular perceptions that alcohol problems are resolutely an issue of personal responsibility/individual weakness shapes policy and clinical endeavour. Thus, the risk of liver cirrhosis for a small group of drinkers who are deemed to have unique vulnerabilities may be less influential in driving public support for effective prevention than perceived threats to personal and public safety from intoxicated individuals. In this context,

Substance Abuse Disorders: Evidence and Experience, First Edition. Edited by Hamid Ghodse, Helen Herrman, Mario Maj and Norman Sartorius.
© 2011 John Wiley & Sons, Ltd. Published 2011 by John Wiley & Sons, Ltd.

policy can be influenced by idiosyncratic and perverse interpretations of the evidence. I share the amazement of Saunders and Latt who draw our attention to a recent claim in a British Government report denying a relationship between the amount of and pattern of alcohol consumption and the nature or level of alcohol-related harm, but acknowledge the perspectives that contribute to such conclusions.

There is a literature on influencing policy (see [6]) and perhaps the alcohol field can learn from such work. Part of the process of better community and political engagement is likely to include the establishment of effective monitoring systems that adequately assess the burden imposed by risky alcohol consumption, not just on individual drinkers, but on the broader community. Impact will be influenced by the current relevance of data – unfortunately the enumeration of adverse outcomes is often historical. Similarly, we need to better communicate how our prevention and treatment investment will secure personal and community-wide benefits. Patra and colleagues offer important guidance in this regard. We should also look to the forthcoming outputs of work being undertaken, for example by Robin Room (Australia) and Sally Caswell (New Zealand) and their respective colleagues, on the secondary costs of risky alcohol use.

As noted by Passetti and Drummond, the psychological and pharmacological treatment options, brief to intensive, which variously aim to manage withdrawal, assist in attaining abstinence or controlled drinking outcomes and focus on avoiding relapse have informed the development of a number of clinical guidelines. But, much of the focus has remained on the more acute presenting issues and on drinking outcomes. This is possibly why enduring treatment impact is elusive [7] suggesting that more attention should focus on post-treatment 'quality of life.' (e.g. see [8]). The key challenge is to '... ensure therapeutic gains are maintained over time ... low key interventions aimed at keeping people well after the end of active treatment may be beneficial' (Passetti and Drummond p.). In a review of relapse-prevention strategies, this important element has been neatly summed up by Connors and colleagues:

> In simple language, the secret to helping people prevent relapse is to keep them happy [7].

This may also apply to preventive effort. Risky drinking sometimes develops in a context of intolerable physical, economic and social conditions. This means that miserable abstinence or reduced alcohol use, which in all probability will be short lived, should not be accepted as sufficient prevention or treatment outcomes. While stepped-care approaches may mean simple alcohol-focused interventions (for example, controlling access to alcohol) will suffice for some clients and communities, others will require more intensive, integrated and enduring interventions that address factors such as housing, psychological well-being, family life, employment, social networks and so on.

With the notable exception of brief intervention research, delivered in a range of settings, from primary health-care services to emergency departments (e.g. see [9]) we have had limited influence on those who do not enter or are not retained in alcohol treatment services. Given the prevalence of risky alcohol use in many countries and the observation that only a minority of people perceive the need for and receive treatment (see [10]) it is important to broaden the reach of interventions. This might involve trialling innovative approaches to engage nontreatment populations, such as using mobile phone and web-based technology (e.g. [11]) addressing the slow uptake of brief interventions (see [12]) and adopting more assertive outreach methods to enhance treatment engagement and retention (see [13]). Possibly driven by models that emphasized the importance of intrinsic client motivation, the alcohol field has been slower than other domains, such as mental-health services, to adopt assertive outreach. Poor treatment engagement and retention have sometimes been interpreted as indicative of individual symptom rather than service design flaws. Adopting assertive outreach strategies, such as providing appointment reminders, using electronic media, following up missed appointments, investing in practical changes to enhance treatment access, extending hours of service, providing home visits, community-based interventions and better service integration (including enhancing case management practices) might improve client engagement and retention.

Finally, changing population demographics and patterns of alcohol use, cultural evolution and industry deregulation create new research, prevention and treatment challenges. Many governments, contrary to evidence on how to reduce alcohol-related harm, are adopting policies of deregulation and liberalization, which, along with changes in population demographics, influence the cultural drivers of alcohol consumption. Some countries are being confronted by increasing heavy episodic drinking amongst young people, while many developed countries have ageing populations, who have drunk more and for longer than their predecessors. Despite a potential public-health challenge, many of those in the alcohol field, and their counterparts in gerontology, are yet to assess the nature or extent of this emerging issue, let alone describe effective interventions.

REFERENCES

1. Trotter, T. (1981/1804) *An Essay, Medical, Philosophical and Chemical on Drunkenness*, Arno Press, New York.
2. Babor, T., Caetano, R., Casswell, S. *et al.* (2010) *Alcohol: No Ordinary Commodity – Research and Public Policy*, 2nd edn, Oxford University Press, Oxford.
3. Loxley, W., Toumbourou, J., Stockwell, T.R. *et al.* (2004) *The Prevention of Substance Use, Risk and Harm in Australia: A Review of the Evidence*, National Drug Research Institute and the Centre for Adolescent Health.
4. Miller, W.R. and Wilbourne, P.L. (2002) Mesa Grande: a methodological analysis of clinical trials of treatments of alcohol use disorders. *Addiction*, **97** (3), 265–277.
5. Raistrick, D., Heather, N. and Godfrey, C. (2006) *Review of the Effectiveness of Treatment for Alcohol Problems*, National Treatment Agency for Substance Misuse, London.
6. Kingdon, J. (1995) *Agendas, Alternatives and Public Policies*, 2nd edn, Longman, New York.
7. Connors, G.J., Longabaugh, R. and Miller, W.R. (1996) Looking forward and back to relapse: implications for research and practice. *Addiction*, **91** (12 Supp 1), S191–S196.
8. Gladis, M.M., Gosch, E., Dishuk, N.M. and Critz-Christoph, P. (1999) Quality of life: Expanding the scope of clinical significance. *Journal of Consulting and Clinical Psychology*, **67** (3), 320–331.
9. Moyer, A., Finney, J.W., Swearingen, C.E. and Vergun, P. (2002) Brief interventions for alcohol problems: a meta-analytic review of controlled investigations in treatment-seeking and non-treatment-seeking populations. *Addiction*, **97** (3), 279–292.
10. SAMHSA (2006) 2005 National survey on drug use and health. Substance Abuse and Mental Health Services Administration (SAMHSA), Office of Applied Studies, US Department of Health and Human Services.

11. Hallett, J., Maycock, B. and Kypri, K. *et al.* (2009) Development of a web-based alcohol intervention for university students: Processes and challenges. *Drug and Alcohol Review*, **28** (1), 31–39.

12. Roche, A.M., Hotham, E.D. and Richmond, R.L. (2002) The general practitioner's role in AOD issues: overcoming individual, professional and systemic barriers. *Drug and Alcohol Review*, **21** (3), 223–230.

13. Mueser, K.T. and Drake, R.E. (2002) Integrated dual disorder treatment in New Hampshire (USA), in *Substance Misuse in Psychosis: Approaches to Treatment and Service Delivery* (eds. H.L. Graham, A. Copello, M.J. Birthwood and K.T. Mueser), John Wiley & Sons, West Sussex, pp. 93–105.

8.2 Implementing the Evidence Base

Duncan Raistrick, MBChB, MPhil, FRCPsych

Leeds Addiction Unit, Leeds, UK

One of the attractions of the addiction field is that it cuts across many disciplines ranging from the neurochemistry of receptors through to public policy and the three preceding chapters illustrate the point. The evidence required to inform public policy, choice of treatment strategies, and the means to measure the effectiveness and cost effectiveness of all these strategies is available. This commentary selects clinically important issues in order to ask why there is a failure to implement the evidence and to consider what more practitioners might do.

It may be that the science is not as clear cut or as easy to understand as those immersed in the study of alcohol problems suppose. The impact of alcohol varies markedly across different geographical regions. Take, for example, alcohol attributable deaths across World Health Organisation regions: as a proportion of all deaths, Europe has the highest rate at 11.0% of men and 1.8% of women, the Eastern Mediterranean is lowest at 0.8% of men and 0.1% of women. These mortality data are matched by overall consumption figures, 11.9 litres per adult across Europe and 0.7 litres per adult for the Eastern Mediterranean. In all parts of the world men drink more than women but most of the world-wide population, 45% of men and 66% of women, abstain from drinking alcohol and there is much less variation in the amount consumed by drinkers in different countries than there is in the total number of abstainers who, therefore, account for the different rates of per capita consumption [1]. This huge variability gives an insight into the complexities that underpin alcohol problems, but crucially is a reminder of the need for population-level interventions to which clinicians can contribute.

There are some 30 disorders where, by definition, alcohol is the cause, for example alcoholic cardiomyopathy or alcoholic liver cirrhosis, and some 200 more where alcohol is one of a number of causative factors, for example cancers or cardiovascular disease (www.who.int/en). Different disorders are associated with different patterns of drinking that are of clinical relevance. Thus, the risk of a chronic alcohol-related disorder has a more or less linear relationship with lifetime exposure to alcohol, whereas acute disorders and accidents are related to the frequency of intoxication and the risk increases exponentially

Substance Abuse Disorders: Evidence and Experience, First Edition. Edited by Hamid Ghodse, Helen Herrman, Mario Maj and Norman Sartorius.
© 2011 John Wiley & Sons, Ltd. Published 2011 by John Wiley & Sons, Ltd.

dependent on the amount consumed on a given occasion [2]. These World Health Organi-zation estimates of alcohol-related disease and disability do not include many of the social problems related to alcohol such as domestic violence, dysfunctional family relationships, criminal activity, employment problems and general nuisance. Social problems are difficult to measure and even more difficult to cost but they should not be forgotten when summing up the total cost of alcohol to society.

Policy makers are generally not scientists, rather they are politicians or they service political machines. Politicians want simple answers to complex problems, so, when the science is unclear or difficult to understand, they worry less about the long-term health of the population and much more about short-term employment, tax revenues and popularity. There is no single alcohol message. Even if it was thought desirable, prohibition has not worked. Moreover, modest levels of drinking bring health benefits; it is unlike smoking that is unambiguously detrimental to health. The response of government has been to support weak population-level measures and to demonize subgroups of drinkers such as 'the alcoholic', 'the binge drinker', or 'the young person'. The drinks industry and the general public are more than happy to collude with this approach and to support or lobby for action to curtail the 'demons'. Public opinion data are available from a survey in Ontario that sought views on eight alcohol policy measures rated according to expected impact, from high to low: alcohol taxes; minimal legal drinking age; monopoly system of alcohol retailing; restricted outlet density; restricted hours of sale; stopping service to intoxicated patrons; advertising bans; and warning labels. Those policies that might be considered to be personally intrusive or inconvenient received low support and *vice versa* [3] in other words, given the choice, the public support ineffective policies. It is understandable that policy makers will opt for simplistic and popular solutions, particularly so where these can be targeted at groups where the link between drinking and harmful consequences is self-evident. It is up to scientists, including clinicians who are not natural campaigners, to organize better and lobby more effectively for sensible alcohol policies that are suited to their particular culture.

Over the last decade there has been increasing interest in the use of brief interventions. Unfortunately, there has been confusion as to exactly what constitutes a brief intervention and what its purpose might be. Brief intervention has been used to refer to i) opportunistic interventions for hazardous drinkers delivered by primary care staff and typically lasting 5–30 minutes over 1–3 sessions; ii) interventions for help seekers delivered by alcohol specialists, typically over 1–5 therapy sessions – referred to as less-intensive treatment by Raistrick *et al.* ([4], pp. 79–101). When applied opportunistically brief interventions are a secondary prevention measure expected to impact at a population level. Kaner *et al.* [5] found that brief interventions produced a reduction in alcohol consumed of 4–5 units per week when compared with no intervention or simple advice. The reductions found were from baseline levels ranging from 8 to 50 units weekly but it was not possible to pinpoint whether lower levels of drinking were the result of reduced frequency or reduced intensity of consumption. There was some suggestion that the longer, albeit still brief, the intervention the greater the reduction in alcohol consumption. Importantly, those trials in real-world primary care delivered equally good results as those set up under optimal research conditions. This is a significant finding since the briefer the intervention the more difficult the staff training: brief interventions require staff to be competent at using a motivational delivery style, giving accurate feedback and information and rapidly assessing risk. This size of effect can only be significant if delivered on a large scale to the hazardous end of the drinking spectrum.

Widespread use of brief interventions will deliver results in the medium term but will also increase the need for specialist services in the short term. Specialist treatment will vary in duration and intensity depending on motivation, availability of support and complexity. The active ingredients of effective treatment include structure, goal agreement and therapeutic alliance [6] and were brought together in a novel intervention called Social Behaviour and Network Therapy [7] for the UK Alcohol Treatment Trial. Practitioners need familiarity with pharmacological therapies that can be used to enhance the psychosocial element of treatment and treatment needs to be followed by an effective aftercare arrangement.

A lot of attention has been given to refining specific treatments and, in the main, treatment outcome trials, such as, Project Match in the United States or the UK Alcohol Treatment Trial, compare one intervention against another. The problem with this approach is that effective treatments, even those that appear quite different such as Twelve-Step Facilitation and Motivational Enhancement Therapy, actually have much in common [8]. Trials of treatment effectiveness will attempt to control for therapist behaviours and yet many consider it is the therapists' delivery of treatment that is much more important than the treatment itself. There is a tension between allowing therapists free expression and the need for adherence to validated treatment protocols. Treatment manuals have been developed as one solution. The evidence suggests that a flexible adherence to treatment manuals delivers better outcomes, but that building a strong therapeutic alliance is even more important than adherence [9]. It follows from this that experience will be an important part of being a successful therapist. Whatever the experience of practitioners, supervision of video-recorded practice is the only way of assuring effective treatment delivery.

At a time when health-care resources are ever more stretched it is important carefully to assess the cost effectiveness of treatment. It is also important that clinicians can justify the cost effectiveness of their own services. One area of concern is prescribing for people who misuse alcohol. There is a culture in the treatment of addiction of 'prescribing against the evidence' that to a degree is understandable since often there is little evidence and, almost by definition, prescribing will not follow formulary guidance. Guidelines are available, for example from the British Association of Psychopharmacology [10], and yet it is common to see polypharmacy, in particular anti-depressants, anti-psychotics, anti-convulsants, vitamin supplements and anxiolytics or hypnotics prescribed without justification. Unsurprisingly, service users often see medication as a solution to their problems but, to work effectively with people who have addiction problems, practitioners must be competent to use motivational skills [11] and engage them in change. This is more difficult than being content to pursue a harm-reduction goal only, and is one reason for extending specialist services.

A slightly different question of resources arises with detoxification. While the pharmacological aspects of detoxification are well worked out, evidence on the optimal setting is sparse. Service users prefer to have home detoxification but this is considerably more expensive than an outpatient or day-patient arrangement, though both are considerably less expensive than in-patient or residential treatment. Some of the traditional criteria for inpatient detoxification, for example, a history of seizures or delirium, need not be a barrier to home detoxification. There are, of course, situations that require inpatient care, notably people with medical or psychiatric complications or those taking a cocktail of drugs such that the course of a detoxification is difficult to predict. That said, detoxification can often be delivered safely and effectively at home if attention is given to the medical risks, the efficacy risk – particularly social support and relapse risk.

Specialist services should always be concerned to look at outcomes from treatment and increasingly this will become a requirement of funding. An extensive range of assessment and outcome measurement tools are available: a menu of these can be found on the University of Washington, Alcohol and Drug Abuse Institute web site (www.lib.adai. washing.edu/instrustments/selected.html). The RESULT Project (www.leedspft.nhs.uk/our_services/leeds_addiction_unit/RESULT) has combined validated scales into a single package that can be tailored to individual service need. The guiding principles are:

- where possible to use measures that are self-reported by service users;
- to use a package capable of integration into routine practice;
- to use scales with properties that have been shown to have internal consistency, reproducibility, content and construct validity, responsiveness and are interpretable;
- to summarize complex information clearly and simply for professionals;
- to use measures that are of value to service users.

Measures are selected to be an integral part of treatment collected at 3 months (this is when most change is expected) and then at 12 months (to test the sustainability of change) and thereafter annually:

Level 1 data – universal health measures

Two internationally recognized measures

EQ5D – measures quality of life; used to generate QALYs;
ICD-10 – categorical codes for substance use.

Level 2 data – key addiction domains

These are the key domain measures that are validated as independent scales

LDQ – Leeds Dependence Questionnaire: dependence;
CORE – Clinical Outcomes Routine Evaluation: psychological well-being;
SSQ – Social Satisfaction Questionnaire: social well-being;
Substance use – detailed QF and route.

Level 3 data – specific problem measures

These are the scales and measures that should be selected to suit a particular service, e.g. self-harming, occupational activity, anxiety rating.

Level 4 data – personal measures

These are the personal, possibly idiosyncratic or aspirational, outcome goals agreed by each service user with their key worker.

In conclusion, there is an abundance of evidence to support effective policy and treatment. Implementation of evidence-based policy is often in conflict with political expediencies and therefore fails; supervision of treatment and measurement of its effectiveness is often seen as a threat to clinicians and so also fails. The public and the drinks industry collude with token efforts to deal with alcohol-related problems and so there is no pressure for change. At an individual level, however, there are no such constraints on becoming a first-class practitioner.

REFERENCES

1. Rehm, J., Mathers, C., Popova, S., *et al.* (2009) Global burden of disease and injury and economic cost attributable to alcohol use and alcohol-use disorders, Alcohol and Global Health 1. *Lancet*, **373**, 2223–2233.

2. Anderson, P., Chisholm, D. and Fuhr, D. (2009) Effectiveness and cost-effectiveness of policies and programmes to reduce the harm caused by alcohol, Alcohol and Global Health 2. *Lancet*, **373**, 2234–2246.

3. Giesbrecht, N., Ialomiteanu, A. and Anglin, L. (2005) Drinking patterns and perspectives on alcohol policy: results from two Ontario surveys. *Alcohol & Alcoholism*, **40**, 132–139

4. Raistrick, D., Heather, N. and Godfrey, C. (2006) *Review of the Effectiveness of Treatment for Alcohol Problems*, National Treatment Agency, London.

5. Kaner, E.F., Dickinson, H.O., Beyer, F.R. *et al.* (2009) Effectiveness of brief alcohol interventions in primary care populations (Review), *The Cochrane Collaboration*.

6. Moos, R. (2007) Theory-based active ingredients of effective treatments for substance use disorders. *Drug and Alcohol Dependence*, **88**, 109–121.

7. Copello, A., Orford, J., Hodgson, R. and Tober, G. (2009) *Social Behaviour and Network Therapy for Problem Drinkers*, Routledge, London.

8. Tober, G. (2002) Evidence based practice – still a bridge too far for addiction counsellors? *Drugs: Education, Prevention and Policy*, **9**, 7–9.

9. Martino, S., Ball, S.A., Nich, C., *et al.* (2008) Community program therapist adherence and competence in motivational enhancement therapy. *Drug and Alcohol Dependence*, **96**, 37–48.

10. Lingford-Hughes, A., Welch, S. and Nutt, D. (2004) Evidence based guidelines for the pharmacological management of substance misuse, addiction, and co-morbidity: recommendations from the British Association for Psychopharmacology. *Journal of Psychopharmacology*, **18**, 293–335.

11. Tober, G. and Raistrick, D. (eds.) (2007) *Motivational Dialogue: Preparing Addiction Professionals for Motivational Interviewing Practice*, Routledge, London.

8.3 Further Insights into the Burden of Alcohol Use on Mental Illness

Nady el-Guebaly, MD

Addiction Division, Department of Psychiatry, University of Calgary, Calgary, Alberta, Canada

The three excellent reviews addressing the epidemiology, prevention and management of alcohol problems make reference to their impact on neuropsychiatric disorders.

I will further detail the association between alcohol-use disorders (AUDs) and mental illness.

DEFINITIONS

In psychiatry, the term *co-morbidity* describes the presence of any additional coexisting disorder in an individual with a given index disorder. The terms *co-occurring or concurrent disorders* are common terms in the addiction research literature used to describe patients with AUDs and one or more additional disorders, including the full spectrum of non-AUD Axis I disorders, personality disorders, mental retardation and medical problems.

AETIOLOGICAL MODELS

Several models have been hypothesized about the association of AUDs and mental illness, including [1]:

- A shared vulnerability or risk factors for both disorders ranging from the genetic to sociocultural. So far, no common gene has been identified. The best evidence so far is limited to the anti-social personality disorder acting as a common risk factor for both mental illness and AUDs.
- The self-medication hypothesis posits that addicted patients select substances including alcohol according to their specific psychopharmacological properties to treat symptoms

Substance Abuse Disorders: Evidence and Experience, First Edition. Edited by Hamid Ghodse, Helen Herrman, Mario Maj and Norman Sartorius.
© 2011 John Wiley & Sons, Ltd. Published 2011 by John Wiley & Sons, Ltd.

of mental disorders [2]. The majority of data gathered so far does not support this specific hypothesis. There is evidence, however, that substances may be used to medicate unpleasant, nonspecific dysphoric states across a variety of diagnoses.

- The supersensitivity model whereby patients with mental illness will experience greater negative medical and psychosocial consequences with lower dosages of substance use.
- Primary substance abuse as a risk factor to develop psychiatric illness. Data from longitudinal studies so far remain inconsistent.

THE EPIDEMIOLOGY OF AUD AND MENTAL ILLNESS

Estimates of the alcohol-attributable Disability – Adjusted Life Years (DALYs) point to a significant difference with respect to neuropsychiatric disorders between the impact on disability (38% of alcohol-attributable DALYs) compared to the impact on mortality (5% of alcohol-attributable deaths). Amongst these various disorders, only unipolar depressive disorders and self-inflicted injuries are specifically estimated [3].

In the United States, large, third-generation, epidemiological community studies have been conducted. In the first one, the Epidemiologic Catchment Area (ECA) study, the lifetime prevalence of any substance-use disorder (SUD) in a community sample was 16.7%, whereas 29% of patients with a lifetime history of mental illness met criteria for a lifetime co-morbid SUD. The National Comorbidity Survey and its replication (NCS and NCS-R) studies found an odds ratio of 2.4 for co-morbidity between any lifetime mental illness and any lifetime SUD. In these surveys, 50.9% of individuals with a lifetime mental illness had a history of an SUD, and 51.4% of those with a lifetime SUD met criteria for a lifetime mental illness [4, 5]. The AUDs twelve-month prevalence varied between 4.4 and 9.7% of the population, and the lifetime prevalence varied between 13.5 and 30.3%.

In the ECA study, 34% of persons with schizophrenia had a current AUD. The prevalence of lifetime co-occurring SUDs amongst patients with a major depressive disorder was 17–18%. In treatment settings for SUDs, the lifetime prevalence of major depressive disorder (MDD) in patients with alcohol dependence ranges from 20 to 67%. Amongst anxiety disorders, panic disorders and obsessive compulsive disorders, the rates of AUDs (OR for AUD = 3.3 and 2.5, respectively) were particularly elevated. Post-traumatic stress disorder (PTSD), attention-deficit/hyperactivity disorder, eating disorders, and of course, personality disorders also had elevated rates of AUDs. Anti-social personality had the strongest association with alcohol dependence of any Axis I or II disorder, with an odds ratio of 21 [6].

THE PREVENTION OF AUD AND MENTAL ILLNESS

All preventive strategies in this review article have an implication for the target population suffering from co-morbid mental illness [7]. Screening for substance misuse and brief intervention are the most consistently effective strategies in primary care (4). Assessment of a patient's alcohol intake with feedback can help reduce excessive consumption. There is a paucity of data regarding the impact of these strategies on the population suffering from mental illness [7]. Linkages between drug and alcohol services and mental-health services should be able to reduce, for example, the incidence of suicidal behaviour. An important requirement for screening in busy clinical practices is to have reliable and valid brief assessment tools that measure both psychiatric and SUD domains and estimate their severity. While a number of instruments exist for SUD, the multiplicity of psychiatric disorders has made the drafting of brief screening instruments, for primary care elusive. One such instrument has been PRIME-MD [8], which has not received wide acceptance. Addiction treatment settings using the Addiction Severity Index (ASI) apply an 11-item psychiatric subscale as a screen for potential psychiatric co-morbid disorders [9, 10]. More recently, the Global Appraisal of Individual Needs (GAIN) and its 4–5-item subscreeners (internalizing disorders, externalizing disorders, substance disorders and crime/violence) demonstrates good screening potential for people with co-morbid disorders [11].

In the United States, the latest management strategy promotes inducement of behavioural change through a continuum of Screening, Brief Intervention and Referral to Treatment (SBIRT). Multisite outcome findings report substantial declines in both drug use and heavy alcohol use over a 6-month follow-up [12].

THE TREATMENT OF AUD AND MENTAL ILLNESS

In the review of the management of alcohol-use disorders, their high prevalence in psychiatric populations requires for mental health services to be an important treatment setting. A crucial issue is to ensure that alcohol-use disorders are identified by psychiatric staff. Interventions aimed at reduced drinking may improve the overall outcome of psychiatric treatment. Compared to the general population, lower levels of drinking amongst psychiatric populations may carry significant health consequences, and more extended interventions may be required. To address the co-morbid substance misuse and psychiatric disorders, three organizational models have been identified: serial, integrated, or shared care. The review promotes a shared-care model assigning individuals with dual diagnosis to either mental-health or addiction services, depending on the relative severity of mental-health and substance-misuse problems and leaving the other agency to take an advisory role. It is acknowledged that the model preferred may also depend on the particular overall health system [13].

Clinically, it is recognized that patients with co-occurring mental illness and AUD across a broad spectrum of diagnostic types and combinations have greater severity of illness and worse longitudinal course of illness in multiple domains, including increased risk for psychiatric and substance-use relapses; higher rates of criminal recidivism; higher levels of psychological distress; poorer psychosocial functioning; worse treatment retention; poor medication compliance; higher rates of violence, suicide, legal difficulties, medical problems, and family stress; higher utilization of health-care services such as emergency department and inpatient services [14, 15].

A vital factor to consider is the severity of each concurrent illness. Patients who have the same diagnoses (e.g., schizophrenia and marijuana dependence) will have very different courses of illness due to the relative severity of either disorder. These relative differences dictate different biological and psychosocial interventions and require varying intensity of levels of care. One helpful model of subcategorization that addresses the continuum of severity as a factor in the heterogeneity of patients with both mental illness and AUDs divides patients into four quadrants, that is, Low or High severity of AUD matching with Low or High severity of mental illness [16].

The current realization is that co-morbidity is so common that it should be expected rather than considered an exception. Outcomes depend on the extent to which support at the system level is provided. Consensual standards have recently been developed to address managed care needs in the US [17].

One such example is the ASAM criteria for use of the substance-abuse network, which identifies two levels of program capability in handling individuals with concurrent disorders: a) dual diagnoses capable (DDC) programs (i.e. programs accommodating admissions with somewhat stabilized psychiatric disorders and with a primary focus on the treatment of substance-related disorders); b) dual diagnoses enhanced (DDE) programs (i.e. programs accommodating more unstable or disables psychiatric admissions short of requiring 24 hours supervision) [18].

The Dual Diagnosis Capability in Addiction Treatment (DDCAT) Index, is being used to assess public and private-sector addiction-treatment services at agency, regional and state system levels. The DDCAT method is based on observational, interview, and material review data gathered during a site visit. These data are then used to complete ratings on 35 benchmarks along seven dimensional or scale scores: Program Structure; Program Milieu; Clinical Practice; Assessment; Clinical Practice: Treatment; Continuity of Care; Staffing; and Training. Programs receive scores and a graphic profile on these dimensions. Based upon overall performance, they are categorized as: Addiction Only Services (AOS), Dual Diagnosis Capable (DDC) or Dual Diagnosis Enhanced (DDE). The index was developed and tested in community addiction treatment programs and systems and psychometric studies have been conducted. Presently, applications of the DDCAT are in progress in at least 20 state systems and internationally [19].

In conclusion, just as individuals with AUDs often use other drugs, the presence of other co-morbidities is increasingly the norm, at least in clinical populations. These factors are recognized in epidemiological surveys, although the data is mostly from developed countries. By comparison, empirically based preventive and treatment strategies are still at the pioneering stage. A major effort is required to further investigate these challenging needs.

REFERENCES

1. Mueser, K.T., Drake, R.E. and Wallach, M.A. (1998) Dual Diagnosis: a review of etiological theories. *Addictive Behaviors*, **23**, 717–734.

2. Khantzian, E.J. (1997) The self-medication hypothesis of substance use disorders: a reconsideration and recent applications. *Harvard Review Psychiatry*, **4**, 231–244.

3. Patra, J., Samokhvalov, A.V. and Rehm, J. (2011) Alcohol epidemiology: extent and nature of the problem, in *Substance abuse: Evidence and Experience in Psychiatry* (eds. H. Ghodse, H. Herman, M. Maj and N. Sartorius), Wiley-Blackwell.

4. Kessler, R.C., Nelson, C.B., McGonagle, K.A. *et al.* (1996) The epidemiology of co-occurring addictive and mental disorders: implications for prevention and service utilization. *American Journal of Orthopsychiatry*, **66**, 17–31.

5. Kessler, R.C. (2004) The epidemiology of dual diagnosis. *Biological Psychiatry*, **56**, 730–737.

6. Regier, D.A., Farmer, M.D., Rae, D.S. *et al.* (1990) Comorbidity of mental disorders with alcohol and other drug abuse. Results from the Epidemiologic Catchment Area (ECA) Study. *Journal American Medical Association*, **264**, 2511–2518.

7. Saunders, J.B. and Latt, N.C. (2011) The prevention of alcohol problems, in *Substance abuse: Evidence and Experience in Psychiatry* (eds. H. Ghodse, H. Herman, M. Maj and N. Sartorius), Wiley-Blackwell.

8. Spitzer, R.L., Williams, J.B.W., Kroenke, K. *et al.* (1994) Utility of a new procedure for diagnosing mental disorders in primary care. The PRIME-MD 1000 Study. *Journal of the American Medical Association*, **272**, 1749–1756.

9. McLellan, A.T., Kusher, H., Metzger, D. *et al.* (1992) The fifth edition of the Addiction Severity Index: Historical critique and normative data. *Journal Substance Abuse Treatment*, **9**, 199–213.

10. Hodgins, D. and el-Guebaly, N. (1992) More data on the Addiction Severity Index. Reliability and validity with the mentally ill substance abuser. *Journal Nervous and Mental Disease*, **180**, 197–201.

11. Dennis, M.L., Chan, Y.-F. and Funks, R.R. (2006). Development and validation of the GAIN Short Screener (GSS) for internalizing, externalizing, and substance use disorders and crime/violence problems among adolescents and adults. *American Journal on Addictions*, **15**, 80–91.

12. Madras, B.K., Compton, W.M., Avula, D. *et al.* (2009) Screening, brief interventions, referral to treatment (SBIRT) for illicit drug and alcohol use at multiple healthcare sites: comparison at intake and 6 months later. *Drug Alcohol Dependence*, **99**, 280–295.

13. Passetti, F. and Drummond, C. (2011) Alcohol use disorders – Treatment and management, in *Substance Abuse: Evidence and Experience in Psychiatry* (eds. H. Ghodse, H. Herman, M. Maj, and N. Sartorius), Wiley-Blackwell.

14. Hser, H., Grella, C., Evans, E. *et al.* (2006) Utilization and outcomes of mental health services among patients in drug treatment. *Journal Addictive Disorders*, **25**, 73–85.

15. Ziedonis, D. (2004) Integrated treatment of co-occurring mental illness and addiction: clinical intervention, program, and system perspectives. *CNS Spectrum*, **9**, 892–904, 925.

16. Ries, R.K. (1993) The dually diagnosed patient with psychotic symptoms. *Journal Addictive Disorders*, **12**, 103–122.

17. el-Guebaly, N. (2004) Concurrent substance-related disorders and mental illness: the North American experience. *World Psychiatry*, **3** (3), 182–187.

18. Mee-Lee, D. (2001) *ASAM Patient Placement Criteria for the Treatment of Substance Related Disorders*, 2nd ed-revised, American Society of Addiction Medicine, Chevy Chase.

19. McGovern, M.P., Matzkin, A.L. and Giard, J. (2007) Assessing the dual diagnosis capability of addiction treatment services: The Dual Diagnosis Capability in Addiction Treatment (DDCAT) Index. *Journal Dual Diagnosis*, **3** (2), 111–123.

8.4 Alcohol Issues – What Next?

Griffith Edwards, C.B.E., D.M., D.Sc., F.R.C.P., F.R.C.Psych, F.Med.Sci

National Addiction Centre, Institute of Psychiatry, King's College London, London, UK

It is a privilege to be asked to comment on the three excellent foregoing contributions to the alcohol section of this text. Those statements are highly authoritative and comprehensive, and speak for themselves. It would be inappropriate for any commentator to come in at this juncture and attempt to put a gloss upon them. Instead, this short addendum will take those chapters as the starting point from which to explore some 'what next' types of question. Those chapters between them outline most of what is today known about the epidemiology of drinking problems within the burden of disease perspective, about the treatment of those problems, and about their prevention. But what don't we know? And what to do next?

WHAT FUTURE FOR TAKING ALCOHOL PROBLEMS SERIOUSLY?

The chapter by Patra *et al.* [1] speaks to the capacity of modern epidemiological methods to quantify and rank the adverse impact on the world's health of specified causes of illness. These authors present data that shows that tobacco accounts for 4.1% of the world's burden of disease, with alcohol in very near fifth place; three conditions only rank in damage ahead of these two legal and recreational drugs. One might expect such data to galvanize a vociferous public outcry, and energetic political action. And that follow through would seem all the more probable given that as Saunders and Latt [2] demonstrate in their chapter, the range of evidence-based prevention strategies that could readily be implemented.

But test that hopeful expectation globally against happenings in the real world, and they seem surprisingly seldom to be met. Take as just one small poignant recent example the fact that when the Chief Medical Officer for England advised the government that the price of alcohol should be raised in the health interest, that advice was rejected instantly at the political level with the argument that a tax would unfairly burden moderate drinkers [3].

From the deeper history there are lessons to be learned bearing on how governmental neglect of the drink problem has at times been overcome. When drinking problems of the kind easily discernible on the street become flagrant, a popular movement demanding action has quite often evolved. Such happened in the nineteenth century when in the wake of the industrial revolution America was stigmatized as 'the Alcoholic Republic' [4]: in Britain 'drunk for a penny, dead drunk for twopence' had become the street reality. At the community level in Europe and North America a variety of local initiatives emerged that coalesced into the Temperance Movement with calls for restriction on the number of license premises and ultimately in some countries, prohibition [5]. What needs to be emphasized is the grass-roots nature of that response – it was not in its origins a policy response imposed by high authorities but a matter for instance of praying women gathering on the pavements outside the taverns. Public opinion and popular action are often vital pressures that catalyse political response.

If one surveys present responses to alcohol in the light of that historical experience, the Temperance Movement is still active in some countries but has generally lost its nineteenth-century power. Prohibition is unlikely to be favoured as a response option other than in Islamic countries. Mothers Against Drunk Driving provides an interesting example of a spontaneously-generated pressure group successfully campaigning for action on a specific alcohol-related problem. There are examples of local action by indigenous communities in North America to curb access to drink. An important line of research has explored the effectiveness of community level responses to alcohol-related problems [6].

By and large, however, what stands out from a review of the contemporary scene is the lack of any considerable evidence that people themselves are demanding that something be done about the drink problem. That is the missing link between the evidence-based public-health policies identified by Saunders and Latt, and any follow through to commitment at the political level.

What can be done to strengthen this linkage? That is a large and complex question with no simple, unitary answer. The scientific community has a responsibility to ensure that the relevant scientific evidence is presented in an accessible manner to decision makers, and since 1976 a series of scientific reports have sought directly to meet that need [7]. But that is an example of experts talking to government more than to the people at large. Specialized national professional organizations that take alcohol and drug problems as their remit usually, but with some exceptions, offer a forum for professionals to talk to professionals rather than attempting a reaching out.

One possible strategy for energizing popular support for a public-health response to alcohol would be to encourage those working in the array of treatment services identified by Passetti and Drummond [8], more often to take the catalysing of community action to be part of their business. At present, it seems probable that most alcohol-treatment agencies will in most countries see working on prevention with their local communities, as off limits. If there is in the future to be a widening in their responsibilities, not only will the rule book have to be revised, but new types of skill will have to be learned. What is needed is the capacity to stimulate and mobilize community action that is truly owned by the community, and that enables the community to find its own voice rather than the experts being in charge. One might in due time hope to see collaboration between local initiatives giving rise to a significant national voice that would have to be listened to by politicians.

The cause of alcohol and public health has over recent years at times been actively impeded by the alcohols and beverage industry that has set out numerous so-called 'public interest' organizations as a front for resistance to any tightening of controls over the liquor supply. It has been suggested that alcohol problems related harm can be viewed as an industrial epidemic [9], along with for instance health damages done by asbestos, tobacco and junk food. At present the industry tends to deny the close relationship between per capita consumption and population-level alcohol-related harm.

ALCOHOL PROBLEMS: THINKING ONE WORLD

Responses to alcohol problems world-wide are predominantly modelled on Western perceptions of what should be done about this drug. Western ideas on treatment and prevention of these problems are exported, and that is inevitable given the fact that it is the richer countries that have the long history here of alcohol-treatment experience, and also the power base for the relevant research. An important African journal on addiction is now published and there is certainly some relevant alcohol research emanating from low- and middle-income (LAMI) countries.

Let us, however, examine the validity of the Western exports in this particular arena, while being careful that in raising questions nothing destructive is accidentally done. It could be argued that the two-hundred-year alliance of Western medical professions with the concept of alcoholism as a disease [10], has usefully legitimized damaging drinking as a professional treatment concern. If compassion proposes that treatment should be on offer for the victims of such a disorder, the research reviewed by Passetti and Drummond [8], confirms that such treatment, whether at primary-care or specialist level, is often cost effective. The message of that review chapter is clearly also that intervention can be usefully directed at early-stage excessive drinking, as well as at alcohol dependence. The Western world thus has something to offer toward understanding of appropriate service organization as well as its having a research base bearing on the relative efficacy of different treatment modalities.

If the conclusions outlined above are acceptable, one should on that basis clearly hope to see this knowledge applied and exploited toward the development of alcohol-related treatment in LAMI countries. The aim, however, must be to identify how Western models are to be modified to meet very different cultural, social and economic conditions from those of the countries that originated the treatment technology. Possibilities and problems relating to that kind of technology transfer have so far been little researched in this particular field, but it seems likely that in poorer countries the emphasis should be predominantly on primary-care responses to alcohol with the interventions provided by generalists rather than specialists.

Having acknowledged the potential relevance with the western experience to treatment of drinking problems beyond the base that originated these methods, it may then be appropriate to ask a further and testing question about their export of the wider, overall policy approach to alcohol problems developed in the west to very different national situations. Are we in danger of inviting a recapitulation of our own fundamental policy error in terms of the frequent favouring of treatment provision as a salient response, with prevention relatively neglected? The inappropriateness of that western formula is very evident in countries where support for the development of treatment services at any level lacks resources, but where meanwhile alcohol consumption enjoys progressive and uncontrolled expansion. The relevant public-health situation for those countries is often further harmed by the marketing practices of an industry that refers to vulnerable populations experiencing the disruptions of rapid socioeconomic change, simply as 'expanding markets'. There is again a need to evolve mechanisms that will allow the voice of the people to be heard.

INTERNATIONAL ORGANIZATIONS AND THE WORLD RESPONSE TO DRINKING PROBLEMS

A line of work on drinking problems emerged early in WHOs history and now stretches back for nearly sixty years [11]. Numerous contributions have been made to such activity in terms of Technical Reports and other publications, from teaching and manpower development, advice to governments and research. WPA has also for many years exerted an influence in this field. Those contributions deserve acknowledgement and one cannot doubt that when dealing with those 'what next?' questions and in particular with how the voice of local communities, nations and the world community are to be better heard on what to do about alcohol, WHO and WPA will continue in the future to play an important role.

ACKNOWLEDGEMENTS

I am grateful to Louisa Strain and Jean O'Reilly for expert technical support in preparing this text.

REFERENCES

1. Patra, J., Samokhvalov, A.V. and Rehm, J. (2010) Alcohol consumption, alcohol use disorders, and Global Burden of Disease, in *Substance Abuse: Evidence and Experience in Psychiatry* (eds. H. Ghodse, H. Herrman, M. Maj, and N. Sartorius), Wiley-Blackwell, London.
2. Saunders, J.B. and Latt, N.C. (2010) The prevention of alcohol problems, in *Substance Abuse: Evidence and Experience in Psychiatry* (eds. H. Ghodse, H. Herrman, M. Maj, and N. Sartorius), Wiley-Blackwell, London.
3. The Iguana column (2009). *Addiction*, **104**, 1773–1774.
4. Rorabauch, W.J. (1979) *The Alcoholic Republic: An American Tradition*, Oxford University Press, New York.
5. Blocker, J.S. (1984) *American Temperance Movements: Cycles of Reform*, Twayne, Boston.
6. Holder, H.D. (1998) *Alcohol and the Community: A Systems Approach to Prevention*, Cambridge University Press, Cambridge.
7. Babor, T.F., Caetano, R., Casswell, S. *et al.* (2010) *Alcohol: No Ordinary Commodity*, 2nd edn, Oxford University Press, Oxford.
8. Passetti, F. and Drummond, P. (2010) Alcohol use disorders: Treatment and management, in *Substance Abuse: Evidence and Experience in Psychiatry* (eds. H. Ghodse, H. Herrman, M. Maj and N. Sartorius), Wiley-Blackwell, London.
9. Jahiel, R.I. and Babor, T.F. (2007) Industrial epidemics, public health advocacy and the alcohol industry: Lessons from other fields. *Addiction*, **102**, 1335–1339.
10. Moser, J. (1991) Joy Moser, WHO, interviewed by Griffith Edwards, in *Addictions: Personal Influences and Scientific Movements* (ed. G. Edwards), Transaction, New Brunswick, NJ, pp. 3–24.
11. Edwards, G. (2010, forthcoming) The trouble with drink: Why ideas matter. *Addiction*, **105**, pp. 797–804.

8.5 The Evolving Global Burden of Disease from Alcohol

Joshua Tsoh, MRCPsych and Helen Fung-Kum Chiu, FRCPsych

Department of Psychiatry, Faculty of Medicine, The Chinese University of Hong Kong (CUHK), China

The three chapters in this section are devoted to an examination of the current global epidemiology of diseases and deaths attributable to alcohol, approaches to preventing alcohol-related health harm and the principles of treating and managing alcohol-use disorders.

In the first chapter, Patra *et al.* describe variations of alcohol consumption around the world. Countries are grouped into 6 'World Health Organisation (WHO) regions' according to their geographical location. The prevalence of male/female alcohol abstention and per capita alcohol consumption (officially recorded and unrecorded) for each region in 2003 was retrieved from the WHO online database. The authors describe the disease burdens expressed as disability-adjusted life years (DALYs) and mortalities resulting from various types of diseases and injuries that are attributable to alcohol.

Globally, the leading cause of death attributable to alcohol during 2004 was from accidents (unintentional injuries), which occurred mostly in younger adults. The leading cause of disease burden from alcohol use was neuropsychiatric disorders. Within each region, per capita alcohol consumption was strongly related to the prevalence of AUDs, and the mortality rate and DALYs from a number of major diseases and injuries. Most of the net effects of alcohol consumption on mortalities were grossly negative (like those from cancer, cirrhosis, neuropsychiatric disorders, intentional or unintentional injuries, etc.) with the notable exception that a number of deaths from diabetes mellitus and cardiovascular disorders amongst women within a specified WHO subregion in Europe were prevented. The detrimental effect of alcohol on disease burden was many times higher than the beneficial effect across all regions.

The authors conclude that alcohol continues to be one of the most important risk factors for mortality and burden of disease in the world. With current trends in both exposure to and increases of alcohol consumption in very populous nations such as India and China, a major impact on public health outcomes is expected 'if no additional interventions are introduced'.

Substance Abuse Disorders: Evidence and Experience, First Edition. Edited by Hamid Ghodse, Helen Herrman, Mario Maj and Norman Sartorius.
© 2011 John Wiley & Sons, Ltd. Published 2011 by John Wiley & Sons, Ltd.

In the second chapter, Saunders and Latt outline potential public-health measures to reduce alcohol-related harm at the population level and address the merits and shortcomings of 'universal' and 'targeted' interventions. They note that there is substantial evidence that the total extent of alcohol-related harm can be significantly reduced via successful control measures at the population level, despite the diversity of drinking patterns (e.g. episodic binge drinking vs. chronic heavy drinking as in alcohol dependence). The authors propose that this might verify Ledermann's 'single distribution' model theory of alcohol consumption, which identifies alcohol as a 'socially infectious commodity' and an individual's consumption is considerably influenced at the societal level. In targeted approaches, resources are provided to groups of people who might be the most susceptible to alcohol-related harm, for example drivers, young people and people with pre-existing diseases. They also address the difficulty of implementing such public-health measures as the alcohol industry is a major employer and powerful political lobbyist in the Western world, and its products are a considerable source of tax revenue. Furthermore, alcohol itself is traditionally valued in many cultures; to change this collective view would not be an easy task.

Based on their review of available evidence of studies conducted in the US and Europe, the authors argue that there are six most effective approaches towards reducing alcohol-related harm in society: 1. legislation for a minimum alcohol purchase age; 2. regulation of alcohol's physical availability (by reducing the number and opening hours of outlets); 3. taxation; 4. drunk-driving countermeasures; 5. early (screening) and brief interventions for people with AUDs; and 6. treatment programmes for those people (e.g. self-help groups like Alcoholics Anonymous, and formal psychological and drug therapies). In contrast, convergent evidence has shown that community education (e.g. of school children) and advice and media campaigns are generally ineffective as public-health measures.

Of those interventions listed, measures 1–4 are universal ones. The authors point out that measure 2 often succumbs to commercial/political pressures in free-market economies. The price inelasticity of cheaper alcoholic beverages might reduce its effectiveness of measure 3. Measures 5 and 6 are typical targeted interventions. Evidence of the effectiveness of the former is strong, and it has been applied in a wide range of health and social care settings. For the latter, there are controversies over whether management of the selected group of people identified to have AUDs and willing to be treated could actually bring down alcohol-related health and social harm for the population-at-large in a quantifiable way.

In the final chapter, Passetti and Drummond comprehensively review the treatment and management principles for AUDs that are practiced and substantiated by evidence collected in the heath settings of the Western world. They emphasize that diversified treatment approaches, intensities and settings should be made available to match the spectrum of patients with different degrees of alcohol-related problems, and a 'stepped-care approach' would be a pragmatic and cost-effective way to enable delivery of care in the stated manner.

Moreover, the authors point out that evidence generally defies the notion that treatment intensity and outcomes are directly related. Emphasis should be placed more on the 'extensity' rather than intensity of conditions like alcohol dependence, which is a chronic relapsing disorder and where difficulties with patient engagement and revolving-door phenomenon are commonplace.

The authors also argue that to drive government investment, the beneficial effects of alcohol treatment must be quantified and translated into an 'assessment of potential costs and costs savings', and that the evidence is generally favourable for both psychotherapies and drug treatments (including acamoprosate, naltrexone and disulfiram) across the spectrum of alcohol-misuse and dependence conditions. Finally, they address treatment arrangements for special groups like homeless people, youngsters, ethnic minorities and people with co-morbid psychiatric disorders ('dual diagnosis'). For the latter group, service organization models such as 'integrated care pathways' and 'shared care' have their advocates, but there is insufficient evidence to give preference to one over the other. The authors call for further research into the major cost-effectiveness implications of this area.

THE EVOLVING GLOBAL BURDEN OF DISEASE FROM ALCOHOL

There is substantial evidence that AUDs and the alcohol-related disease burden increase with per capita consumption of alcohol [1]. At the global level, alcohol consumption has increased in recent decades, mainly through decreased alcohol abstention in developing nations. Many of such nations have little tradition of alcohol use at the population level, and few have adequate infrastructure for the prevention, control or treatment of AUDs and the related physical and psychosocial problems. The widespread consumption of unrecorded alcohol (please see the latter part of this commentary) further compounds the problem [2]. In fact, in the low-mortality developing countries, AUDs already rank as the top risk factor for the total disease burden in terms of the aggregate DALYs.

One should also be aware that developed nations have the highest numbers of drinkers (e.g. the average rate of abstention from alcohol in the UK, USA and Australia is only 19% for males and 35% for females), and that 60% of the total amount of alcohol consumed globally (including recorded and unrecorded figures estimated by the WHO) is attributable to these parts of the world. Consumption of unrecorded alcohol is relatively uncommon (except in some of the Nordic nations that have long traditions of producing alcohol at home, but this apparently diminished after those nations joined the European Union (EU) and state production monopolies and high taxation were removed due to EU trade treaties [3]). AUDs are currently the third largest risk factor for disease burden in these nations. The WHO predicted that by 2030, AUDs would surpass ischaemic heart diseases (IHDs) to become the greatest cause of DALYs amongst men in the developed world. The anticipated enormity of the economic impact from health and social costs is a perturbing cause for concern and a strong call for action in both developing and developed nations [1, 2, 4, 5].

PREVENTION IN DEVELOPED NATIONS

Saunders and Latt outline the details of the most evidence-based measures for alcohol-related disease prevention in developed nations. However, there are strong barriers against scaling these measures up to effective levels (as evidenced by, for example rises in the use of alcohol amongst young people in mature markets according to Casswell and Thamarangsi [6]). As Saunders and Latt illustrate, 9 of 12 listed developed countries have no explicitly stated goal of reducing overall alcohol consumption in their public-health policies. In the UK, taxation and pricing measures were scraped despite the strong evidence of their effectiveness. Casswell and Thamarangsi [6] argued that the very unhelpful participation of the alcohol industry in the policy process and the increase in free-trade environments make it difficult for governments to respond adequately at a national level.

Saunders and Latt quote early screening and brief interventions (SBI) and effective treatment of persons with AUDs as the most useful targeted approaches to preventing alcohol-related harm. Boland, *et al.* [7] also commented that there is strong evidence for SBI as a screening and treatment tool and an important first step in the stepped-care approach to problem drinking. However, for such intervention to be effective it should be implemented in a wide range of venues; apart from the primary-health setting, SBI should be performed in general hospital wards, casualty departments, various outpatient settings and even educational and social establishments and the workplace, especially in nations where the prevalence of AUDs are high as in the UK. However, encouraging provision in these settings has been a major challenge; SBI and other AUD treatments have not been priorities for statutory services, which do not regard them as part of their business. The impact of SBI on public health in the UK is also very dependent on political will and the availability of funding.

The notion that effective treatment programmes for high-risk drinkers could have beneficial effects at the population level might appear to be less controversial than Saunders and Latt illustrate, as highlighted by the series of large-scale studies conducted in the past decade (e.g. [8]).

The chapter by Passetti and Drummond is highly commendable in relation to its coverage of the theory, delivery, practice and cost-effectiveness of modern modalities of assessment and treatment for persons with AUD who have multifaceted, varying and often fluctuating medical needs. To this we would like to add that drinkers with co-morbid psychiatric disorders ('dual diagnosis'), identified as the last 'special groups' in the chapter, are actually very common. According to a WHO review of major epidemiological studies undertaken in high-income European countries over 15 years, co-morbidity between mental diseases and AUDs is highly prevalent across countries. There is strong evidence that alcohol is a casual factor of depression; in some European countries it accounts for up to 10% of male depression [2, 9].

More importantly, the US National Epidemiologic Survey on Alcohol and Related Conditions (NESARC) of 43 093 adults found that 40.7% of individuals with a current AUD who sought treatment had at least 1 current independent mood disorder [10]. Mental co-morbidity in people with AUDs within the clinical treatment context appears to be almost the rule rather than the exception. Thus, a comprehensive assessment to screen for such mental disorders should be part of the routine assessment of people with AUDs who seek treatment. We agree that further research into the most cost-effective mode of delivery for mental services (e.g. shared/integrated care) for this group would be very worthwhile in helping to curb the disease burden of AUDs. This is especially the case in light of reviews that have found contrasting or incompatible philosophies and treatment methods across the systems that have led to multiple service gaps for people with dual diagnoses [11].

Furthermore, despite the trend of global population greying, the chapter does not mention the assessment and treatment of elderly people with AUD. Although there is a general impression of an apparently lower rate of problem drinking in late life as compared to youth, standard screening tests in primary health (e.g. the AUDIT [12]) might be less sensitive for the elderly populations [13].

Moreover, experts in the field have predicted that with the current prevalence of alcohol use amongst baby boomers, related problems will escalate as they enter old age. This was at least partially confirmed by the 2005 and 2006 National Surveys on Drug Use and Health (NSDUH) in the US, which assessed a total of 10 953 subjects aged 50 years and older (6 717 subjects aged 50–64 years and 4 236 subjects aged over 65). Nearly 60% of the subjects used alcohol during the past year and alcohol use was far more frequent in subjects aged 50–64 years than grouping those aged over 65 [14]. Specialized service for older drinkers should be considered because the suicide rate is highest in late life in most developed nations, and there is ample evidence that alcohol-related problems, especially with co-morbid depression, are a potent predictor of self-destructive acts amongst the elderly [15], which might indirectly add to the mortality attributable to alcohol.

ALCOHOL USE AND AUDs IN DEVELOPING NATIONS

In the chapters on prevention and treatment, the recommended practices and the supporting evidence are almost all derived from developed Western healthcare settings. Although aggregate alcohol consumption is fast escalating in the developing world, limited research data are available on the regional prevalence and patterns of alcohol use in a vast number of countries. Such data would aid in the formulation of cost-effective treatment strategies within the respective medical and social infrastructures of those countries [6]. The impact of alcohol misuse is worst amongst poor populations and in low- and middle-income countries (LMICs) where the disease burden attributable to per litre alcohol consumed is greater than in high-income countries [16]. Compared with the average volume of alcohol consumed per capita, the highest prevalence of AUDs is in the western Pacific region (with China as the most populated country), South Asia (with India as the most populous nation) and in the Americas [17]. The ecology for the development of AUDs and the underpinning risk and protective factors are poorly understood, which limits evidence-based preventive efforts for AUDs and related health and social harms.

The total consumption of alcohol in a nation and the drinking pattern of its people have multiple determinants [18]. In general, there is a close and reverse association between the alcohol abstention rate and the rise in gross domestic product (GDP) in a country (up to a purchasing-power parity (PPP)-adjusted level of US$7 000). The rapidly rising consumption of alcohol in China and India is likely to be most closely related to economic improvement [1]. Apart from affluence, local alcohol policies, the marketing prowess of global alcohol brands, the proliferation of local alcohol beverage industries, cultural influence, social (including religious) factors, health beliefs and genetic characteristics concerning alcohol metabolism regulation are at play [1, 18]. The degrees to which these potential determinants could be significant remain poorly understood in the developing world, and within vast countries like India and China there might be many regional differences as well, especially between their respective urban and rural areas. However, their elucidation is important because per capita alcohol consumption in pure alcohol for adults is an essential predictor of alcohol-related health and social problems [1].

Holistic estimation of the aggregate level of alcohol use at the national or regional level is compounded by the problem of unrecorded alcohol (defined as alcohol not taxed as beverage alcohol or registered in the jurisdiction where it is consumed), which has a strong presence in countries with lower to middle levels of average income [19, 20]. Acknowledging the inherent difficulty of obtaining a precise figure, unrecorded alcohol is estimated to account for near 80% of the total alcohol consumption in India and some nearby Southeast Asian countries. In Africa the proportion exceeds 50%, and in the Russian Federation and the Ukraine the figure is close to 40% [21]. A five-area study in China yielded a figure of 15% [22].

Rehm *et al.* [19] identified four main categories of unrecorded alcohol: 1. unrecorded legal alcohol products (e.g., the home-brewed alcohol that is legal, or tolerated, in some nations); 2. unrecorded illegal alcohol products (e.g., from illegal production and/or smuggling); 3. surrogate alcohol not originally made for human consumption; 4. recorded alcohol from a different jurisdiction (e.g., as the result of cross-border shopping).

The health and socioeconomic ramifications of unrecorded alcohol are complex and often underestimated. Unrecorded alcohol has social costs in terms of decreased revenue from taxation, reduced employment in domestic alcohol-related businesses, and organized crime being involved in the smuggling and distribution of the product in many nations [3]. Extra health costs derive from a multitude of factors. In India, Russia and African countries, unrecorded alcohol mostly takes the form of home-fermented liquors or distilled spirits made from locally available crops and fruit; quality control is often poor and adulteration (e.g. with industrial methylated spirits, heavy metals, pesticides, etc.) is not uncommon, which has led to mass poisonings [19, 23, 24]. In Russia and adjacent nations, the unrecorded consumption of surrogate alcohols (e.g., from cosmetics, tinctures, or medicinal alcohol) is also particularly widespread; chronic exposure to the variety of hydrocarbon compounds often leads to toxicity in multiple organs [19]. Furthermore unrecorded products are generally higher in alcohol concentration and an elevated risk for hepatotoxicity and cirrhosis is thus anticipated. Overall, unrecorded alcohol is associated with a more sizeable and often underestimated disease burden than the recorded counterpart in low- to middle-income countries (interested readers could refer to Rehm *et al.* [19] for a complete review).

A study of the disease burden attributable to alcohol (both recorded and unrecorded) conducted in 2004 showed that amongst all countries, China topped the list in terms of DALYs (14.9 million), followed by India (8.1 million) [17]. For both countries, the disproportionately high DALYs are attributable to alcohol causing unintentional and intentional injuries that involve young men and women [17].

The overall rate of alcohol dependence in China according to a WHO-sponsored study involving nearly 25 000 adults in five regions during 2001 was 3.8%, and the overall rate of alcohol abuse was 1.1% [22]. The particularly high prevalence of genetic polymorphism of the aldehyde dehydrogenase gene ALDH2 (about one-third of Han Chinese possess at least one ALDH2*2 allele) and the alcohol dehydrogenase gene ADH1B (84 to 92% of Han Chinese possess at least one ADH1B*2) was taken to explain the relatively lower rate of alcohol use in Chinese as compared to people of other ethnic origins (e.g. [25]). The resultant dysfunctional enzymes slow the metabolism of alcohol, lead to the rapid accumulation of aldehyde in the body that manifests as facial flushing and autonomic disturbances and possibly aversion to alcohol. However, the relative contribution of genetic effects to alcohol consumption should be viewed in parallel with the substantial rise in the per capita alcohol consumption in the past three decades, up from 1.0 in the 1970s to 4.5 litres/adult/year in 2001. This growth was simultaneous with the rapid social and economic change of increased urbanization, Westernization and changes towards a free-market economy, especially in the coastal areas, which provided a new and vast market for alcohol beverages for importers and local producers (China is now the second largest producer and one of the biggest consumers of beer in the world) [26]. More recently, research conducted on over 5 000 adults in Shanghai and Beijing revealed that alcohol abuse has become the most common mental disorder, at the rate of 4.7% [27]. The increased sociocultural acceptance of alcohol might have attenuated the 'protective' effect from the prevailing population genotype and might be seen as a form of gene–environment interaction [28]. Studies in Japan show that individuals who are homozygous or heterozygous for the enzyme deficiency and go on to drink have elevated risk of gastrointestinal disorders, particularly oesophageal carcinoma (e.g. [29]).

A review of alcohol use in India conducted during 2005 reported a wide range of prevalence from 7 to 75% in the various states, but there was an overall steady and significant rise in the per capita consumption of alcohol (counting in unrecorded figures) over the years that reached 4 litres/adult/year upon 2005. That growth appears to have paralleled the rapid increase in socioeconomic development, affluence and alcohol marketing in the country, especially its south. More young people and urban women drank than ever before. The proportion of hazardous drinkers in the adult population had reached a sizeable 20%, and the dependence rate was about 4% in the male population [30].

A step towards meeting the colossal public-health challenge was the endorsement and adoption by 37 countries (including China and India) in September 2006 of a set of WHO Western Pacific regional strategies aimed at reducing alcohol-related harm through raising awareness of and advocacy on the issue, the enhancement of the implementation of harm-reduction measures by the health, welfare and law-enforcement sectors, regulation of the production and sale of alcoholic products, and the establishment of mechanisms to facilitate the strategies with relevant data collection and analyses that facilitate the development of nationally appropriate alcohol policies [6].

Moreover, understanding the determinants of the prevalent use of unrecorded alcohol is pivotal to the formulation of evidence-based and cost-effective public-health solutions. Socioeconomic analyses have revealed that its use is particularly common when legal products are expensive (relative to the local living standard), heavily taxed, or limited in availability. Other factors might include the availability of natural resources, labour and technology for small-scale, local production, local economic value (e.g., as a source of employment), public attitudes and the degree of ease with which local producers can gain entry to the market. Also of relevance is the extent to which laws related to alcohol production and taxation are enforced [3, 31]. The restriction of sales or heavy taxation on alcohol as a public-health policy, when used alone, might carry the risk of boosting the 'moonshine' market; they should be coupled with the strict abolition of illegal production and trades, the use of tax stamps on legal products, and public education about responsible drinking and the harm caused by alcohol-related disorders [23, 32]. Taxation policy could also be adjusted so that consumers favour the use of products with lower alcohol content, or unrecorded products become less attractive. The economic principles and models involved are complex, and interested readers might refer to Nordlund and Osterberg [3] or Single [31] for further details. Surrogate alcohol (e.g. that used in industrial products) could be pretreated with strong bittering agents. The sale of medicinal alcohol should be tightly regulated in places where its use as surrogate alcohol are prevalent. Moreover, the complete removal of methanol from denatured spirits would also be a key measure in reducing morbidity and mortality from its toxicity [32].

Health and social packages of care for AUDs designed for developing countries (e.g. [16]), which emphasize both universal and targeted measures to reduce alcohol-related harm, the early detection of AUDs and the stepped-care model of service delivery, await regional adoption, modification and evaluation.

Furthermore, for each region concerned, the health and economic effects from both recorded and unrecorded alcohol should be further studied to inform locally relevant policies. To this end, the local determinants of consumption, volume and patterns of use, and the biochemical content of the alcohol consumed require indepth examination. This is particularly urgent in areas characterized by a disproportionately high rate of cirrhosis [19].

Other than their local contributions, such projects might help to build a knowledge base for other localities and societies in similar situations (e.g. via the Global Information System on Alcohol and Health [GISAH] of the WHO), and may require support and input from international agencies and developed countries [33].

CONCLUDING REMARKS

Pathways for the development and the economic impacts of alcohol-related disorders are still poorly understood in many localities, and further reviews are merited to drive evidence-based alcohol policies. On the other hand, the aggregate health benefit at the population level for moderate drinking is still a contestable subject; further research should be undertaken given the potential to modulate the size of the disease burden attributable to alcohol [2, 34, 35].

In the era of globalized economies, more intensive international collaboration is needed to control the burgeoning disease burden and mortalities from alcohol misuse. The WHO could be a key facilitator in these processes, and information exchanges amongst experts in the field through regional professional organizations like the Pacific Rim College of Psychiatrists (PRCP), and international professional associations such as the World Psychiatric Association will be of particular relevance.

REFERENCES

1. WHO (2007) *Second report/WHO Expert Committee on Problems Related to Alcohol Consumption*, World Health Organization, Geneva, Switzerland.
2. WHO (2004) *WHO Global Status Report on Alcohol 2004*, Department of Mental Health and Substance Abuse, World Health Organization, Geneva, Switzerland.
3. Nordlund, S. and Osterberg, E. (2000) Unrecorded alcohol consumption: its economics and its effects on alcohol control in the Nordic countries. *Addiction*, **95** (Suppl-4), S551–564.
4. WHO (2005) *Updated Projections of Global Mortality and Burden of Disease, 2002–2030: Data Sources, Methods and Results*, Evidence and Information for Policy, World Health Organization, Geneva, Switzerland.
5. Baumberg, B. (2006) The global economic burden of alcohol: a review and some suggestions. *Drug & Alcohol Review*, **25** (6), 537–551.
6. Casswell, S. and Thamarangsi, T. (2009) Reducing harm from alcohol: call to action. *The Lancet*, **373**, 2247–2257.
7. Boland, B., Drummond, C. and Kaner, E. (2008) Brief alcohol interventions – everybody's business. *Advances in Psychiatric Treatment*, **14**, 469–476.
8. Smart, R.G. and Mann, R.E. (2000) The impact of programs for high-risk drinkers on population levels of alcohol problems. *Addiction*, **95**, 37–51.
9. Jane-Llopis, E. and Matytsina, I. (2006) Mental health and alcohol, drugs and tobacco: a review of the comorbidity between mental disorders and the use of alcohol, tobacco and illicit drugs. *Drug & Alcohol Review*, **25**, 515–536.
10. Grant, B.F., Stinson, F.S., Dawson, D.A. *et al.* (2004) Prevalence and co-occurrence of substance use disorders and independent mood and anxiety disorders: results from the national epidemiologic survey on alcohol and related conditions. *Archives of General Psychiatry*, **61**, 807–816.

11. Sciacca, K. and Thompson, C.M. (1996) Program development and integrated treatment across systems for dual diagnosis: mental illness, drug addiction, and alcoholism (MIDAA). *Journal of Mental Health Administration*, **23** (3), 288–297.

12. WHO (2001) *Brief Intervention for Hazardous and Harmful Drinking Manual for Use in Primary Care*, Department of Mental Health and Substance Abuse, World Health Organization, Geneva, Switzerland.

13. Babor, T.F., Higgins-Biddle, J.C., Saunders, J.B. and Monteiro, M.G. (2001) *AUDIT: The Alcohol-use disorders Identification Test. Guidelines for Use in Primary Care*, 2nd edn, Department of Mental Health and Substance Abuse, WHO, Geneva, Switzerland.

14. Blazer, D.G. and Wu, L.T. (2009) The epidemiology of substance use and disorders among middle aged and elderly community adults: national survey on drug use and health. *American Journal of Geriatric Psychiatry*, **17**, 237–245.

15. Conwell, Y., Duberstein, P.R. and Caine, E.D. (2002) Risk factors for suicide in later life. *Biological Psychiatry*, **52**, 193–204.

16. Benegal, V., Chand, P.K. and Obot, I.S. (2009) Packages of care for alcohol-use disorders in low- and middle-income countries. *Public Library of Science Med*, **6**, e1000170.

17. Rehm, J., Mathers, C., Popova, S. *et al.* (2009) Global burden of disease and injury and economic cost attributable to alcohol use and alcohol-use disorders. *Lancet*, **373**, 2223–2233.

18. Moussas, G., Christodoulou, C. and Douzenis, A. (2009) A short review on the aetiology and pathophysiology of alcoholism. *Annals of General Psychiatry*, **8**, 10.

19. Rehm, J., Kanteres, F. and Lachenmeier, D. W. (2010) Unrecorded consumption, quality of alcohol and health consequences. *Drug and Alcohol Review*, Advance online publication. Doi: 10.1111/j.1465-3362.2009.00140.x.

20. Lachenmeier, D.W. (2009) Reducing harm from alcohol: what about unrecorded products? *Lancet*, **374**, 977.

21. Rehm, J., Rehn, N., Room, R. *et al.* (2003) The global distribution of average volume of alcohol consumption and patterns of drinking. *European Addiction Research*, **9**, 147–156.

22. Hao, W., Su, Z., Liu, B. *et al.* (2004) Drinking and drinking patterns and health status in the general population of five areas of China. *Alcohol and Alcoholism*, **39**, 43–52.

23. Gaunekar, G., Patel, V. and Jacob, K.S. (2004) Drinking patterns of hazardous drinkers: a multicenter study in India, in *Moonshine Markets: Issues in Unrecorded Alcohol Beverage Production and Consumption* (eds. A. Hawton and R. Simpson), New York: Brunner-Routledge, pp. 125–144.

24. Haworth, A. (2004) Local alcohol issues in Zambia, in (eds. A. Hawton and R. Simpson), *Moonshine Markets: Issues in Unrecorded Alcohol Beverage Production and Consumption*, Brunner-Routledge, New York, pp. 41–66.

25. Eng, M.Y., Luczak, S.E. and Wall, T.L. (2007) ALDH2, ADH1B, and ADH1C genotypes in Asians: a literature review. *Alcohol Research & Health: the Journal of the National Institute on Alcohol Abuse & Alcoholism*, **30**, 22–27.

26. Cochrane, J., Chen, H., Conigrave, K.M. and Hao, W. (2003) Alcohol use in China. *Alcohol and Alcoholism*, **38**, 537–542.

27. Lee, S., Tsang, A., Zhang, M.Y. *et al.* (2007) Lifetime prevalence and inter-cohort variation in DSM-IV disorders in metropolitan China. *Psychological Medicine*, **37**, 61–71.

28. Luczak, S.E., Glatt, S.J. and Wall, T.L. (2006) Meta-analyses of ALDH2 and ADH1B with alcohol dependence in Asians. *Psychological Bulletin*, **132**, 607–621.

29. Brooks, P.J., Enoch, M.A., Goldman, D. *et al.* (2009) The alcohol flushing response: an unrecognized risk factor for esophageal cancer from alcohol consumption. *Public Library of Science Medicine/Public Library of Science*, **6**, e50.

30. Benegal, V. (2005) India: alcohol and public health. *Addiction*, **100**, 1051–1056.

31. Single, E. (2004) Key economic issues regarding unrecorded consumption, in *Moonshine Markets: Issues in Unrecorded Alcohol Beverage Production and Consumption* (eds. Hawton A. and Simpson R.), Brunner-Routledge, New York, pp. 163–117.

32. Anderson, P., Chisholm, D. and Fuhr, D. C. (2009) Effectiveness and cost-effectiveness of policies and programmes to reduce the harm caused by alcohol. *The Lancet*, **373**, 2234–2246.

33. WHO (2002) *Alcohol in Developing Societies : a Public Health Approach*, Department of Mental Health and Substance Abuse, World Health Organization, Geneva, Switzerland.

34. Collins, M.A., Neafsey, E.J., Mukamal, K.J. *et al.* (2009) Alcohol in moderation, cardioprotection, and neuroprotection: epidemiological considerations and mechanistic studies. *Alcoholism: Clinical & Experimental Research*, **33**, 206–219.

35. Freiberg, M.S. and Samet, J.H. (2005) Alcohol and coronary heart disease: the answer awaits a randomized controlled trial. *Circulation*, **112**, 1379–1381.

8.6 A Timely Review of Alcohol Related Disorders

Nasser Loza, MSc, DPM, FRCPsych and Waleed Fawzi, Dip. Ger., M.Sc., MRCPsych, M.D.

Ministry of Health, Egypt

Providing clinicians with an evidence-based compendium on epidemiology, prevention and approaches to treatment of alcohol misuse is a welcome step. Clinicians and policy makers have had variable views on the definition and management ethos of alcohol use. In many parts of the world addiction is still perceived as a social deviance rather than an illness. Alcohol misuse is sometimes particularly stigmatized due to culture and religion. It is therefore heartening to find this timely publication when many countries are reviewing their mental-health policies and legislations. This is an objective review on alcohol and related disorders.

Patra, Samokhvalov and Rehm in their chapter on epidemiology have pointed to the global increase in the consumption of alcohol over the last decade. A worrying trend, yet there remains significant regional variation with the Eastern Mediterranean Region (EMRO) showing the lowest rates of consumption. As a result, the global burden of disease and mortality show similar regional variation, but remain significant worldwide. A comprehensive review discusses the morbidity wholly attributed or contributed to by alcohol, this data empowers policy makers and clinicians in influencing change and reducing alcohol-related harm on a population level. The burden to society is the important message to the reader, necessitating immediate global action. This is an appropriate introduction to the ensuing chapters.

In their review on prevention Saunders and Latte discussed the compelling evidence in support of universal measures for reducing alcohol-related harm. Government policies do not necessarily follow the evidence. History has shown that policies are influenced by public perception of the substances in question, cannabis being the obvious example, and the furore in the UK over the classification of drugs is a case in point.

Key approaches to prevention, interestingly occur naturally in certain regions of the world due to cultural and societal attitudes. Prohibition is clearly not the answer, but legislation remains a crucial weapon in controlling alcohol-related harm. Availability, cost and other regulatory measures are the main factors discussed. There appears to be less evidence to

Substance Abuse Disorders: Evidence and Experience, First Edition. Edited by Hamid Ghodse, Helen Herrman, Mario Maj and Norman Sartorius.
© 2011 John Wiley & Sons, Ltd. Published 2011 by John Wiley & Sons, Ltd.

support media campaigns and public awareness efforts in prevention of alcohol-related disorders.

In the chapter on treatment Passetti and Drummond outlined principles of management of the spectrum of alcohol problems, whereas earlier clinical guidelines focused on the more severe end of alcohol misuse in an all or none approach. The review of the literature on pharmacological and psychological interventions was extensive and highlights that diversity still exists amongst clinicians as to the most effective approach to managing alcohol-related disorders. Psychological and psychosocial approaches are crucial for preventing relapse and must be tailored to patient needs. The authors discussed the therapies supported by the strongest evidence and highlighted the importance of a pragmatic approach utilizing available resources and tailoring them to individual patient needs. Attempting to review the relationship between alcohol problems and the family on a global scale must be difficult in a world where the definition of family is variable and family breakdown and early independence are on the rise. The authors have successfully summarized various priorities for marital and family interventions. The role of different pharmacological interventions in withdrawal states and relapse prevention was provided and service provision was discussed, highlighting the importance of providing services in the community in different settings as an integral part of an alcohol service.

In conclusion, this global review of the alcohol problem, its magnitude, approaches to prevention and treatment is a timely contribution supporting clinical efforts in the field. Professionals need to standardize their approaches and use the evidence base available, while tailoring treatments to suit individual patients. It is now clear that brief interventions are an important and cost-effective component of a successful prevention and treatment strategy. Furthermore, politicians and legislators will find this section invaluable in supporting their efforts to combat this global problem.

Tobacco

CHAPTER 9

Epidemiology of Tobacco Use

Ilana B. Crome[1], MD FRCPsych and Marcus R. Munafò[2], PhD

[1]*Academic Psychiatry Unit, Keele University Medical School,
St George's Hospital, Stafford United Kingdom*
[2]*School of Experimental Psychology, University of Bristol,
Bristol, United Kingdom*

9.1 HISTORICAL OVERVIEW

The use of tobacco began in the Americas, possibly several thousand years ago, and was introduced to Europe in the late 1400s and early 1500s. The methods of delivery used by Native Americans included smoking, inhaling and drinking of various tobacco preparations, and was associated with medical and religious rituals. In Europe, a ban on the use of tobacco was included in a Papal decree of 1586, although this was on the grounds of preventing the contamination of Christian rituals by Native American religious rituals, rather than as a result of any health considerations. Indeed, tobacco was initially supposed to confer healing properties, and was widely regarded as a medicinal plant. However, health concerns have existed since the 1600s.

Patterns of tobacco consumption in Europe changed from its introduction in the 1500s, where the delivery device of choice was the pipe, through the 1700s, when snuff was commonly used, and the 1800s, when snuff-taking declined and cigar smoking became popular. In the 1900s cigarette smoking became the most common form of tobacco consumption, and this continues to the present day. The invention of the manufactured (as opposed to hand-prepared) cigarette resulted in tobacco smoking becoming a habit adopted by the majority of the population, to the extent that cigarettes were included as part of the daily rations issued to soldiers in the First World War.

There are currently two approaches to reducing smoking rates – a disease-centred approach, and a population approach [1]. The former emphasizes smoking cessation interventions at an individual level, which may be pharmacological or behavioural in nature. The latter emphasizes public health and policy strategies designed to reduce the prevalence of tobacco use within a country (or perhaps across countries, in the case of World Health Organization or European Union initiatives). These two approaches are complementary, and any comprehensive tobacco control strategy will incorporate elements of best practice in both [2].

Substance Abuse Disorders: Evidence and Experience, First Edition. Edited by Hamid Ghodse, Helen Herrman, Mario Maj and Norman Sartorius.
© 2011 John Wiley & Sons, Ltd. Published 2011 by John Wiley & Sons, Ltd.

The recent Framework Convention on Tobacco Control promises to accelerate the adoption of comprehensive tobacco control policies throughout the world [3], emphasizing harm reduction, demand reduction, denormalization of tobacco use (in particular amongst health workers in nations where use in this subgroup remains high), and regulation of the tobacco industry.

Despite these promising advances, however, the global burden of tobacco-related morbidity and mortality remains extremely high. If current trends continue, tobacco use will kill 1000 million people prematurely during this century [2]. This chapter provides an overview of tobacco epidemiology, including smoked and smokeless tobacco product use both developed and developing countries. The recent literature since 2004 was reviewed systematically by searching the Medline and Embase indexing services, which generated approximately 100 references that met inclusion criteria. These were augmented by earlier key references.

9.2 TOBACCO PRODUCTS

9.2.1 Smoked Tobacco

The manufactured cigarette is a highly engineered and efficient delivery device for tobacco and nicotine. Tobacco-industry documents reveal the intention of tobacco manufacturers in designing the cigarette:

> The cigarette should be conceived not as a product but as a package. The product is nicotine. Think of the cigarette pack as a storage container for a day's supply of nicotine. . . .. Think of the cigarette as the dispenser for a dose unit of nicotine. . . . Smoke is beyond question the most optimised vehicle of nicotine and the cigarette the most optimised dispenser of smoke.

A cigarette consists primarily of a paper tube that contains chopped tobacco leaf and 'filler' (stems and other parts of the tobacco plant that are essentially waste, although they do contain nicotine) and a filter made of cellulose acetate. Filler content (i.e. density of tobacco leaf), filter design (i.e. number and size of perforations) and type of paper used can all influence machine-measured tar delivery and how much air is drawn into the cigarette, thereby diluting the smoke. The filter also traps some of the particulate content of cigarette smoke and cools the smoke, making it easier to inhale.

As well as the physical construction of the cigarette, the chemical engineering of the content contributes to its effectiveness. Several additives are permissible in the manufacture of cigarettes, which include sugars to make the smoke milder and, therefore, easier to inhale and flavourings to improve the taste of the smoke. Another group of additives commonly used are ammonia compounds, which raise the alkalinity of cigarette smoke, thereby increasing the concentration of unbound nicotine in cigarette smoke and increasing the speed with which nicotine is absorbed. There are around 600 additives permitted, contributing to around 10% of the cigarette by weight, although the actual number of additives used in different brands and their exact function, is often unknown.

Various changes to the manufacture of cigarettes were introduced in the 1970s by voluntary agreement between governments and the tobacco industry in response to the growing concern about the health effects of cigarette smoking. These led to the introduction of 'low-tar' cigarettes, which resulted in lower tar yields in the particulate phase of cigarette smoke, for example by using filters that drew in more air, thereby diluting the smoke. In 1970 tar yields were typically 20 mg per cigarette, whereas a limit of 12 mg per cigarette was set by the European Union to be achieved by 1997. These figures for tar yield (and corresponding nicotine yield) are generated from data on machine-smoked cigarettes, however and there is strong evidence that these data say little about nicotine and tar yields in cigarettes smoked by humans, since smoking behaviour can be modified to achieve the desired intake. For example, tar and nicotine yields can be increased by puffing on a cigarette more often, by inhaling more deeply or by blocking the filter holes with one's fingers. Such compensatory behaviour suggests that the health benefits of changing to low-tar cigarettes may be less than anticipated. This is supported by evidence showing that the nicotine and tar yields from machine-smoked cigarettes are poor predictors of nicotine intake (and, therefore, tar intake, since the two are highly correlated) in smokers [4].

Tobacco smoke consists of both volatile and particulate phases; the volatile phase includes several hundred gaseous compounds (e.g. carbon monoxide), while the particulate phase is composed of several thousand compounds. Absorption of nicotine from burning tobacco is dependent on the acidity or alkalinity of the smoke. This, in turn, depends on the method of curing the tobacco; smoke from cigar and pipe tobacco, for example, is alkaline and is readily absorbed in the mouth; it is also harsher and therefore less likely to be inhaled deeply. Smoke from cigarette tobacco, however, is more acidic and must be inhaled into the lungs to be effectively absorbed; it is also less harsh, in part because of additives introduced during the curing process.

Menthol cigarettes allow deeper inhalation because they are less harsh, which results in a risk of adenocarcinoma of the peripheral lung rather than squamous cell carcinoma of the bronchus. The nicotine in cigarette smoke, therefore, is inhaled and deposited in the airways and alveoli. It is then rapidly absorbed into systemic arterial blood and reaches the brain within 10–20 seconds. Arterial blood levels of nicotine concentration can be up to six times those found in venous blood levels. This is relevant in understanding the addictive properties of nicotine from cigarette smoke, since while venous blood levels of nicotine after smoking a single cigarette peak after around 10 minutes and then gradually decline, the concentration of nicotine in arterial blood peaks and drops sharply following each inhalation. This strengthens the addictive properties of nicotine absorbed in this way. Tobacco-industry documents reveal two types of cigarette smoker at which menthol cigarettes were targeted; the first includes those for whom menthol reduces negative sensory characteristics of tobacco smoke, while the second includes established menthol smokers who actively seek enhanced sensory attributes, including higher menthol levels [5].

9.2.2 Smokeless Tobacco

Smokeless tobacco (i.e. tobacco that is not burnt as part of the consumption process) contains and delivers quantities of nicotine comparable to cigarette smoking, although lacking the high concentration arterial bolus resulting from inhaling tobacco smoke. The time course and symptoms of withdrawal from smokeless tobacco are also broadly similar to those of cigarette smokers. Nicotine from oral products (e.g. chewing tobacco) and nasal products (e.g. snuff) is absorbed through the mucosa, and nicotine levels rise more slowly than in cigarette smoking. The different rates of absorption from such products means that the addiction potential of these products is probably less than that offered by cigarettes. In addition, the rapid delivery offered by cigarette smoking allows for the fine titration of the level of plasma nicotine in order to achieve the desired effect.

There are different types of smokeless tobacco in use around the world and the health risks related to their use vary considerably. Smokeless tobacco comes in two main forms: snuff (finely ground or cut tobacco leaves that can be dry or moist, loose or portion packed in sachets and administered to the mouth, or the dry products to the nose or mouth) and chewing tobacco (loose leaf, in pouches of tobacco leaves, 'plug' or 'twist' form). When administered orally, the tobacco can also be mixed with other psychoactive ingredients.

There is considerable ongoing debate regarding the capacity for smokeless tobacco products to achieve harm reduction if existing cigarette smokers could be encouraged to switch to smokeless products. Although the harms associated with smokeless tobacco are acknowledged to be less than those associated with smoked tobacco (although certainly not trivial), the argument is complicated by complexities such as whether smokers may instead initiate dual use (thereby increasing total exposure), or whether the promotion of smokeless products may lead to confusing public health messages [6]. Currently the evidence base for the promotion of smokeless tobacco products is mixed [7], but this is largely due to the general lack of evidence. New smokeless products with lower toxicant levels are currently being developed [6], which may have a place in any future harm-reduction strategy, but such strategies remain highly controversial.

9.3   CURRENT PATTERNS OF TOBACCO USE

One in three adults worldwide, equating to over one billion individuals, use tobacco, with the majority using cigarettes (although a substantial minority use other tobacco products, in particular smokeless products). While tobacco production and consumption has declined dramatically in developed countries over the last thirty years, it has more than doubled in developing countries over the same period [8].

Smoking commonly begins in adolescence and about half of those who do not quit will die of smoking-related disorders. Smoking history within an individual can be characterized as consisting of distinct phases including, for example, early experimentation, progression to regular use, development of dependence, cessation and (possibly) relapse. Of course, there is considerable variation within these phases – in particular, many individuals do not progress to regular use and continue as irregular, nondependent smokers (sometimes called 'chippers').

At a population level, cigarette use tends to increase once it is introduced into a society, to a maximum point when public-health strategies then begin to reduce the prevalence of smoking and treatments for cessation become available. Trends for women typically lag behind those of men – for example, in many countries the prevalence of smoking amongst men has peaked, while amongst women it continues to climb [9]. However, these general patterns may differ considerably between countries, in particular between those in the developed and developing world.

9.3.1   Developed Countries

Recent estimates of smoking prevalence in the USA indicate that approximately 20% of the adult population are current cigarette smokers, the majority of which (approximately

80%) are daily smokers, and the remainder (approximately 20%) nondaily smokers. These figures vary considerably by ethnicity (see below), and is socially patterned by, for example, socioeconomic status and educational level. Amongst current smokers, a large proportion (approximately 50%) have stopped smoking for at least one day in the preceding year in an attempt to stop smoking and a majority (approximately 70%) express a desire to stop smoking. These figures represent a considerable decline from the peak prevalence of cigarette smoking, in the 1960s, when almost half of the adult population were current smokers.

These figures are broadly representative of the smoking prevalence in developed countries generally, although in many the prevalence of cigarette smoking in the adult population is higher. For example, countries in Europe, and in particular southern Europe, typically have higher rates of current smoking, and lower rates of attempted cessation (and correspondingly lower rates of expressed desire to stop smoking). For example, the prevalence of current smoking in the United Kingdom is approximately 25%, in Germany it is approximately 27%, while in Greece it is approximately 50%. Indeed, Greece is noteworthy for having the highest smoking prevalence amongst members of the European Union, and all members of the OECD [10]. The reasons for these local variations are often poorly understood, and are likely to result from a complex mixture of societal influences and norms. Nevertheless, the general pattern in developed countries is one of a secular trend for smoking prevalence to be declining over time, as the health effects of smoking have become widely known and evidence-based interventions for smoking cessation more widely available.

It is worth noting that individual countries will demonstrate peculiarities in the prevalence and nature of cigarette smoking that are beyond the scope of this chapter to describe in detail. For example, due to the innovative nature of Japanese society, the tobacco industry was able to strongly capitalize on the introduction of 'light' cigarettes in the 1970s, leading to the very high popularity of low-tar cigarettes (marketed as 'light' or 'mild', despite evidence that they confer no health benefits) in this society [11].

A recent development in some developed countries, including certain cities and states in the USA, has been a ban on smoking in public places. While there have been concerns raised about these policies (such as the potential loss of revenue in restaurants and bars), the impact has generally been regarded as positive, certainly from a public-health perspective. For example, in Italy (one of the first countries to enact a nationwide ban on smoking in public places) the prevalence of smoking declined by over 7% between 2004 (shortly before the ban was introduced, in 2005) and 2006 [12]. The number of countries enacting these bans is growing, and they are increasingly seen as an important and broadly acceptable method of reducing smoking prevalence. Indeed, a recent Cochrane Review on the impact of legislation on second-hand smoke and health outcomes has demonstrated that there is a reduction of second-hand smoke in some groups, a trend for reduction in active smoking and admissions for acute coronary syndrome [13]. However, although the review highlights the possible association, many variables are at play, so there is a need for more epidemiological studies over the next few years to establish the true level/degree of the contribution the ban has made.

9.3.2 Developing Countries

One difficulty with assessing the level of tobacco use in developing countries is that it is in these countries that the use of smokeless tobacco products is greatest, but high-quality data on tobacco consumption only exist for smoked tobacco. Therefore, the best estimates available are likely to be a substantial underestimate of the overall prevalence of tobacco use in many countries (in particular for those in southern Asia and the Indian subcontinent). Therefore, higher-quality data on overall rates of tobacco consumption, incorporating both smoked and smokeless tobacco, are required, although this is complicated by the sheer range and variety of smokeless-tobacco products available in different countries.

In general, rates of cigarette smoking are higher in developing countries than in developed countries. However, these overall rates mask substantial variation in the patterns of cigarette smoking *within* these countries. One common theme that emerges is that sex differences in the prevalence of smoking are considerably greater in developing countries, generally reflecting considerably higher rates amongst males than females. For example, in many countries in the Middle East, the prevalence amongst men may be 50% or higher, but in women may be marginal (less than 5%). Much of the social patterning observed in developed countries is also observed in developing countries, such as the tendency for high rates of tobacco use amongst groups with lower levels of education [14].

Cigarette smoking in the Middle East, Asia and South America may be considered a relatively mature problem, with prevalence rates as high or higher than in developed countries, albeit with considerably more variation between subgroups (e.g. males and females, as described). China, in particular, remains both the largest producer and consumer of tobacco countries in the world. Prevalence in these countries appears to be close to peaking (although not necessarily for females), and there is evidence that public-health campaigns and smoking-cessation initiatives are beginning to have an impact. The Framework Convention on Tobacco Control has contributed positively to tobacco control initiatives in these countries, such as the eastern Mediterranean [15, 16].

The situation in Africa is somewhat different, with prevalence still relatively low in many countries. There is evidence that the tobacco industry regards African countries as a developing market, where tobacco use may increase considerably over the next few years or decades. Although there are attempts to initiate public health campaigns to slow or halt this increase, these are frequently limited by lack of resources. Unfortunately, high-quality data on the prevalence of smoking in African countries is often limited [17], hindering attempts to assess the scale of the problem and, critically, any change in prevalence over time.

One factor that can hinder the implementation of tobacco control strategies in developing countries (and some developed countries, in particular the USA) is the contribution of tobacco production to that country's economy. For example, many economies in South and Central America have become dependent on tobacco production [18]. Finding alternative crops for tobacco countries may therefore be considered an integral part of any comprehensive tobacco-control strategy.

9.4   MORTALITY AND MORBIDITY

The World Health Organization estimates that one third of the global adult population smokes, and tobacco use is the leading cause of preventable death in developed countries [19]. The fact that smoking is unhealthy is now well established in both the scientific and popular literature. For example, approximately 30% of deaths from cancers of all kinds in developed countries can be attributed to cigarette smoking. In particular, there is now convincing evidence that smoking is associated with the development of several specific cancers, and the nature of this association is becoming increasingly understood at the cellular level. This has been shown to be primarily a consequence of the components of the particulate phase of tobacco smoke.

A meta-analysis of cigarette smoking and excess mortality has recently been carried out [20]. Smoking was stratified into light, medium and heavy use, although the description of each varied between studies. For example, light included <10 to <21 cigarettes per day, while medium could cover 10–25 cigarettes per day. Exclusion for illnesses related to smoking might resulted in lower relative risks, whereas confounding factors such as age, sex, race, education, weight, cholesterol, blood pressure, heart disease and cancer resulted in higher relative risks. Combined estimates of the relative risks for light, medium and heavy smokers in men were 1.47, 2.02 and 2.38, respectively, and were very similar for women at 1.50, 2.02 and 2.66, respectively. This clearly indicates that all smokers have substantially higher mortality than average, and that this increases with heaviness of smoking. However, this study did not take account of the severity of dependence and other substance misuse.

The harm associated with smoking is considerable. For example, smoking doubles the risk of cough and wheeze and increases the risk of respiratory infections [21]. Nonspecific symptoms such as tiredness, pain and headache are also more common [22]. Moreover, as a recent review highlighted, smoking exacerbates the clinical course of conditions such as asthma by producing more severe symptoms, worse indices of health status, decline in lung function, and resistance to the beneficial effects of steroid medication [23].

The prevalence of smoking is higher in certain subgroups within the population, and there is accumulating evidence that mental-health problems also increase the likelihood of smoking, as do other factors (e.g. young people, ethnic minority status). The well-established co-morbidity between cigarette smoking and psychiatric illness is a matter of ongoing debate regarding the direction of causation underlying this relationship.

9.5   SPECIAL POPULATIONS

9.5.1   Young People

By age 11 years about one-third of children in England have tried a cigarette, although only 1% smoke every week, and by age 15 years about two-thirds have tried [22]. A more recent survey in the UK showed that amongst 11–16 year olds 20% smoked regularly [24], with more girls now smoking than boys. This has obvious implications for the future. The majority of adults who are nicotine dependent started smoking as teenagers [25]. In the UK alone it is estimated that 3000 teenagers a week start to smoke [21]. Those who start early are more likely to smoke as adults and are least likely to stop. Despite the overall decline in smoking over the last 3 decades, in the UK cigarette smoking is highest in the age group 20–24 year olds. It is estimated that 38% of males and 35% of females in this age group are smokers [26].

It is important to try to understand the predictors of smoking initiation, such as peer pressure, experimentation, mood regulation and familial example, so that these can be influenced in public-health campaigns. Experimentation usually commences between the ages of 11 and 13 years, and a complex mixture of factors determines tobacco use behaviour. These include biological (genetic, gender, age, ethnicity), behavioural or attitudinal (attitudes to substance misuse, religious affinity, educational aspiration), interpersonal (family relationships and friends) and environmental and economic factors (socioeconomic status, neighbourhood unrest). These may operate at any time, and some are more susceptible to change than others. Mental-health problems (e.g. depression and anxiety, impulsivity and sensation seeking, attention deficit hyperactivity disorder, eating disorders and other substance use) also increase the risk of smoking [27,28]. Teenagers who smoke appear to come from disadvantaged backgrounds with poor educational attainment and social difficulties.

Dependence develops rapidly and it has been suggested that the adolescent brain may be more sensitive to the effects of nicotine. Young people who smoke are at substantial risk of developing dependence and achieve dependence at lower smoking rates than adults, which results in a lower probability of quitting smoking in adulthood, and is more likely to lead to medical complications [29–32]. Even those who do not smoke daily can still have difficulty with withdrawal symptoms and quitting.

9.5.2 Pregnant Women

Tobacco dependence poses particular health risks for women, and the rate of lung cancer amongst women has been increasing in the last 50 years. Not only has the number of women taking up smoking increased rapidly, but the rate of decline of smoking has also been slower in women.

If mothers smoke, their babies have increased risk of preterm birth, intrauterine growth restriction, low birth weight, small size for gestational age, small head circumference, digital abnormalities, cardiac septal defects, oral clefts, and cyanotic episodes. Offspring also have 40% increased rate of perinatal death [33]. In the developing world, where the mother's health is compromised by poverty and malnutrition, the impact is even greater. Exposure to environmental smoke is an added consideration [34].

In industrialized countries, between 20 and 30% of pregnant women report smoking [35]. Between 11 and 48% of pregnant smokers quit at some stage during pregnancy [36,37], and in the UK an estimated 27% of pregnant women continue to smoke throughout pregnancy [38]. Up to a quarter of women who smoke before pregnancy are likely to stop before their first antenatal visit without professional help. A further 10% are likely to stop following their first antenatal visit. However, the majority of those who do not quit prior to becoming pregnant continue to smoke. That 27% of women may continue to smoke during pregnancy is confirmed by a recent report in the USA [39]. While many women reduce the use of alcohol, cigarettes and illicit drugs in the third trimester, a sizable proportion report recent use of cigarettes (21%) in the first trimester, and one in seven women use cigarettes in the second and third trimester. In addition, many women resume their use of tobacco after childbirth and resumption is rapid. After 18 months, cigarette use is almost as high as prior to pregnancy.

Schnieder and Schutz [40] conducted a systematic review of population-based studies, identifying those factors that differentiated between women who did and did not smoke during pregnancy. Women of younger age, lower social status, with a large number of children, without a partner, or with a partner who smokes, are more likely to smoke during pregnancy. Whether a woman stops depends on the extent of her habit. Women who smoke during pregnancy are more likely not to attend for screening and early booking. However, many studies relied on self-reported smoking data, which imposes a limitation on the validity of these data – estimates that are biologically validated are approximately 3% higher than those derived by self-report.

9.6   RACE AND ETHNICITY

Consideration of different and dynamic patterns of smoking behaviour amongst ethnic groups is important to inform policy. For example, in the USA Hispanics and African Americans appear to be more responsive to taxation and price control policies [41]. The 'elimination of tobacco related disparities amongst racial and ethnic minority groups represent[s] a major goal in the campaign to reduce the health and economic burden of tobacco use' [42].

Between 1900 and 1964 the use of cigarettes increased from 54 cigarettes per year per capita to 4345, but by 2004 it had fallen to 1747. In line with this, smoking prevalence decreased from 40% in the 1960s to 25% by the 1990s. However, this rate of decline has decelerated – it was 7% between 1983 and 1993, but only 3.4% between 1993 and 2003. The most striking trends have been in adolescents and adolescents and adults in different ethnic groups. For example, in 1976, European, Hispanic and African Americans adolescents had similar smoking rates, but by 1991, the 30-day prevalence rates for European, Hispanic and African Americans were 32%, 11% and 24%, respectively, and by 2004, 28%, 10% and 19%, respectively, were current smokers in the Monitoring the Future Study [43].

For adults, the 2005 National Interview Surveys reported prevalence of current smoking amongst American Indians/Alaskan Natives, European Americans, African Americans, Hispanics and Asians were 32%, 22%, 22%, 16% and 13%, respectively, although the decline was inversely related to the prevalence [44]. The low smoking prevalence amongst Asians is due to a very low rate in women and in African American and European American females it is similar, although the decline has been greater amongst African Americans [45]. The mean number of cigarettes per day varies from 16 in European American to 9 in Hispanics. Age of initiation also varies with ethnicity with more Hispanics (32%) starting before the age of 16, than Asians (13%) [46]. It is recognized that acceptance of smoking and acculturation also influence prevalence and these have to be taken into account when designing control policies.

Cigarette smoking amongst American Indian youth in Minneapolis-St Paul was examined because this population comprises about 40% of American Indians in Minnesota [47]. Since the prevalence is higher than other racial minorities, an understanding of the factors surrounding tobacco use was considered central to appreciation of the impact of control policies. For instance, ban on smoking at home and in public places, enforcement of the law regarding access to youth and tax increases are effective measures.

Tobacco use and cessation has been examined amongst Somalis in Minnesota because half of all Somalis – estimated to be about 25 000 – in the USA live in Minnesota. They are bedevilled by similar problems to other refugee groups such as no health insurance, low literacy rates and poor educational achievement, transportation, difficulty in accessing services [48]. Information was accrued from key informant interviews and focus-group discussions in an effort to estimate the prevalence of tobacco use in Somali adolescents and adults and identify appropriate interventions. Focus-group discussants estimated the prevalence to be between 5–70% for adults and 30–100% for adolescents. Key informants estimated prevalence to be between <1 and 70%. Women were perceived as smoking less, though it was acknowledged that their smoking might be hidden. The Somali community accepts that there is a need to target interventions taking account of psychosocial factors, including for example, water-pipe smoking amongst women.

Smoking prevalence is especially problematic in the Upper Midwest of the USA, where American Indians smoke cigarettes earlier, at higher levels with more severe health problems [47]. In 2006 a cross-sectional study on self-identified American Indians aged 11–18 years was carried out where traditional tobacco use, recreational tobacco use, social exposure (the smoking behaviour of siblings, close friends, adults and households rules), second-hand smoke exposure and policy awareness was investigated. This survey indicated that 37% reported use in the previous 30 days. Use in the 16–18 year olds was three times that in the 11–13 year olds. The overall prevalence in 16–18 year olds was about three times higher than in this age group than in Minnesota overall. While 63% used tobacco for traditional, that is ceremonial purposes, they mostly used commercial tobacco for this. Forty per cent had friends who smoked, 78% lived with an adult who smoked and 44% had a sibling who smoked. Seventy five per cent reported second-hand exposure during the previous week. Twenty five per cent bought cigarettes from a store, while 50% smoked on school property, and 75% heard of someone getting caught at school smoking. Number of friends who smoked was predictive of smoking. However, there was less likelihood of smoking if there were household rules or bans against smoking, or hearing of someone who got caught smoking at school. It is suggested that these estimates may be conservative and not representative of American Indian youth from other areas. Furthermore, the study is cross-sectional and therefore does not describe trends that are necessary to inform policies. Yet these findings suggest points of intervention for example reduction in adults, establish smoke-free environments, enforcement in schools and at point of purchase and use of traditional tobacco for rituals.

Tobacco use and misuse in Aboriginal people is another study outlining the staggering rates of tobacco use in so-called 'First Nations People' in Canada where, at 59%, it is estimated to be 3 times that of the overall population at 20% [49]. Aboriginal youth smoking and use of smokeless tobacco can begin as early as 7 or 8 years of age, that is several years earlier than in the general population. Low income and high unemployment are problems that affect Aboriginal people living in and off reserves. In addition, cigarettes may be bought tax free on reserves. First Nations Elders maintain that the 'recreational' use as opposed to the spiritual, medicinal and traditional use of tobacco, is disrespectful. In the Inuit culture, 70% adults smoke daily and the women have one of the highest rates of lung cancer in the world. As a result, a range of recommendations reached by consensus and aimed at both community-orientated and individual levels have been proposed.

Acculturation and smoking patterns amongst Hispanics in the USA have been studied in a systematic review that yielded 11 studies, all cross-sectional, which met inclusion criteria [50]. Four were nationwide and seven on specific states (e.g. Colorado, California, Arizona, Texas and New Mexico). The term 'acculturation' describes the modification in values, attitudes and behaviours by people in an ethnic group consequent upon their contact with another ethnic group. This model would predict that smoking in Hispanics would adopt the smoking patterns of the host culture. Hispanics comprise 35 million of the USA population, with 40% having been born abroad. The eleven studies had sample sizes between 76 and 8882. Three studies analysed women only, and eight investigated men and women. Acculturation was scrutinized in different ways, for example formal scales, country of birth, language spoken. The findings demonstrated that men (range 24.5–45.8%) smoked twice as much as women (range 11.5–26.1%). A positive association was found between acculturation and smoking in women, that is English language use was associated with higher rates of smoking than Hispanic language use. In men, using this measure, no association was found. When formal scales were used, similarly, a consistent association with acculturation and higher smoking rates was found in women but not in men. It was suggested that the low smoking rates in women Mexico may help to explain this association as women may use cigarette smoking to demonstrate independence and equality. Since rates of smoking are high in men in Mexico, this may explain why there is an apparent absence of association. It is recognized that there are limitations in the assessment of acculturation and that this study may not generalize across the whole of the Hispanic population in the USA. However, the study indicates that specific account should be taken of gender and immigrant status.

Tobacco use and dependence in Asian Americans was also the subject of a systematic review [51]. It is postulated that since the tobacco epidemic has affected Asian countries, this might impact on Asian American immigrants and their children. It is estimated that smoking in Korea and China is about 67% with increasing mortality. From 1980 to 2000, the Asian population in the USA tripled from 3.5 million to 11.9 million. 'Asian' encompasses Chinese, Filipinos, Japanese, Asian Indians, Koreans and Vietnamese who account for 87% of Asian Americans. Asian Americans generally smoke cigarettes and the smoking prevalence rate in 2003 was estimated to be 11.7% compared with 21.6% in the general population [44]. Asian American men (17.5%) are more likely to smoke than women (6.5%). This low rate may be explained by the socioeconomic and educational level of immigrants. The review was undertaken to identify predictors of smoking in this group and enlighten treatment approaches. The review established that publication on American Asians had increased from 1 in 1970–4 period to 94 in 2000–4. Thirty nine studies met inclusion criteria and covered smoking prevalence, correlates and treatment. Most studies were population-based studies with response rates of 43–89%. The rates varied from 0.9 to 56% and were higher for men than for women, regardless of country of origin. South East Asian men had much higher rates than the 17.5% in the 2003 National Health Interview Survey. Chinese Americans had rates ranging from 14.3 to 33.6%. There was also variation amongst women, but when biological corroboration was used, the rates were higher.

In Asian Indian, Pakistani and Thai Americans no relationship with acculturation has been reported. Amongst Chinese American men, there was an inverse relationship between acculturation and smoking, but in women there was a positive relationship between smoking and acculturation. A similar finding was reported for Korean men and women. In Japanese American men there was also an inverse relationship with acculturation and smoking behaviour. There are some inconsistencies in findings which may be related to measures utilized.

When other correlates, for example co-morbid depression, anxiety and alcohol use are examined, some associations emerged. For example, alcohol use has been found to be associated with smoking in Chinese American men and Korean American men [52–54]. Stress and anxiety has been shown to be associated with higher smoking rates in Korean American men [55] and depression in Vietnamese American men [56].

Since co-morbid psychiatric and physical illness plays such a significant role in smoking behaviour, either as a precursor or as a consequence, or both, the next section considers this relationship.

9.7   CO-MORBID CONDITIONS

Key areas that have generated interest over the last few years are chronic ill health in adolescents, psychiatric co-morbidity including other substance misuse, and physical health problems.

9.7.1   Co-Morbidity with Alcohol and Other Drug Problems

It is now well documented that psychoactive substance misuse increases in the high school or teenage years. Tobacco and alcohol are the substances that are the first that children and teenagers try, and use regularly as they are easily available and cheap. In the USA more than 60% of young people try tobacco and about one third will become daily smokers [57]. This is because addiction rapidly develops in young people [58]. However, adolescents experience more positive and fewer negative effects than adults after their first smoking episode. Once they are addicted smokers experience relaxation, arousal, relief from stress and anxiety from smoking [59].

Young people who smoke are more likely to use alcohol and illicit drugs [60]. Adolescents who drink and smoke have a variety of problems such as difficulties at school, deviant behaviour, violence, use of other drugs [61, 62]. In a state-wide survey, whereas one third of current drinkers smoked, 95% of current smokers used alcohol [62]. It was noted by Orlando et al. [61] that 'it is common to drink and not smoke, it is very unusual to smoke and not drink' (i.e. smoking is a marker of alcohol use).

Myers and Kelly [63] reviewed the relationship between cigarette smoking and psychiatric problems and other substance misuse. The association with depressive disorder and disruptive behaviour is a recurrent theme [64]. In clinical samples of adolescents treated for substance misuse, 85% reported current smoking behaviour: 75% were daily smokers and 60% smoked 10 or more cigarettes daily [65] which was more than the general population. Heavier smokers were more likely to report respiratory problems, indicating the rapidity with which health problems emerge. Although rates reduced following treatment, they still remained very high. In a later publication, at 4 years after treatment, 80% of those who smoked at the time of treatment were still smokers. Nonsmoking was related to lower rates of substance misuse [66]. Myers and Kelly concluded that adolescents in treatment for substance misuse are heavy smokers and that this persists after treatment. This is not because adolescents do not want to stop. Indeed, a study by Myers and Macpherson [67] established that two thirds had attempted to quite but 70% started smoking within a month of stopping. These findings emphasize the need for smoking interventions that attach importance to the developmental needs of young people, peer influences, the development of dependence at lower levels of use than adults, perception of the health problems associated with cigarettes in comparison with other substances and the desire to stop. Treatment research is limited in this vulnerable group [68].

A recent review by Littleton and colleagues has highlighted several similar issues by drawing attention to the need to treat nicotine dependence in alcohol 'co-dependence' since it is smoking that is responsible for the development of cancer and cardiovascular conditions, which in turn lead to death [69]. In an alcohol-dependent population smoking is estimated to be in excess of 80% [70] and about 40% heavy smokers develop alcohol-use disorders [71].

The strong relationship between alcohol use in early adolescence and adult smoking prevalence, as well as the association of foetal alcohol exposure with later substance misuse including nicotine, raises the question about the mechanism by which alcohol use during development might influence the development of nicotine use [72,73]. Adult alcohol users are reported to have higher levels of nicotine dependence, greater difficulty in stopping smoking, greater severity of craving [74–76].

There is also evidence that personality traits influence smoking behaviour. A meta-analysis by Munafò et al. [77] indicated consistent positive associations between the likelihood of being a current smoking and both extraversion (reflecting sociability and sensation seeking) and neuroticism (reflecting anxiety) traits. Although observational studies of this kind are not informative with respect to direction of causation, it is notable that the strength of the relationship between these traits and smoking behaviour was comparable, despite these traits being relatively independent of each other. This suggests that different mechanisms may underpin these relationships (for example, sociability and peer pressure for extraversion traits and self-medication of negative affect for neuroticism traits).

9.7.2 Psychiatric Co-Morbidity in Adults

People with mental illness smoke heavily [71,78,79]. The National Comorbidity Survey revealed that whereas the prevalence of current smoking amongst those with no mental illness was 22.5%, the prevalence amongst those reporting a mental illness was 40% [78]. The odds ratio for cigarette smoking those with mental illness compared to no mental illness is 2.7. Current smokers without mental illness smoke 22.6 cigarettes per day compared with 26.2 for those with mental illness.

Anxiety and depressive disorders predict first onset of smoking and the development of dependence [80]. Smoking prevalence also increases with the number of mental-illness diagnoses [78]. This high prevalence leads to adverse health outcomes and adverse events during medical and surgical hospitalizations [81].

In schizophrenics tobacco use is especially high and estimates range from 50 to 80%. A study investigated what role the tobacco industry played in perpetuating the view that this particularly vulnerable group were less inclined to stop smoking because nicotine was used to self-medicate, that psychiatric symptoms would worsen, they were not motivated and even that they had some immunity from tobacco-related illness [79]. Two hundred and eighty records, which had been secret, from 1955 to 2004 were analysed. Three areas were of interest: health effects, the self-medication hypothesis and maintenance of tobacco use in psychiatric settings.

It appears that research on health effects was denied funding or the research that was funded, for example on psychosomatic causes of cancer, was a 'smoke-screen'. Indeed, recent governmental research has clearly demonstrated that schizophrenics are at elevated risk from cancer, cardiovascular and respiratory disorders and are therefore not immune as had been proposed. Similarly, research that sought to demonstrate the advantages of smoking in schizophrenia were funded but it is of interest that they were not published in the scientific literature. In addition, the industry directly and indirectly promoted the use of nicotine even in nonsmoking patients. In short, there is evidence that the industry aimed to influence practice and policy so that the notion that smoking was harmful would be undermined.

[82] reviewed smoking and obesity in individuals with serious mental illness because of the 'enormous public health burden' [83, 84]. Compared to patients without a current mental illness, those who were mentally ill were twice as likely to be smokers and 50% more likely to be overweight.

9.7.3   Physical Health Problems

A systematic review of tobacco smoking and total cancer risk amongst Japanese populations reported in 2005 [85]. A total of eight cohort studies were identified and concluded that current tobacco smoking moderately increased the risk, that is about 1.5 times of total cancer in the Japanese population compared with never-smoking Japanese.

A particular interest has revolved around chronic illness in teenagers [86–88]. This is not only because the normal physical, social and psychological development may be undermined and that may render the young person more susceptible to tobacco use, but also because professionals already tend to be involved in the management of the young person, and therefore are centrally situated to intervene.

Although there are myths that there is a reduced likelihood that teenagers with chronic illness will smoke, prevalence studies suggest that, at the very least, they resemble their peer group in this regard. Although the risk factors may be the same or similar, the overall context in which they come about differ because of the anxieties and the stresses created by the presence of a serious chronic disorder in children and for their parents. For instance, post-traumatic stress disorder is more common amongst cancer survivors than their healthy peers [89]. Studies on asthmatics were contradictory in terms of a positive relationship between distress and smoking [90–92].

Young people with chronic illness may, on the other hand, be more independent since they have to learn how to handle living with a medical condition. Part of this may involve the need to miss school and interact less with children of their own age and thus may not be exposed to the pressure of peers. Perceived risk of vulnerability to the adverse effects of smoking is not always related to self-report of smoking. Poor problem-solving skills and decision making may also influence substance use in adolescents by having an effect on behavioural choices. This is perhaps especially relevant to those with brain tumours, for instance, and the impact of treatment. They may also come to rely on health providers for advice and guidance about aspects of their lives that are not directly related to their illness. Thus, there remains a gap in the specific environmental and personal risk factors for fragile or adolescents at high risk due to chronic illness.

It is noted that advances in medical science and technology has meant that young people with diseases such as cystic fibrosis, sickle cell disease, autoimmune diseases such as rheumatoid arthritis, diabetes and cancer live on into adulthood. This is problematic in that all these diseases have an enhanced vulnerability to cardiovascular or respiratory dysfunction resulting from the disease or its treatment. Adolescent smokers experience slower rates of lung growth and reduced lung function, airway obstruction, increased phlegm production, increased shortness of breath, higher rates of cough and other respiratory symptoms than nonsmokers [93, 94].

As noted by [86] tobacco poses significant health risks. In general, tobacco use may lead to poor nutrition, reduced functional status and poor quality of life [95, 96]. For example, cigarette smoking damages airway cilia and irritates respiratory mucosa, which serve as important barriers against respiratory pathogens for youngsters on immunosuppressive therapy. Smoking may precipitate a decline in pulmonary function in those with cystic fibrosis or sickle cell anaemia. Furthermore, these risks become more severe with advancing age.

Despite insufficient research, it is estimated that the prevalence of smoking amongst at-risk youth is comparable to their healthy peers [88]. Smoking in teens with physical health problems may be 1.5 times more than their health peer group [92]. Smoking in adolescents with asthma range between 20 and 55%, in between 8–31% of those with diabetes smoke and in 15% of those with juvenile arthritis (see [88] for more detailed information). This is an area that requires more research because it is not clear whether the trajectory of development of smoking follows that of health peers. Teenage asthmatics have started smoking at a significantly younger age than those without asthma. Teenagers with cystic fibrosis, sickle cell disease and cancer survivors, however, report smoking at lower rates than their healthy peers. These studies have many methodological problems, for example small samples, age range, lack of control groups, so need to be considered cautiously.

In the USA it is estimated that there are 40 million adolescents between the ages of 10 and 19 [97], that 30% have one or more chronic health condition [98], and that about 20% of high-school students smoke [99]. If it is assumed that this group with chronic conditions smoke less than average, if low-intensity smoking cessation interventions were implemented, about 70 000 teenagers would quit smoking if treated in health facilities.

Healthy teenagers do try to quit: 70% of high-school students have tried once in the preceding year and 44% have tried twice [100]. Encouragingly, health concerns are the top reasons for quitting [101]. However, relapse rates are disappointingly high, with 80% who quit relapsing within a year perhaps because the strategies that they use are not sufficiently focused that may reflect a general feature of adolescent development (see [87]). A better understanding of these issues are vital to inform the best prevention and treatment strategies.

9.8 PROFESSIONAL GROUPS

9.8.1 Health Professionals

Several systematic reviews have been undertaken in healthcare professional groups primarily doctors, dentists and nurses. There are a number of reasons why it is considered important that the nature and extent of smoking behaviour in these groups is understood. By virtue of their training and position, healthcare professionals have a frontline role in preventive and intervention aspects. Since they are knowledgeable about the consequences of early initiation and chronic illness related to tobacco use, it is assumed that they are competent to intervene to prevent or reduce harm at an individual or community level. They are perceived as having a potentially vital leadership role and model for their colleagues, patients and the public. Thus, the extent of their personal use of tobacco and how this might influence their professional role is of great interest. Data on predictors of uptake and cessation in this specific group may inform and influence policy makers on the predicted decline of smoking and associated medical conditions in the general population.

However, despite the fact that health professionals should have access to information about the risks of smoking and a key role in the management of smoking and the morbidity associated with smoking, this knowledge does not inevitably translate into a lower prevalence of use. Smith and Leggat [102,103] conducted an international systematic review on tobacco-smoking habits in medical students. Prevalence varies widely in male students from 3% in the USA to 58% in Japan, with Spain and Greece having rates of about 40%. Males usually show higher rates than females, and in some countries (e.g. China, Thailand, Malaysia and India) no females reported smoking at all. These generally reflect current population trends. Rates tend to increase as students progress through their course. The authors discerned two trends: most developed countries have witnessed a decline, while most developing countries have faced an increase. It is not clear precisely what determines use whether it be social, cultural or parental patterns of use. Understanding of the determinants in this group is important to inform public health policy. Education is an important first step and it is not being comprehensively undertaken in medical schools.

Physicians appear to give up smoking before other health professional groups, and fewer smoke compared with dentists and nurses. There may be some differences between grades and specialities in medicine, although this evidence is not been consistent [104–111]. Whether smoking influences the physician's propensity to give anti-smoking advice is an important issue and some studies have acknowledged that there is a positive relationship between nonsmoking status and taking a smoking history and providing advice, although this is not always the case [102, 103]. As discussed later in relation to nursing students, cross sectional studies indicate wide variation in smoking prevalence [112, 113, 114, 115].

Despite the fact that health professionals should have access to information about the risks of smoking and a key role in the management of smoking and the morbidity associated with smoking, this knowledge does not inevitably translate into a lower prevalence of use. Smith and Leggat [102,103] conducted an international systematic review on tobacco smoking habits in medical students. Sixty six papers met inclusion criteria the most common countries where research was conducted being India, USA, Australia, Japan, Pakistan Turkey and the UK. Median number of students was 407 and median response rate was 90%. Prevalence varies widely in male students from 3% in the USA to 58% in Japan, with Spain and Greece having rates of about 40%. Males usually predominate over females and in some countries (e.g. China, Thailand, Malaysia and India) no females were reported at all. These generally reflect current population estimates. Rates tend to increase as students progress through their course though there were some fluctuations. It is not clear precisely what determines, use whether it be social, cultural or parental patterns of use. Understanding of the determinants in this group is important to inform public-health policy. Education is an important first step and it is not being comprehensively undertaken in medical schools, price increases and support for students.

Research indicated that from 1959 to the mid-1990s, the prevalence of smoking in physicians in the USA decreased from 40% to under 10%, as it did in the Scandinavian countries over a similar period [103]. A classic and unique study on British doctors contributed substantially to the epidemiology of smoking behaviour and consequences [117, 118]. Smith and Leggat [103], who described the longitudinal study by Doll and Hill [117] as 'pioneering' that 'researchers would do well to follow', carried out an international systematic review of tobacco smoking in the medical profession from 1974 to 2004. Eighty one studies met inclusion criteria. Response rates varied from 27 to 100%. Sample sizes ranged from 49 to 10 807. The majority of studies (52/81) were conducted from 1990. The USA produced the most, that is 18 studies; 7 emanated from Japan, 6 from Italy, 5 each from the UK and Australia and 3 from New Zealand. The authors discerned two trends: most developed countries have witnessed a decline, while most developing countries have faced an increase. However, this is not straightforward. For example, while rates in the USA, Australia and New Zealand are lower than 10%, in the UK the Doll and Hill study revealed that British physicians continued to use pipes and cigars and thus the decline in overall tobacco use from 1951 to 1990 was from 62 to 18%. The lowest rates reported were between 2 and 3% in the USA, UK and Australia. Yet in Italy, Japan and France the rate is consistently over 25%. However, in China, Estonia, Bosnia/Herzegovina and Turkey rates are high and increasing. Rates between 40 and 49% are reported from Greece, China, Japan and India and about one third in Kuwait and United Arab Emirates.

The gender profile is worthy of note: smoking prevalence rate was found to be 61% of male physicians in China and 34% of female physicians in Italy. Twenty-five per cent of French female physicians smoke, but smoking amongst female physicians is virtually unknown in China, Hong Kong, Wales and Malaysia, but in Italy more women than men smoke and in the USA, Australia and Israel there appears to be no difference between the genders.

Physicians appear to give up smoking before other professional groups and fewer smoke compared with dentists and nurses. There may be some differences between grades and specialities in medicine as there have been a series of reports some of which have not been consistent. Consultants may smoke more than trainees [104], general practitioners smoke more than specialists [105, 106], but some reports suggest that psychiatrists [107, 108], obstetricians [109, 110] and surgeons [110, 111] were more likely to smoke. Whether smoking influences the physician's propensity to give anti-smoking advice is key and some studies have acknowledged that there is a positive relationship between nonsmokers and taking a smoking history and provision of advice, although this is not always the case [102, 103].

In comparison with other health professionals, doctors appear to smoke less, as do dentists. Smith and Leggat [116,119] also studied dental students and dentists using systematic review methodology. Twenty seven studies from 19 countries, two of which were longitudinal in design. The studies covered 1970–2006. Eight studies were undertaken in Europe, five in the US, 3 in the UK, two from Canada and India and one from Australia, Bagladesh, Brazil, Ireland, Jordan, Saudi Arabia and Japan. Sample sizes varies from 41 to 1266 and response rates from 50 to 99%. In some countries smoking rates were low, for example Canada (3%), USA (4%), Brazil (6%) and UK (7%), whereas in India (10%), and Australia (13%) rates were under 20%. Almost half the students smoked in Greece (47%), Serbia (43%), and a third in Hungary (34%) and France (33%). Studies have identified a decrease in some countries (e.g. US, Canada, Norway and India). Men smoked more than women in Asian and Middle Eastern countries but in Greece and Serbia women smoked more than men. Although some studies identified a trend to increase smoking with year of study, this was not uniform and some studies demonstrated a decline as students progressed through their course Newbury Birch et al. [120]. In Australia, Canada, UK and USA smoking rates were lower than in the general population where it is about 25%, in contrast to Greece, Serbia, Hungary and France where smoking rates for the general population are about 35%.

The study on dentists [119] reviewed 35 studies, half of which were published since 2000. Ten manuscripts were from the USA, 9 from Europe, 7 from Britain, 5 from Australia and four from other countries. Sample sizes were 33–2628 and response rates 8–90%. The lowest rate was in the USA (1%), and rates were also low in Thailand (2%), Finland (3%), Australia (3%) and Canada (4%). In Jordan and Italy rates were high in that one third of dentists were smoking. It should be noted that the general population rates are high in these countries at 29 and 25%, respectively. Never smokers ranged from 55 to 82% but 22% smokers had no intention of stopping. Males smoked at higher rates than females and older dentists smoked more than younger dentists.

Smith's [121] study in nursing students was based on the rationale that nurses have a crucial role to play in advice, information and intervention. Nurses' willingness to be proactively involved in catalysing change is related to their own smoking behaviour. Thirty five articles met inclusion criteria. Eleven were cross-sectional, 16 on single or multiple grades of students that is did not target the whole school and 5 were longitudinal. Studies were conducted in developed countries in the main.

Cross-sectional studies demonstrated wide variation in smoking prevalence. Although sample sizes ranged from 96 to 3866, 6/11 studies had sample sizes of over 400. Response rates above 69% were seen in all except 2 studies. Some studies indicate that smoking increased with year of study and some that it decreased. Prevalence was lowest in students who replied to the first mailing [115]. Strangely, 75% students considered smoking cessation interventions would be successful [115] and asthmatic nurses smoked more than nonasthmatic control students [115].

Single-grade or multiple-grade studies had sample sizes between 100 and 914 and response rates from 47 to 100%. Similarly, there was wide variation in smoking rates depending on the country and year of study. While in Australia 65% of nursing students were smokers [122], in Italy approximately half of nursing students smoke [123, 124] and in Nigeria hardly any (1%) [125]. Interestingly, public-health nursing students had lower rates than midwifery students in Japan [126]. These studies highlighted some relationships with nursing students who smoked, that is initiation of smoking prior to commencement of studies, friends who smoked, lack of conviction that nurses were role models and less likelihood of participation in harm reduction or cessation.

Of the 5 longitudinal studies identified, 4 demonstrated an increase (range 2–10% over one to two years) in smoking and one a decrease of 2% [127]. Clement et al. [127] also reported that between 10 and 12% nursing students smoked so that nonsmokers were considerably higher than in the general population. The review concluded that standardization of definitions of smoking would aid future work on this topic given the importance of prevention of initiation and cessation in nursing students, their potential role as health professionals and the relationship between their own behaviour and reluctance to intervene. The spectrum of nonsmoking policies, support peer as well as the availability of interventions was required.

9.8.2 Military Groups

Another professional group subjected to stress are the military [128]. Bachman et al. [129] had described how high-school students who entered the military were over twice as likely to smoke compared with those who entered college. Although initially perceived as a luxury item, soldiers under traumatic conditions used cigarettes to cope with the unpalatable aspects of war. Indeed, cigarettes were part of rations, although this practice was eventually stopped.

Nelson and Pederson [128] reviewed all types of tobacco in active duty USA military personnel from 1991 to 2006. Forty one studies met the inclusion criteria, twenty nine of which were on prevalence and factors associated with tobacco use. This study reported that cigarette smoking declined from >50% in 1980 to about 33% in 2005, though there had been an increase between 1998 and 2002. While the prevalence of current smokers aged 18–25 in the general population was 28%, amongst the military it was 41%. Furthermore, alternative forms of tobacco use may be increasing, especially in cigarette smokers. As in the general population, the use of tobacco is associated with having peers who smoke, and risky behaviours such as binge drinking and unprotected sex. European Americans were more likely to smoke, as were males, younger members, and those with less formal education. The fact that many young tobacco users start use after entering the military raises concerns about the impact of the range of stresses (separation, conflict, anxiety, exposure to combat) inherent in the role might precipitate or exacerbate smoking. Further research into the prevalence, pathways to use, prevention, intervention and current policies was recommended, which is of substantial relevance to the general population and professional groups working under unpredictable and stressful conditions.

9.9 METHODOLOGICAL ISSUES – CONSIDERATIONS FOR FUTURE RESEARCH

There are some common themes that resonate throughout the research described above.

The limitations of cross-sectional research are emphasized, as are studies with small sample sizes. Samples are sometimes convenience rather than random with differing length of follow up periods. The definition of what constitutes a 'current' smoker varies as does the type and quantification of cigar, pipe and smokeless tobacco use. Problematic too, are the fact the self-report and the ability to recall information that may affect the validity of data collection. Lack of biochemical validation of usage is a major contributor to inaccuracies in assessment of smoking status. Furthermore, the importance of differentiating varying degrees of dependence on tobacco is acknowledged. Thus, quantity, frequency and severity need to be integrated into any assessment of use. Tobacco use can no longer be studied in isolation from other substances of misuse given the high levels of co-morbidity. Finally, since only publications in the English language were included, a bias against developing countries, many of which have been encumbered by increasing trends, may result. Consideration of these drawbacks is essential if methodologies are improved, thus generating enhanced capacity to discern trends and predictors of smoking behaviour. This, in turn, will offer top-quality prevention and intervention initiatives linked to variations in subgroups within diverse communities, countries and continents.

REFERENCES

1. Frohlich K. (2008) Is tobacco use a disease? *Canadian Medical Association Journal* **179**, 880–882.
2. Frieden TR, Bloomberg MR (2007) How to prevent 100 million deaths from tobacco. *Lancet* **369**, 1758–1761.

3. Chapman S. (2008) Global perspective on tobacco control. Part II. The future of tobacco control: making smoking history? *International Journal of Tuberculosis and Lung Disease* **12**, 8–12.

4. Jarvis, M. J., R. Boreham, *et al.* (2001) Nicotine yield from machine-smoked cigarettes and nicotine intakes in smokers: evidence from a representative population survey. *Journal of the National Cancer Institute* **93**, 134–138.

5. Kreslake JM, Wayne GF *et al.* (2008) The menthol smoker: tobacco industry research on consumer sensory perception of menthol cigarettes and its role in smoking behavior. *Nicotine and Tobacco Research* **10**, 705–715.

6. Hatsukami DK, Ebbert JO *et al.* (2007) Changing smokeless tobacco products new tobacco-delivery systems. *American Journal of Preventive Medicine* **33**, S368–378.

7. Tomar SL (2007) Epidemiologic perspectives on smokeless tobacco marketing and population harm. *American Journal of Preventive Medicine* **33**, S387–S397.

8. Davis RM, Wakefield R *et al.* (2007) The Hitchhiker's Guide to Tobacco Control: a global assessment of harms, remedies, and controversies. *Annual Review of Public Health* **28**, 171–194.

9. Slama K. (2008) Global perspective on tobacco control. Part I. The global state of the tobacco epidemic. *International Journal of Tuberculosis and Lung Disease* **12**, 3–7.

10. Vardavas CI, Kafatos AG, (2006) Greece's smoking policy: another myth? *The Lancet*, **367**(9521):1485–1486.

11. Assunta M, Chapman S (2008) The lightest market in the world: light and mild cigarettes in Japan. *Nicotine and Tobacco Research* **10**, 803–810.

12. Gorini G, Chellini E *et al.* (2007) What happened in Italy? A brief summary of studies conducted in Italy to evaluate the impact of the smoking ban. *Annals of Oncology* **18**, 1620–1622.

13. Callinan, JE, Clarke A, Doherty K, Kelleher C, (2010) Legislative smoking bans for reducing secondhand smoke exposure, smoking prevalence and tobacco consumption The Cochrane Collaboration. Published by John Wiley & Sons, Ltd

14. Gupta PC, Ray CS (2007) Tobacco, education & health. *Indian Journal of Medical Research* **126**, 289–299.

15. El Awa F (2008) Tobacco control in the Eastern Mediterranean Region: overview and way forward. *Eastern Mediterranean Health Journal* **14**, S123–131.

16. Sussman SP, Pokhrel P *et al.* (2007) Tobacco control in developing countries: Tanzania, Nepal, China, and Thailand as examples." *Nicotine and Tobacco Research* **9**, S447–S457.

17. Nturibi EM, Kolawole AA *et al.* (2009) Smoking prevalence and tobacco control measures in Kenya, Uganda, the Gambia and Liberia: a review. *International Journal of Tuberculosis and Lung Disease* **13**, 165–170.

18. Muller F, Wehbe L (2008) Smoking and smoking cessation in Latin America: a review of the current situation and available treatments. *International Journal of Chronic Obstructive Pulmonary Disease* **3**, 285–293.

19. Dani JA, Harris RA. (2005) Nicotine addiction and co-morbidity with alcohol abuse and mental illness. *Nature Neuroscience* **8**, 1465–1470.

20. Shavelle RM, Paculdo DR, Strauss DJ *et al.* (2008) Smoking habit and mortality: a meta-analysis. *Journal of Insurance Medicine* **40**, 170–178.

21. Royal College of Physicians (1992) *Smoking and the Young*. Royal College of Physicians: London.

22. Woodhouse K. (2004) Young people and smoking. In Crome I, Ghodse H, Gilvarry E *et al.* (eds) *Young People and Substance Misuse*. Gaskell: London, pp 114–128.

23. Thomson NC, Chauduri R, Livingston E. (2004) Asthma and cigarette smoking. *European Respiratory Journal* **24**, 822–833.

24. Action on Smoking and Health (2009) *Essential Information on Young People and Smoking*. At http://www.ash.org.uk/files/documents/ASH_108.pdf (Accessed 21 August 2009).

25. Holden D, Hund LM, Gable JM. (2003) *Youth Tobacco Cessation: Results from the 2000 National Youth Survey*. At http://www.youthtobaccocessation.org/publications/reports.asp#pub7 (Accessed 21 August 2009).

26. ONS (2008/9) Living in Britain

27. Tyas SL, Pederson LL. (1998) Psychosocial factors related to adolescent smoking: a critical review of the literature. *Tobacco Control* **7**, 409–420.

28. Patton GC, Carlin JB, Coffey C *et al*. (1998) Depression, anxiety and smoking initiation. *American Journal of Public Health* **90**, 1518–1522.

29. DiFranza JR, Savageau JA, Fletcher K *et al*. (2002) Measuring the loss of autonomy over nicotine use in adolescents: the DANDY study. *Archives of Pediatric and Adolescent Medicine* **156**, 397–403.

30. Wellman RJ, DiFranza JR, Savageau JA, *et al*. (2004) Short term patterns of early smoking acquisition. *Tobacco Control* **13**, 251–257.

31. Khuder SA, Dayal HH, Mutgi AB. (1999) Age at smoking onset and its effect on smoking cessation. *Addictive Behaviors* **24**, 673–677.

32. Karp I, O'Loughlin J, Paradis G *et al*. (2005) Smoking trajectories of adolescent novice smokers in a longitudinal study of tobacco use. *Annals of Epidemiology* **15**, 445–452.

33. Tobacco Control Resource Centre (2006) *Smoking and Child Health: A review for paediatricians*. TCRC: Edinburgh.

34. Samet JM, Yang G. (2001) Passive smoking, women and children. In: *Women in the Tobacco Epidemic*. World Health Organisation: Geneva.

35. Lumley J, Oliver SS, Chamberlain C *et al*. (2004) Interventions for promoting smoking cessation during pregnancy. Cochrane Database of Systematic Reviews 4. Art. No.: CD001055. DOI: 10.1002/14651858.CD001055.pub2.

36. Cnattingius S, Lindmark G, Mierik O. (1992) Who continues to smoke while pregnant? *Journal of Epidemiology and Community Health* **46**, 218–221.

37. Isohanni M, Oja H, Moilanen I *et al*. (1995) Smoking or quitting during pregnancy: Association with background and future social factors. *Scandinavian Journal of Social Medicine* **23**, 32–38.

38. Owen LA, Penn GL. (1999) *Smoking and Pregnancy: A Survey of Knowledge, Attitudes and Behaviour, 1992–1999*. Health Education Authority: London.

39. National Survey on Drug Use and Health (NSDUH) (2009) *Substance Use Among Women During Pregnancy and Following Childbirth*. At http://www.oas.samhsa.gov/2k9/135/PregWoSubUse.htm (Accessed 21 August 2009).

40. Schneider S, Schütz J. (2008) Who smokes during pregnancy? A systematic literature review of population-based surveys conducted in developed countries between 1997 and 2006. *European Journal of Contraception and Reproductive Health Care* **13**, 138–147.

41. Tauras JA. (2007) Differential impact of state tobacco control policies among race and ethnic groups. *Addiction* **102**, 95–103.

42. US Department of Health and Human Services (2000) *Reducing Tobacco Use: A report of the Surgeon General*. US Department of Health and Human Services: Atlanta, GA.

43. Johnston L, O'Malley P, Bachman J *et al*. (2004) Cigarette smoking among American teens continues to decline, but more slowly than in the past. Available at: http://www.monitoringthefuture.org/pressreleases/04cigpr_complete.pdf (Accessed 21 August 2009).

44. Centers for Disease Control and Prevention (CDC) (2005) Tobacco use among adults – United States. *Morbidity and Mortality Weekly Report* **55**, 1145–1148.

45. American Lung Association (2006) *Trends in Tobacco Use Epidemiology and Statistical Unit Research Programme Services*. At http://www.lungusa.org/atf/cf/{7A8D42C2-FCCA-4604-8ADE-7F5D5E762256}/TREND_TOBACCO_JUNE07.PDF (Accessed 21 August 2009).

46. Adams P, Scheonborn CA. (2006) *Health Behaviours of Adults, United States 2002–2004*. At http://www.cdc.gov/nchs/data/series/sr_10/sr10_230.pdf (Accessed 21 August 2009).

47. Forster JL, Widome R, Bernat DH. (2007) Policy interventions and surveillance as strategies to prevent tobacco use in adolescents and young adults. *American Journal of Preventive Medicine* **33**, S335–S339.

48. Giuliani KKW, Mire OA, Jama S *et al.* (2008) Tobacco use and cessation among Somalis in Minnesota. *American Journal of Preventive Medicine* **35**, S457–S462.

49. Canadian Paediatric Society (CPS) (2006) Use and misuse of tobacco among Aboriginal peoples HYPERLINK "http://www.cps.ca/english/statements/II/FNIH06-01.htm" \l "COMMITTEE" \t "_blank" First Nations and Inuit Health Committee, Paediatric Child Health;11(10):681–5.

50. Bethel JW, Schenker MB. (2005) Acculturation and smoking patterns among Hispanics: a review. *American Journal of Preventive Medicine* **29**, 143–148.

51. Kim SS, Ziedonis D, Chen KW. (2007) Tobacco use and dependence in Asian Americans: a review of the literature. *Nicotine and Tobacco Research* **9**, 169–184.

52. Yu ES, Chen EH, Kim KK *et al.* (2002) Smoking among Chinese Americans: behaviour, knowledge and beliefs. *American Journal of Public Health* **92**, 1007–1012.

53. Kim KK, Yu ES, Chen EH *et al.* (2000) Smoking behaviour, knowledge and beliefs among Korean Americans. *Cancer Practice* **8**, 223–230.

54. Juon HS, Kim M, Han H *et al.* (2003) Acculturation and cigarette smoking among Korean American men. *Yonsei Medical Journal* **4**, 875–882.

55. Lew R, Moskowitz JM, Wismer BA *et al.* (2001) Correlates of cigarette smoking among Korean American adults in Alameda County, California. *Asian American and Pacific Islander Journal of Health* **6**, 13–24.

56. Wiecha JM, Lee V, Hodgkins JH. (1998) Patterns of smoking, risk factors for smoking, and smoking cessation among Vietnamese men in Massachusetts (United States). *Tobacco Control* **7**, 27–34.

57. Henningfeld JE, Moolchan ET, Zeller M. (2003) Regulatory strategies to reduce tobacco addiction in youth. *Tobacco Control* **12**, i14–i24.

58. DiFranza JR, Rigotti NA, McNeill AD *et al.* (2000) Initial symptoms of nicotine dependence in adolescents. *Tobacco Control* **9**, 313–319.

59. Benowitz NL. (1999) Nicotine addiction. *Primary Care* **26**, 611–631.

60. Vega WA, Gil AG. (2005) Revisiting drug progression: long range effects of early tobacco use. *Addiction* **100**, 1358–1369.

61. Orlando M, Tucker JS, Ellickson PL *et al.* (2005) Concurrent use of alcohol and cigarettes from adolescence to young adulthood: an examination of developmental trajectories and outcomes. *Substance Use and Misuse* **40**, 1051–1069.

62. Hoffman JH, Welte JW, Barnes GM. (2001) Co-occurrence of alcohol and cigarette use among adolescents. *Addictive Behaviours* **26**, 63–78.

63. Myers MG, Kelly JF. (2006) Cigarette smoking among adolescents with alcohol and other drug use problems. *Alcohol Research and Health* **29**, 221–227.

64. Brown RA, Lewinsohn PM, Seeley JR *et al.* (1996) Cigarette smoking, major depression and other psychiatric disorder among adolescents. *Journal of the American Academy of Child and Adolescent Psychiatry* **35**, 1602–1610.

65. Myers MG, Brown SA. (1994) Smoking and health in substance abusing adolescents: a two year follow up. *Pediatrics* **93**, 561–566.

66. Myers MG, Brown SA. (1997) Cigarette smoking for years following treatment for adolescent substance abuse. *Journal of Child and Adolescent Substance Abuse* **7**, 1–15.

67. Myers MG, Macpherson L. (2004) Smoking cessation efforts among substance abusing adolescents. *Drug and Alcohol Dependence* **73**, 209–213.

68. Myers MG, Brown SA. (2005) A controlled study of a cigarette smoking cessation intervention for adolescents in substance abuse treatment. *Psychology of Addictive Behaviours* **19**, 230–233.

69. Littleton J, Barron S, Prendergast M, *et al.* (2007) Smoking kills (alcoholics)! Shouldn't we do something about it? *Alcohol and Alcoholism* **42**, 167–173.

70. Miller NS, Gold MS. (1998) Comorbid cigarette and alcohol addiction: epidemiology and treatment. *Journal of Addictive Diseases* **17**, 55–66.

71. Grant B, Hasin DS, Chou PS *et al.* (2004) Nicotine dependence and psychiatric disorders in the United States. *Archives of General Psychiatry* **61**, 1107–1115.

72. Paavola M, Vartiainen E, Haukkala A. (2004) Smoking, alcohol use and physical activity: a 13 year longitudinal study ranging from adolescence into adulthood. *Journal of Adolescent Health* **35**, 238–244.

73. Obot IS, Wanger FA, Anthony JC. (2001) Early onset and recent drug use among children of parents with alcohol problems: data from a national epidemiological survey. *Drug and Alcohol Dependence* **65**, 1–8.

74. John U, Meyer C, Rumpf HJ, *et al.* (2003) Probabilities of alcohol high risk drinking, abuse or dependence estimated on grounds of tobacco smoking and nicotine dependence. *Addiction* **98**, 805–814.

75. Novy P, Hughes JR, Callas P. (2001) A comparison of recovering alcoholic and nonalcoholic smokers. *Drug and Alcohol Dependence* **65**, 17–23.

76. Hillemacher T, Bayerlein K, Wilhelm J *et al.* (2006) Nicotine dependence is associated with compulsive alcohol craving. *Addiction* **101**, 892–897.

77. Munafó MR, Zetterler JI, Clark TG. (2007) Personality and smoking status: a meta-analysis. *Nicotine and Tobacco Research* **9**, 405–413.

78. Lasser K, Boyd JW, Woolhamdler S *et al.* (2000) Smoking and metal illness: a population based study. *Journal of the American Medical Association* **284**, 2606–2610.

79. Prochaska JJ, Hall SM, Bero LA. (2008) Tobacco use among individuals with schizophrenia: what role has the tobacco industry played? *Schizophrenia Bulletin* **34**, 555–567.

80. Breslau N, Novack SP, Kessler RC. (2004) Psychiatric disorders and stages of smoking. *Biological Psychiatry* **55**, 69–76.

81. Daumit GL, Pronovost PJ, Anthony CB *et al.* (2006) Adverse events during medical and surgical hospitalizations for persons with schizophrenia. *Archives of General Psychiatry* **63**, 267–272.

82. Compton MT, Daumit GL, Druss BG. (2006) Cigarette smoking and overweight / obesity among individuals with serious mental illnesses: a preventive perspective. *Harvard Review of Psychiatry* **14**, 212–222.

83. Felker B, Yazel JJ, Short D. (1996) Mortailty and medical co-morbidity among psychiatric patients: a review. *Psychiatric Services* **47** 1356–1363.

84. Osborn D.P.J, Nazareth I and King M.B. (2006) Risk for coronary heart disease in people with severe mental illness, cross-sectional comparative study in primary care. *British Journal of Psychiatry.* **188**, 271–277.

85. Inoue M, Tsuji I, Wakai K *et al.* (2005) Evaluation based on systematic review of epidemiological evidence among Japanese populations: tobacco smoking and total cancer risk. *Japanese Journal of Clinical Oncology* **35**, 404–411.

86. Tercyak KP, Britto MT, Hanna KM *et al.* (2008) Prevention of tobacco use among medically at-risk children and adolescents: clinical and research opportunities in the interest of public health. *Journal of Pediatric Psychology* **33**, 119–132.

87. Robinson LA, Emmons KM, Moolchan ET *et al.* (2008) Developing smoking cessation programs for chronically ill teens: lessons learned from research with healthy adolescent smokers. *Journal of Pediatric Psychology* **33**, 133–144.

88. Tyc VL, Throckmorton-Belzer L. (2006) Smoking rates and the state of smoking interventions for children and adolescents with chronic illness. *Pediatrics* **118**, e471–e487.

89. Schwartz L, Drotar D. (2006) Post traumatic stress and related impairment in survivors of childhood cancer in early adulthood compared to healthy peers. *Journal of Pediatric Psychology* **31**, 356–366.

90. Ferero R, Bauman A, Young I, *et al.* (1996) Asthma health behaviours, social adjustment, and psychosomatic symptoms in adolescence. *Journal of Asthma* **33**, 157–164.

91. Tercyak KP. (2003) Psychosocial risk factors for tobacco use among adolescents with asthma. *Journal of Pediatric Psychology* **28**, 495–504.

92. Zbikowski SM, Klesges RC, Robinson LA *et al.* (2002) Risk factors for smoking among adolescents with asthma. *Journal of Adolescent Health* **30**, 279–287.

93. Gold DR, Wang X, Wypij D *et al.* (1996) Effects of cigarette smoking on lung function: I. adolescent boys and girls. *New England Journal of Medicine* **335**, 931–937.

94. Prokhorov AV, Emmons KM, Fallonen, EU *et al.* (1996) Respiratory responses to cigarette smoking among adolescent smokers: a pilot study. *Preventive Medicine* **25**, 633–640.

95. Oeffinger KC, Hudson MM. (2004) Long term complications following childhood and adolescent cancer: foundations for providing risk-based health care for survivors. *Cancer Journal of Clinicians* **54**, 208–236.

96. Verma A, Clough D, McKenna D, *et al.* (2001) Smoking and cystic fibrosis. *Journal of the Royal Society of Medicine* **94**, 29–34.

97. National Center for Health Statistics. (2000) *United States 2000 with Adolescent Chartbook* National Center for Health Statistics: Hyattsville, MD

98. Newacheck PW, McManus MA, Fax HB. (1991) Prevalence and impact of chronic illness among adolescents. *American Journal of Diseases of Children* **145**, 1367–1373.

99. Centers for Disease Control and Prevention (CDC) (2005) Cigarette use among high school students United States 1991–2005. *Morbidity and Mortality Weekly Report* **55**, 724–726.

100. Reidel BW, Robinson LA, Klesges RC *et al.* (2002) Characteristics of adolescents caught with cigarettes at school: implications for developing smoking cessation programs. *Nicotine and Tobacco Research* **4**, 351–354.

101. Reidel BW, Robinson LA, Klesges RC, *et al.* (2002) What motivates adolescent smokers to make a quit attempt? *Drug and Alcohol Dependence* **68**, 167–174.

102. Smith DR, Leggat PA. (2007) An international review of tobacco smoking among medical students. *Journal of Postgraduate Medicine* **53**, 55–62.

103. Smith DR, Leggat PA. (2007) An international review of tobacco smoking in the medical profession: 1874–2004. *BMC Public Health* **7**, 115.

104. Waalkens HJ, Schotanus JC, Adriaanse H *et al.* (1992) Smoking habits in medical students and physicians in Groningen, The Netherlands. *European Respiratory Journal* **5**, 49–52.

105. Jormanaien VJ, Myllykangas MT, Nissinen A. (1997) Decreasing the prevalence of smoking among Finnish physicians. *European Journal of Public Health* **7**, 318–320.

106. Dekker HM, Looman CWN, Adriaanse HP *et al.* (1993) Prevalence of smoking in physicians and medical students, and the generation effect in the Netherlands. *Social Science and Medicine* **36**, 817–822.

107. Roche AM, Parle MD, Stubbs JM *et al.* (1995) Management and treatment efficacy of drug and alcohol problems: what do doctors believe? *Addiction* **90**, 1357–1366.

108. Hughes PH, Baldwin DC Jnr, Sheehan DV *et al.* (1992) Resident physician substance use by speciality. *American Journal of Psychiatry* **149**, 1348–1354.

109. Hay DR. (1980) Cigarette smoking by New Zealand doctors: results from the 1976 population census. *New Zealand Medical Journal* **91**, 285–288.

110. Wells KB, Lewis CE, Leake B *et al.* (1984) Do physicians preach what they practice? A study of physicians' health habits and counseling practices. *Journal of the American Medical Association* **252**, 2846–2848.

111. Polyzos A, Gennatas C, Veslemes M, *et al.* (1995) The smoking cessation practices of physician smokers in Greece. *Journal of Cancer Education*, **10**, 78–81.

112. Ahmadi J, Maharlooy N, Alishahi M. (2004) Substance abuse: prevalence in a sample of nursing students. *Journal of Clinical Nursing* **13**, 60–64.

113. Baron-Epel O, Josephsohn K, Ehrenfeld M. (2004) Nursing students' perceptions of smoking prevention. *Nurse Education Today* **24**, 145–151.

114. Carmichael A, Cockcroft A. (1990) Survey of student nurses' smoking habits in a London teaching hospital. *Respiratory Medicine*, **84**, 277–282.

115. Boccoli E, Federici A, Melani AS *et al.* (1996) Results of a questionnaire about nurse students' smoking habits and knowledges in an Italian teaching school of nursing. *European Journal of Epidemiology* **12**, 1–3.

116. Smith DR, Leggat PA. (2007) An international review of tobacco smoking among dental students in 19 countries. *International Dental Journal* **57**, 452–458.

117. Doll R, Hill AB. (1954) The mortality of doctors in relation to their smoking habits: a preliminary report. *British Medical Journal* **1**(4877), 1451–1455.

118. Doll R, Hill AB. (2004) The mortality of doctors in relation to their smoking habits: a preliminary report. *British Medical Journal* **328**, 1529–1533.

119. Smith DR, Leggat PA. (2006) A comparison of tobacco smoking among dentists in 15 countries. *International Dental Journal* **56**, 283–288.

120. Newbury-Birch D, Lowry R Kamali F. (2002) The changing patterns of drinking, illicit drug use, stress, anxiety and depression in dental students in a UK dental school: a longitudinal study. *British Dental Journal* **192**(11): 646–9

121. Smith DR. (2007) A systematic review of tobacco smoking among nursing students. *Nurse Education in Practice* **7**, 293–302.

122. Adams, A., P. F. Bell, *et al.* (1994). "Nurses and smoking: a comparative study of students of nursing and teaching." *Aust Health Rev* **17**(2): 84–101.

123. Melani AS, Verponziani W, Boccoli E *et al.* (2000) Tobacco smoking habits, attitudes and beliefs among nurse and medical students in Tuscany. *European Journal of Epidemiology* **16**, 607–611.

124. Andrea MS, Walter V, Elena B *et al.* (2001) Comparison of smoking habits, beliefs and attitudes among Tuscan student nurses in 1992 and 1999. *European Journal of Epidemiology* **17**, 417–421.

125. Centers for Disease Control and Prevention (CDC) (2005) Tobacco use and cessation coun-
     seling – Global health professionals survey pilot study, 10 countries, 2005. *Morbidity and
     Mortality Weekly Report* **54**, 505–509.

126. Ohida T, Sakurai A, Kamal AA *et al.* (2001) Smoking among Japanese nursing students: a
     nationwide survey. *Tobacco Control* **10**, 397.

127. Clement M, Jankowski LW, Bouchard L *et al.* (2002) Health behaviours of nursing students: A
     longitudinal study. *Journal of Nursing Education* **41**, 257–265.

128. Nelson JP, Pederson LL. (2008) Military tobacco use: a synthesis of the literature on prevalence.
     Nicotine and Tobacco Research **10**, 775–790.

129. Bachman JG, Freedman-Doan P, O'Malley PM *et al.* (1999) Changing patterns of drug use
     among US military recruits before and after enlistment. *American Journal of Public Health* **89**,
     672–677.

CHAPTER 10

Tobacco Use: Prevention

Adriana Blanco[1], MD, MA,
Vera da Costa e Silva[2], MD, MPH, PhD
and Maristela Monteiro[1], MD, PhD
[1]*Pan American Health Organization, Washington, DC, USA*
[2]*Rua Pinheiro Guimarães, Rio de Janeiro, Brazil*

Disclaimer: This manuscript contains the views of the authors and does not necessarily represent the stated policy of the Pan American Health Organization (PAHO).

10.1 INTRODUCTION

The vast majority of smokers initiate the consumption of tobacco before the age of 18 [1]. According to the World Health Organization (WHO) three out of every five young people who experiment with tobacco will become dependent smokers into adulthood, and half of them will die prematurely [2]. As also noted by WHO, the joint probability of trying smoking, becoming dependent and dying prematurely is higher than for any other substance-use disorder [3].

On the other hand, the survival of the tobacco industry depends on attracting and retaining young people as consumers of its products. Without new, young tobacco users to replace those who quit or die, the tobacco industry could not continue to exist.

Therefore, prevention interventions must consider the huge investment of the tobacco industry to increase youth initiation and overall consumption and need to be more comprehensive than in the past. These measures were addressed in a global treaty negotiated under the auspices of the World Health Organization, the WHO Framework Convention on Tobacco Control (FCTC). The Convention gathers the scientifically proved most effective interventions to curb the tobacco epidemic and is the most reliable tool to be adopted by countries looking forward to decrease the toll of disease and death related to tobacco use.

This chapter will address the several aspects involved on the experimentation, initiation and consumption of tobacco use by young people as well as the key prevention aspects that can reduce taking up and regular use of tobacco products by this population. The same

Substance Abuse Disorders: Evidence and Experience, First Edition. Edited by Hamid Ghodse, Helen Herrman, Mario Maj and Norman Sartorius.
© 2011 John Wiley & Sons, Ltd. Published 2011 by John Wiley & Sons, Ltd.

policies that have an impact on young people's smoking are the ones most effective to prevent initiation of tobacco use in adulthood. Since most people start smoking in their adolescence or young adulthood and most become dependent, the focus of the chapter is on prevention amongst young people. Once anyone starts smoking, dependence is likely to develop and the best supports to cessation efforts are the same policies to prevent tobacco use amongst youth: increase the price and taxes of tobacco products, ban advertising and smoke-free environments.

10.2   YOUTH AND TOBACCO USE

10.2.1   Current Situation

In 1999, a collaborative effort from WHO, the Office of Smoking and Health from the US Centers for Disease Control and Prevention (CDC) and the Canadian Public Health Association (CPHA) with partnership with country governments resulted on the establishment of a Global Youth Tobacco Surveillance System (GYTSS), as part of a broader Global Tobacco Surveillance System (GTSS).

The Global Youth Tobacco Survey (GYTS) is a school-based survey that applies a standardized methodology and core questionnaire to representative samples of students between 13 and 15 years old. It includes data on prevalence of tobacco use, perceptions and attitudes about tobacco use, access to and availability of tobacco products, exposure to second-hand smoke, school curriculum, media and advertising and smoking cessation. From 1999 to 2008, the GYTS had been completed in 154 WHO Member States and 13 other areas. A second round had been completed in 110 countries and a third one in ten. Over two million students, over 11 000 schools around the world had participated in the survey.

Overall, 9.5% of students currently smoked cigarettes, ranging from 19.2% in the countries surveyed in the European Region,* to 4.9% in the Eastern Mediterranean Region. One in ten of the students used tobacco products other than cigarettes (e.g. waterpipes, smokeless tobacco, bidis, etc.) with the highest rate in the Eastern Mediterranean Region (29.8%). Amongst students who had never smoked cigarettes, almost 20% indicated they were susceptible to initiate the consumption next year [4].

At a population level, male uptake generally occurs sooner than female uptake in most countries. Higher socioeconomic status and social norms that include smoking as a rite of passage for boys are predictors of initial uptake [5].

Despite the fact that males still smoke more than females in most countries there are fewer significant gender differences in smoking as time goes by, indicating that the gender gap appears to be closing and the future of tobacco epidemic amongst women may eventually involve more than the actual estimate. These findings are also corroborated by the fact that cigarette smoking is higher amongst girls compared with rates observed amongst adult females in other studies.

For decades the tobacco industry had targeted woman through linking smoking with independence, stylishness, weight control, sophistication and power [6]. Even though women

* WHO Regions see http://www.who.int/about/regions/en/; In the European Region, most countries participants in the GYTSS are from Eastern Europe.

still smoke at a lower rate than men, there are a huge number of them smoking around the world, which is contributing to change the social acceptance of smoking amongst women [7].

10.2.2 Patterns of Tobacco Initiation

Amongst addictive behaviours, cigarette smoking is the one most likely to became established during adolescence. Globally, most people start smoking before the age of eighteen and almost a quarter of these individuals begin smoking cigarettes before the age of ten. People who begin smoking at an early age are more likely to develop severe levels of nicotine dependence than those who start at a later age. Data from the United Kingdom (UK) and United States of America (USA) suggest that between 33 and 50% of people who try cigarettes escalates to regular use [8]. Studies suggest that the symptoms of nicotine dependence can appear within days to weeks of the onset of occasional nicotine use, often before the onset of daily smoking [9]. Recently studies have also shown that once exposure to nicotine had occurred, remarkably few additional risk factors for smoking consistently contribute to individual differences in susceptibility to the development of dependence, suggesting that the process of dependence starts by the first dose of nicotine [10] and the number of cigarettes required before dependence is established in adolescents is less than in adults [11].

Smokeless-tobacco use seems to be as addictive for young people as it is for adults. Tobacco use is also associated with alcohol and illicit drug use and is generally the first drug used by young people who enter into polysubstance use [12, 13].

Regardless of the age at which young people smoke their first cigarette, there is a progression through a sequence of stages that takes them from receptivity to dependence on tobacco [14]. Even though not all young people who try a cigarette become a daily smoker, almost all of those who become daily smokers made it through similar well-defined stages as shown in Figure 10.1.

10.2.2.1 Determinants of Tobacco use Amongst Youth

Many factors may increase the risk of adolescents to experiment a tobacco product and support youth progress to a regular smoking. The life stage of adolescence itself is a predictor of smoking initiation. Adolescence is characterized by three mayor type of developmental challenges: physical maturation (particularly sexual maturation), responses to cultural pressures in order to transit from childhood to adulthood acquiring emotional independence from parents; and the personal challenge of establishing a coherent set of values and sense of self. In order to meet these challenges characteristically adolescents experiment and engage in risk-taking behaviours. Cigarette smoking is a risk behaviour shown by advertisement and role models as a way to be attractive, to have a positive social image, and at the end as a gateway to adulthood [15].

Tobacco use in adolescence is also associated with other health-risk behaviours, including risky sexual behaviour and the harmful use of alcohol or other drugs.

Several studies report that parental and friends smoking, a lack of perception that smoking is harmful and exposure to tobacco products marketing are associated with youth ever

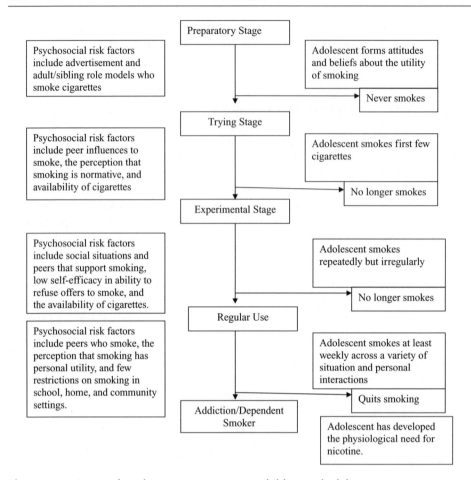

Figure 10.1 Stages of smoking initiation amongst children and adolescents.
Source: US Department of Health and Human Services (1991) SG report. Adapted from Flay (1993).

smoking in developed and developing countries [16, 17]. Other factors associated with youth tobacco use include low socioeconomic status; approval of tobacco use by peers or siblings; accessibility, availability and price of tobacco products; lack of parental support or involvement; low levels of academic achievement; lack of skills to resist influences of tobacco use and lack of self-efficacy to refuse offers of tobacco; lower self-image or self-esteem and belief in functional benefits of tobacco use [18].

The identification of determinants for smoking or using tobacco products should guide the design and implementation of programs aimed to prevent initiation and maintenance of tobacco use amongst young people.

10.3 TOBACCO-INDUSTRY STRATEGIES

In 1998, nine tobacco companies were required by USA courts to make public millions of pages of internal documents. These documents came from the national and international offices of seven cigarette manufacturers and two affiliated organizations doing business in the USA and provided an invaluable opportunity to the public and public-health professionals to get acquainted with what the tobacco industry knew, the sales strategies they used and what they hid from the public about the safety of their product [19].

An analysis of a range of documents released during the course of a governmental enquiry from five advertising agencies that did business with the UK tobacco industry concluded that the tobacco industry focus on a variety of marketing tools and that advertising is only one part of the communications effort, along with, for example, packaging, point of sale materials and direct mail, with all aspects of marketing playing a crucial role in the industry efforts to increase sales [20]. The enquiry has also shown how segments of the market are identified and the product, its price and its distribution are manipulated to maximize consumer satisfaction, uptake and continuation of smoking.

Ultimately, this marketing mix includes: packaging and product features (e.g. use of filters, tar and nicotine contents and emissions, tastes and flavors, pack size, colour, design and brand name), price alternatives (making the product affordable to the consumer), publicity options (e.g. media placements and themes, imagery, brand stretching and sponsorship strategies) and placement opportunities (e.g. accessible channels of distribution, availability) that are developed specifically to appeal to young smokers.

More recently, another legal case in the USA shed more evidence on the use of marketing strategies employed to sell tobacco products. The Final Opinion from US District Judge Gladys Kessler in United States vs. Philip Morris details the tobacco-industry marketing strategies targeted to youth:

> As Bennet Le Bow, President of Vector Holdings Group, stated, 'if the tobacco companies really stopped marketing to children, the tobacco companies would be out of business in 25 to 30 years because they will not have enough customers to stay in business [21]'.

The WHO has recently used the McCathy's marketing tools to illustrate how the tobacco industry is using the marketing mix (Figure 10.2) [22]. This exercise supports the concept that prevention programs need to be comprehensive in order to effectively counteract all the different approaches contained in it.

10.4   A COMPREHENSIVE APPROACH FOR TOBACCO PREVENTION

10.4.1   The WHO FCTC: History, Scope and Governance

The WHO FCTC is the first public-health international treaty developed under the auspices of WHO. It is an evidence-based treaty that reaffirms the right of all people to the highest standard of health. In its Preamble the States underlined their decision to 'give priority to their right to protect public health'.

It represents a paradigm shift in developing a regulatory strategy to address addictive substances; in contrast to previous drug-control treaties, the WHO FCTC asserts the importance of demand reduction strategies as well as supply issues (Figure 10.3).

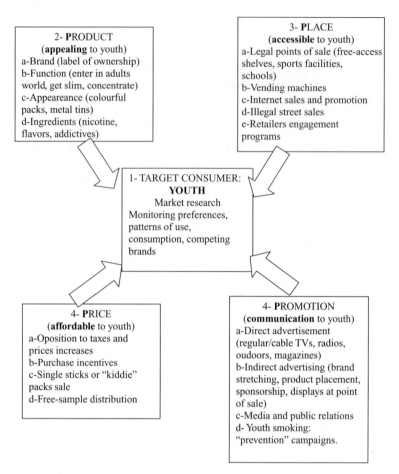

Figure 10.2 The tobacco-industry marketing. Mix to target youth. Based on Mc Carthy's classification of marketing instruments [49].
Source: Costa e Silva, VL Concept paper for WHO WNTD 2008 Unpublished, May 2008.

WHO FCTC CORE MEASURES			
DEMAND-REDUCTION MEASURES		**SUPPLY-REDUCTION MEASURES**	
Price related			
Art. 6	Increase of prices and taxes of tobacco products		
Nonprice related		Art 15	Illicit trade of tobacco products
Art 8	Protection from exposure to second-hand smoke (SHS)		
Art 9 &10	Tobacco products contents and disclosure regulation	Art. 16	Sales of tobacco products to and by minors
Art 11	Packaging and labelling of tobacco products		
Art12	Education, communication, training and public awareness	Art 17	Provision of support for economically viable alternative activities
Art 13	Tobacco advertising, promotion and sponsorship		
Art 14	Tobacco dependence and cessation		

Figure 10.3 Core measures of the WHO Framework Convention on Tobacco Control.

The idea was conceived in May 1995 during the 48th World Health Assembly (WHA) [23], requesting the Director General to report on the Forty-ninth Session of the WHA on the feasibility of developing an international instrument on tobacco control. During the following WHA the Director General was requested to initiate the development of a Framework Convention on Tobacco Control.

On 21 May 2003, the Fifty-sixth WHA, unanimously adopted the WHO FCTC. After its adoption, the WHO FCTC was open for signature until 29 June 2004. One hundred and sixty eight States signed the WHO FCTC during this period expressing their willingness to become a Party to the Convention. After that, the ratification process began, which led to Member States becoming Parties, legally bonded, to the Convention.

The Convention entered into force on 27 February 2005, 90 days after the fortieth State had acceded to, ratified, accepted, or approved it and the Convention currently has more than 170 Parties.[†]

The governing body of the WHO FCTC is the Conference of the Parties (COP) and is comprised of all Parties to the Convention; it shall keep under regular review the implementation of the Convention and take the decisions necessary to promote its effective implementation and may also adopt protocols, annexes and amendments to the Convention. The COP may establish such subsidiary bodies as are necessary to achieve the objective of the Convention. One example is the Intergovernmental Negotiating Body for the elaboration of a Protocol on Illicit Trade in Tobacco Products, the first potential Protocol to the WHO FCTC that will be presented to the forth meeting of the COP for discussion. The COP also established several working groups with the mandate to elaborate guidelines and recommendations for the implementation of the different treaty provisions. So far, guidelines for the implementation of five articles had been approved and others are under discussion.

The Objective of the Convention is *'to protect present and future generations from the devastating health, social, environmental and economic consequences of tobacco consumption and exposure to tobacco smoke by providing a framework for tobacco control measures to be implemented by the Parties at the national, regional and international levels in order to reduce continually and substantially the prevalence of tobacco use and exposure to tobacco smoke'*. It is intended to have the minimum requirements that countries need to put in place in order to curb the tobacco epidemic, and Parties are encouraged to go beyond its mandates in order to protect public health.

10.4.2 Main Components of a Comprehensive Intervention to Prevent Tobacco Use Amongst Young People

For a long time it has been considered that the best way to prevent tobacco use was to focus action on children and youth. Nevertheless, current specific evidence no longer supports children and youth targeted interventions in isolation, and indicates that these strategies should be embedded in a more comprehensive broader strategy including the environment where children and youth live. Without being complemented by other population measures, youth-orientated policies will neither be effective or sustainable and they will only achieve little more than delaying the uptake of smoking [24].

[†] By October 2010.

From a broader public-health perspective, if you only focus in children you will not be able to have benefits for several decades, since most of the tobacco-related deaths that are projected to occur in the first half of the century are amongst today's existing smokers [25].

So, in order to effectively prevent tobacco use, programs should prioritize wider multi-layered societal approaches to tobacco, targeting young people and adults and, including different measures such as:

10.4.2.1   Denormalizing Tobacco Use

Using tobacco products must be seen as a societal problem rather than a youth problem and interventions should include the environment where young people live so that it supports tobacco-free norms. Former WHO Director General Dr. Gro Harlem Brutland states in 1999, that *'the tobacco epidemic is a communicated disease. It is communicated through advertising, through the example of smokers and through the smoke to which non-smokers – especially children – are exposed. Our job is to immunize people against this epidemic [26]'.*

10.4.2.1.1   Implement Smoke-Free Policies

Eliminating smoking in indoor spaces is the only way to fully protect nonsmokers from the second-hand smoke (SHS) exposure. Separating smokers from nonsmokers, cleaning the air and ventilating buildings cannot completely eliminate SHS exposure.

A recent systematic review assessed the results of legislation-based smoking bans in decreasing the exposure to SHS, and its impact in consumption and/or prevalence and its health outcomes. It showed that legislative-based smoking bans do lead to a reduction in exposure to passive smoking. Even though the evidence is limited about the impact in active smoking the trend is downwards and some evidence was also found of an improvement in health outcomes [27].

A thorough review on the effects of smoke-free and clean-air legislation [28] has concluded that teenagers respond to smoke-free environments by decreasing smoking. Teenagers who worked in totally smoke-free workplaces were 68% as likely to ever smoke as those who worked in less restricted workplaces. Smoke-free homes are also associated to lower rates of smoking and the only significant predictor of planning to stop smoking by young people was the belief that passive smoking harms others. These effects, as well as the workplace effects, probably act by reinforcing the social unacceptability of smoking.

According to GYTS, more than seven in ten students thought smoking should be banned in public places, which might be an expression that both information and positive attitudes towards healthier settings are present amongst youth.

10.4.2.1.2   Ban Tobacco Advertising, Promotion and Sponsorship

WHO FCTC defines tobacco advertisement and promotion as: 'any form of commercial communication, recommendation or action with the aim, effect or likely effect of promoting a tobacco product or tobacco use either directly or indirectly'.

In general, promotion is a core part of marketing. It includes all levels of communication with the target group and can vary from direct promotion such as print and TV advertisements to a more indirect appeal to the consumer such as a brand sponsorship of sports and music events and brand stretching. Advertising, direct and indirect, can be alternatively divided on 'above the line' (ATL) and 'below the line' (BTL). ATL refers predominantly to paid advertising, talking to a large audience. It is conventional in nature and considered impersonal to customers (i.e. ads in television, radio, newspapers, internet, etc.). On the other hand, BTL focuses on opportunities to reach the audience on a one-to-one basis, using less conventional brand-building strategies. Examples include the use of direct email, public relations efforts, sales promotion, consumer promotions, consumer incentives, trade incentives, retail promotion. BTL strategies often use highly targeted lists of names to maximize response rates. The tobacco industry frequently uses both ATL and BTL strategies, but in preparation for partial advertising bans, they increase their expenditures on BTL activities [29].

A recent study on existing correlation of promotion and initiation of tobacco use was examined against the Hill criteria to determine causality [30]. The study concluded that exposure to tobacco promotion causes children to initiate tobacco use and meets the Hill criteria of causality.

Furthermore, there is a perception of functionality in the use of tobacco products. Tobacco-industry documents recognize that smoking is a 'rite of passage', with youngsters looking for reassurance and identity. Amongst other beliefs smokers trust cigarettes to help them reduce body weight, improve concentration, and so on. The perception of functionality of tobacco products is one of the determinants of experimentation and initiation. A section of a May 26, 1975 report, prepared for Brown & Williamson titled 'How can we introduce starters and switchers to our brands' stated that *'an attempt to reach young smokers, starters should be based … on the following parameters: [p]resent the cigarette as one of a few initiations into the adult world. Present the cigarette as part of the illicit pleasure category of product and activities…[T]ouch on the basic symbols of the growing-up, maturity process. To the best of your ability (considering some legal constraints) relate the cigarette to "pot", wine, beer, sex, etc. [31]'.*

10.4.2.2   Reducing Accessibility and Affordability of Tobacco Products

Because youth are especially sensitive to tobacco-products prices, strategies counteracting this component of tobacco company's strategies should be considered. Tobacco products should not be affordable to youth in order not to stimulate experimentation, initiation and consumption.

10.4.2.2.1   Increase Taxes and Prices

Price is an essential component of the marketing mix. Prices are calculated after a careful consideration of direct and indirect costs involved in the production and marketing of a product, as well as taxes and potential and target market share.

A basic law of economics states that as the price of a commodity rises, the quantity demanded of that product will fall [32]. This principle also applies to tobacco products and several studies have shown that an increase in price decreases consumption in both developed and developing countries, and that raising tobacco taxes and prices is one of the most effective polices for reducing use. The decrease in consumption may result of reduced initiation of tobacco use, increased cessation, and reduction in the consumption by continuing users.

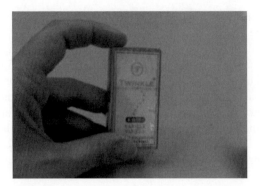

Figure 10.4   Small-size package from Canada.

It is estimated that youth demand is three times more sensitive to price than adults', and this youth sensitivity to high prices may be explained by the lower level of addiction due to lower time of exposure, lower peer smoking and the reduced purchase power of the young smokers [33].

Ideally, taxes should represent two thirds to three quarter of the final retail price. Tax increases may bring substantially higher revenues in the short to medium term, which takes care of governments' concerns of affecting revenues with such a measure. This revenue increases may be earmarked for public health, tobacco control, health promotion, and so on.

10.4.2.2.2   Reducing Youth Access to Tobacco Products

There is a wide range of measures in order to comply with this objective. The most obvious one is the ban of tobacco sales to or by minors. Even though this banning exists in many countries, there is a general lack of enforcement for it. GYTS results shows that five in ten students, who currently smoke cigarettes, usually purchased them in stores; and seven in ten of those who bought cigarettes in stores where not refused purchase of cigarettes during the last month because of their age [34].

Sales of cigarettes individually, in small packages (Figure 10.4), or in packages specifically appealing to children and youth (Figure 10.5), candy and exotic flavors, sales of sweets, snacks, toys or any other objects in the form of tobacco products as well of placing the products in a way that they are directly accessible, such as store shelves or self-service vending machines should not be allowed.

10.4.2.3   Provide Information

In recent decades, studies from several high-income countries had concluded that publicized information about the health effects of tobacco has been responsible for a sustained decline in consumption especially when shocks of information are provided based on the release of studies that confirm the health consequences of using tobacco. Informing consumers can be cost effective in reducing overall consumption [35].

In general, young people appear to be less responsive to information about the health effects of tobacco that older adults, and more educated people respond more quickly to new information than those with no or minimal education. There is evidence that aggressive

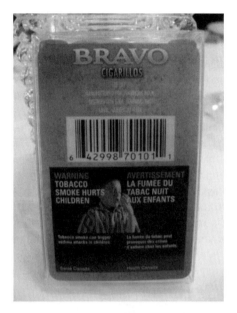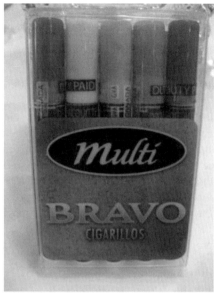

Figure 10.5   Flavoured cigarettes from Canada.

countermarketing campaigns that include strong media elements and highlight the tobacco industry's behaviour have rapid and substantial effects on youth smoking.

10.4.2.3.1   Health-Warning Measures in Packaging and Labelling of Tobacco Products

The package has functions that go beyond the regular use of wrapping and protecting the product. Packs are transformed in brand advertising, as a way to bypass future bans on promotion and advertisement. Packages are seen as the last opportunity of communication with users and also an advertisement in themselves when they are displayed at the points of sale.

The inclusion of big pictorial health warnings in tobacco packages not only provides useful health information regarding health consequences of tobacco use, but also diminishes the appealing of the package. Evidence coming from many countries suggests that warning labels can be effective in reducing consumption, provided they are large, prominent and contain straight and specific factual information. However, one of the weaknesses is that they do not reach some individuals, children and youth amongst them, since they often buy cigarettes by unit rather than by package.

Young people seem to react to health messages in different ways when compared with adults, therefore there is a need to evaluate messages and images to see how they may impact in experimentation and progression to tobacco use.

10.4.2.3.2   Mass-Media Campaigns

Media campaigns play a key role to build knowledge, change attitudes and behaviour in support of a tobacco-free society. They should be culturally and gender sensitive and consider illiteracy rates in the country. Furthermore, messages should be developed for young people and with the help of young people, but should also appeal to adult smokers.

One of the few examples of a successful campaign that targeted young people was the "Truth® campaign" initially implemented by the state of Florida in 1998 and launched at national level by the Legacy Foundation in February 2000 [36]. This campaign was the result of dedicated funds coming from the settlement agreement between the tobacco industry and the states of the USA. Its single focus was to reduce youth-smoking prevalence on the 12–17 year old population. It was conceived as an unconventional campaign with the benefits of all modern marketing tools, the best directors, the creation of a web site with the newest animations and a market research component that has provided relevant information to understand the target-group aspirations and to refine the campaign. An essential component of the Truth® campaign was to create a brand as a piece of identification with the world and its main strategy was to disclose the tobacco-industry manipulation of the information targeted to youth. Moreover, the campaign was run as a business, competing with any other interested group for the best paid time for youth audience. Repeated youth summits to provide insights and feedback were responsible for relevant participation from young people in all stages of the campaign. The message from months of marketing research was that young people didn't want to be told what to do but they rather wanted factual information and decide by themselves.

Furthermore, young people didn't see tobacco as the more relevant problem to them, so the "tobacco kills" message and the life or death tone would not work. In fact young people in Florida were aware of the health damages of tobacco use; but they smoke for emotional reasons and not on the basis of an informed decision and using tobacco was a tool of rebellion and a message that decisions would be made by themselves.

The lessons learnt with this campaign showed that '*generations of well intended social marketers had pounded the airwaves doing everything they could to explain that tobacco kills. What they did not understand (and the tobacco industry did) was that they risked actually making tobacco that much more appealing to youth*'.

The evaluations showed a 92% of brand awareness rate amongst teens, a 15% rise in teens who agree with key attitudinal statements about smoking, a 19.4% decline in smoking amongst middle-school students, and 8% decline amongst high-school students [38]. A more recent study that compared reactions to the Truth® campaign has further concluded that adolescents who live in tobacco-producing regions appear to be as responsive to anti-industry ads as their counterparts in nontobacco-producing regions [39].

Smoking prevalence amongst all students declined from 25.3 to 18.0% between 1999 and 2002 in USA, and the Truth® campaign has accounted for approximately 22% of this decline [40].

10.4.2.3.3   Other Interventions

- **Sports as a preventive tool**: Sports and smoking do not mix. Participation in physical activity and sports can promote social well-being, as well as good physical and mental health, amongst young people. Research had shown those students who participate in interscholastic sports are less likely to be regular and heavy smokers or use drugs, and are more likely to stay in school and have good conduct and high academic achievements. Sports and physical activity can introduce young people to sills such as teamwork, self-discipline, sportsmanship, leadership and socialization. Lack of recreational activity, on the other hand, may contribute to making young people vulnerable to gangs, drugs, or violence [41]. Sports represent great opportunities to reach young people. Young athletes learn to make important health decisions related to tobacco use, physical activity and good nutrition while on a sports team. A smoke-free sports strategy offers good opportunities to inform youth and to create a supportive environment for them not to take up tobacco products. Coaches, teachers and parents can have substantial influence in this regard [42]. Recent studies have found that youth that participated in organized sports were 25% less likely to be current cigarette smokers [43]. Sponsorship of sports events by the tobacco industry would also undermine the value of sports as a preventive tool.

- **Smoke-free schools**: School settings and sports facilities need to have policies that are consistent with a smoke-free society and will support smoke-free youth. Recent studies suggest that students' perceptions of policy enforcement significantly predicted school prevalence. Some studies suggest that school policies banning smoking by teachers and other school personnel within and outside the school should be an important component of comprehensive adolescent smoking-prevention programs. Furthermore, when considering implementing smoke-free schools, policy intention and implementation will only be effective if perceived as strongly enforced [44, 45].

- **School-based programs**: School anti-smoking programs are widespread, particularly in the high-income countries. However, they appear to be less effective than many other types of information dissemination. Even programs that have initially reduced the uptake of smoking appear to have only a temporary effect; they can delay the initiation of smoking but not prevent it. Also need to be taken into account that tobacco companies had created and financed school based interventions.

- **Youth initiatives**: Promoting youth activism is an innovative component that had helped to catalyse health action in tobacco control. In 2006 the First Global Youth Meet on Health [46] took place in India promoting the concept that youth activism can be specially crafted to bring about social or political change. The initiative empowered 225 youth from 35 countries through enhanced health awareness and strengthened health advocacy skills including tobacco control aspects. Other examples of Youth initiatives includes Teens Against Tobacco Use®, a youth empowerment program from West Virginia, supported by the American Lung Association and the Youth Action Committee from Canada, which was formed to advise the government on anti-tobacco programs targeted to youth and how strategies to reach youth audience [47]. More recently, during the 14th World Conference on Tobacco or Health, the Global Youth Meet on Tobacco (GYM) has taken place bringing together more than 160 participants from all over the world to expand the youth role in promoting smoke-free societies and their global network.

10.4.2.4   Product Regulation

The tobacco industry has a long history of manipulating the contents of its products in order to increase use and dependence. For example, chocolate and its derivatives are added to indirectly facilitate the development of dependence by contributing flavour and mouth sensations [48]. Certain additives (i.e. menthol in cigarettes, eugenol in kreteks) are added specifically to reduce the smoke harshness and enable the smoker to take in more dependence-causing and toxic substances.

One of the tobacco industry recent tactics is the introduction of candy and exotic-flavoured cigarettes and smokeless tobacco. These flavoured brands and brand extension are marketed in ways to appeal to youth with colourful and stylish packaging, and flavours that mask the harsh and toxic properties of tobacco.

10.5 CONCLUSION

The smoking epidemic remains a global public-health concern. Despite the efforts governments and civil society are making to reduce the burden of tobacco use, tobacco consumption continues to increase with special impact on developing countries where young people are the key target of the tobacco-industry marketing strategies.

Tobacco control strategies focus basically on four core aspects: preventing tobacco use, protecting people from the consequences of second-hand smoke; promoting smoking cessation amongst smokers and tobacco users and regulating tobacco products. All these strategies are interlinked and are addressed by the core measures of the WHO Framework Convention on Tobacco Control. The first WHO-sponsored treaty provides the best opportunities for governments, the civil society and the world to curb the tobacco epidemic and especially to protect future generations from the consequences of this deadly product.

The main conclusion of this chapter is that no single youth-focused intervention will be effective if the society as a whole does not address tobacco use as a social problem. Therefore, the main recommendation for public-health decision makers and activists is to concentrate efforts in changing the environment in parallel with any youth-orientated strategy in order to ensure adherence of this population to the concept that the best life option is to be or become a nonsmoker.

REFERENCES

1. US Department of Health and Human Services (1994) Preventing tobacco use among young people: A Report of the Surgeon General. Atlanta, Georgia: US Department of Health and Human Services, Public Health Service, Centers for Disease Control and Prevention, National Center for Chronic Disease Prevention and Health Promotion, Office on Smoking and Health.

2. Pan American Health Organization (2000) Tobacco-free youth: A "life-skills" primer. Washington DC. Scientific and Technical Publication No. 579.PAHO.

3. World Health Organization (1999) The World Health Report 1999: Making a difference. WHO, Geneva.

4. Centers for Disease Control and Prevention (2008) Global youth tobacco surveillance, 2000–2007. Surveillance summaries, 2000–2007. *Morbity and Mortality Weekly Report*, **57** (SS-1).

5. Greaves, L. (2005) *Sifting the Evidence: Gender and Global Tobacco*, WHO (IDRC), Geneva, Switzerland. Available from: http://www.who.int/tobacco/resources/publications/WHO_Gender_Sifting.pdf (Accessed 15 October 2009).

6. Campaign for Tobacco-Free Kids (2007) *Tobacco Industry Targeting of Women and Girls*, CTFK Factsheet, May 7, 2007. Available from http://www.tobaccofreekids.org/research/factsheets/pdf/0138.pdf (Accessed 15 October 2009).

7. Waldron, I., Bratteli, G., Carriker, L. *et al.* (1988) Gender differences in tobacco use in Africa, Asia, the Pacific and Latin America. *Social Science and Medicine*, **27**, 1269–1275.

8. US Department of Health and Human Services (1994) Preventing tobacco use among young people: A Report of the Surgeon General. Atlanta, Georgia: US Department of Health and Human Services, Public Health Service, Centers for Disease Control and Prevention, National Center for Chronic Disease Prevention and Health Promotion, Office on Smoking and Health.

9. DiFranza, J.R., Rigotti, N.A., McNeill, A.D. *et al.* (2000) Initial symptoms of nicotine dependence in adolescents. *Tobacco Control*, **9**, 313–319.

10. Di Franza, J.R. *et al.* (2007) The development and assessment of nicotine dependence in youth. *Pediatrics*, **120** (4) e974–e983.

11. Prokhorov, A.V. *et al.* (2006) Youth Tobacco Use: A global perspective for child heath care clinicians. *Pediatrics*, **118** (3), e890–e893.

12. US Department of Health and Human Services (1994) Preventing tobacco use among young people: A Report of the Surgeon General. Atlanta, Georgia: US Department of Health and Human Services, Public Health Service, Centers for Disease Control and Prevention, National Center for Chronic Disease Prevention and Health Promotion, Office on Smoking and Health.

13. Shenghan, L., Hong, L., Page, J.B. and McCoy, C.B. (2000) The association between cigarette smoking and drug abuse in the United States. *Journal of Addictive Diseases*, **19** (4). 11–24

14. Leventhal and Cleary 1980 cited in US Department of Health and Human Services (1994) Preventing tobacco use among young people: A Report of the Surgeon General. Atlanta, Georgia: US Department of Health and Human Services, Public Health Service, Centers for Disease Control and Prevention, National Center for Chronic Disease Prevention and Health Promotion, Office on Smoking and Health, Chapter 4. p. 124.

15. Pan American Health Organization (2000) Tobacco-free youth: A "life-skills" primer. Washington DC, Scientific and Technical Publication No. 579. PAHO.

16. Siziya, S., Rudatsikira, E., Muula, A.S. and Rt Ntnata, P. (2007) Predictors of cigarette smoking among adolescents in rural Zambia: results form a cross sectional study from Luangwa district. *Rural Remote Health* **7** (3), 728 17900223.

17. Lenney, W. and Enderby, B. (2008) Blowing in the wind. A review of teenage smoking. *Archives of Disease in Childhood* 2008; **93**: 72–75.

18. CDC Smoking and tobacco use web site. Youth Tobacco Prevention. Available from: http://www.cdc.gov/tobacco/youth/index.htm (Accessed 15 October 2009).

19. WHO/TFI (2003) The tobacco industry documents: what they are, what they tell us, and how to search them. Geneva, Switzerland. Available from: http://www.who.int/tobacco/communications/TI_manual_content.pdf (Accessed 15 October 2009).

20. Hastings, G. and MacFadyen, L (2000) Keep Smiling no one's going to die: an analysis of internal documents from the tobacco industry's main UK agencies. Available from: http://www.tobacco.org/resources/documents/001004keepsmiling.html (Accessed 15 October 2009).

21. Tobacco Control Legal Consortium (2006) The Verdict is in: Findings from US v Philip Morris, Marketing to Youth. Available from: http://papers.ssrn.com/sol3/papers.cfm?abstract_id=1004323 (Accessed 18 August 2010).

22. World Health Organization (2008) Break the tobacco marketing net. World no tobacco day 2008 material. Available from: http://www.who.int/tobacco/wntd/2008/en/index.html (Accessed 15 October 2009).

23. World Health Organization. The history of the WHO Framework Convention on Tobacco Control. Available from: http://www.who.int/fctc/about/history/en/index.html (Accessed 15 October 2009).

24. EU Commission and Italian Presidency of the Council (2003) Tobacco, Youth prevention and Communication. Rome 13–15 November 2003. Final Recommendations. Available from: http://ec.europa.eu/health/ph_determinants/life_style/Tobacco/conference_prevention_en.htm (Accessed 18 August 2010).

25. World Bank Curbing the Epidemic (1999) *Government and the Economics of Tobacco Control*, The World Bank, Washington DC.

26. WHO's General Director (1999) Available from http://www.who.int/director-general/speeches/1999/english/19990318_international_policy_conference.html (Accessed 15 October 2009).

27. Callinan, J.E., Clarke, A., Doherty, K. and Kelleher, C. (2010) Legislative smoking bans for reducing second-hand smoke exposure, smoking prevalence and tobacco consumption. *Cochrane Database of Systematic Reviews* 4, Art. No.: CD005992. DOI: 10.1002/14651858. CD005992.pub2.

28. Fichtenberg, C.M. and Glantz, S.A. (2002) Effect of smoke free workplaces on smoking behaviour: a systematic review. *British Medical Journal*, **325**, 188–191.

29. Carter, S.M. (2003) Going below the line: creating transportable brands for Australia's dark market. *Tobacco Control*, **12**, 87–94. doi: 10.1136/tc.12.suppl_3.iii87.

30. Di Franza, J.R., Wellman, R.J., Sergeant, J.D. *et al.*, for the Tobacco Consortium, Center for Child (2006) Health Research of the American Academy of Pediatrics – Tobacco promotion and the initiation of tobacco use: Assessing evidence for causality. *Pediatrics*, **117** (6) pp. e1237–e1248 (doi 10.1542/peds.2005-1817).

31. Tobacco Control Legal Consortium (2006) The Verdict is in: Findings from US v Philip Morris, Marketing to Youth. Available from: http://papers.ssrn.com/sol3/papers.cfm?abstract_id=1004323 (Accessed 18 August 2010).

32. World Bank Curbing the Epidemic (1999) *Government and the Economics of Tobacco Control*, The World Bank, Washington DC.

33. Frank J. Chaloupka, The-Wei Hu, (2000) Kenneth E. Warner *et al.* The taxation of tobacco products. In Tobacco Control in Developing Countries. Jha P., Chaloupka F. editors. Oxford University Press, Inc New York. The World Bank 2000.

34. Centers for Disease Control and Prevention (2008) Global youth tobacco surveillance, 2000–2007. Surveillance summaries 2008;. *Morbidity and Mortality Weekly Report 2008*, **57** (SS-1). 1

35. World Bank Curbing the Epidemic (1999) *Government and the Economics of Tobacco Control*, The World Bank, Washington DC.

36. Hicks, J.J. (2001) The strategy behind Florida's "Truth" campaign. *Tob Control*, **10** (1), 3–5.

37. Legacy for longer healthier lives. The "truth" factsheet (2000). Available at http://www.legacy forhealth.org/PDF/truth_Fact_Sheet.pdf (Accessed 18 October 2010).

38. Zucker, D., Hopkins, R.S., Sly, D.F. *et al.* (2000) Florida's Truth campaign a counter marketing, antitobacco media campaign. *Journal of Public Health Management and Practice*, **6** (3), 1–6.

39. Niederdeppe, J., Farrelly, M.C. *et al.* (2004) The impact of anti-tobacco industry prevention Thrasher JF, messages in tobacco producing regions: evidence from the US truth Campaign. *Tob Control*, **13** (3), 283–288.

40. Farrelly, M.C., Davis, K.C., Haviland, M.L. *et al.* (2005) Evidence of a dose-response relationship between "Truth" antismoking ads and Youth Smoking prevalence. *American Journal of Public Health*, **95** (3), 425–431.

41. USDHHS Physical Activity Fundamental to Preventing Disease. (2002) Available from: http://aspe.hhs.gov/health/reports/physicalactivity (Accessed 18 August 2010).

42. Centers for Disease Control and Prevention web site. Available from: http://www.cdc.gov/tobacco/youth/sports/index.htm (Accessed 15 October 2009).

43. Castrucci, B.C., Gerlach, K.K., Kaufman, N.J. and Orleans, C.T. (2004) Tobacco Use and cessation behavior among adolescents participating in organized sports. *American Journal of Health Behavior 2004*, **28** (1), 63–71. 14977160.

44. Poulsen, L.H., Osler, M., Roberts, C. *et al.* (2002) Exposure to teachers smoking and adolescent smoking behaviour: analysis of cross sectional data from Denmark. *Tobacco Control*, **11**, 246–251.

45. Barnett, T.A., Gauvin, L., Lambert, M., *et al.* (2007) The influence of school smoking policies on student tobacco use. *Archives of Pediatric and Adolescent Medicine*, **161**, 842–848.

46. First Global Youth Meet on Health (GYM) (2006) November 14–19, 2006 (New Delhi-Agra) available from: http://www.hriday-shan.org/hriday/gym.html (Accessed 15 October 2009).

47. Health Canada/Healthy living Youth engagement. Available from: http://www.hc-sc.gc.ca/ahc-asc/media/nr-cp/_2010/2010_13-eng.php (Accessed 18 August 2010).

48. WHO Scientific Report Series 945 (2007) The scientific basis of tobacco product regulation: report of a WHO study group, Geneva.

49. Quick MBA Marketing: web page – Available from: http://www.quickmba.com/marketing/mix (Accessed 15 October 2009).

CHAPTER 11

Tobacco Abuse: Treatment and Management

Susanna Galea, M.D., MRCPsych, MSc (Addictive Behaviour), Dip. (Forensic Mental Health)

Community Alcohol & Drug Services, Auckland, Pitman House, Auckland, New Zealand

11.1   INTRODUCTION

The widespread cross-cultural use of tobacco across various age groups is associated with a wide range of health and social problems. Tobacco use is a risk factor for 6 out of the 8 leading causes of death worldwide. In 2005 tobacco was estimated to be responsible for 5.4 million deaths. This figure is projected to increase to 6.4 million by 2015 and to 8.3 million by 2030 [1,2], making tobacco the *'single most preventable cause of death'* [3]. Current and projected mortality figures are mainly attributable to significant tobacco-related mortality rates in low-income and middle-income countries.

The global prevalence of adult tobacco smoking is estimated at around 25% [4] – with the majority of adult smokers (more than 1 billion) living in low-income to middle-income countries. Worldwide, tobacco use has been linked to low socio-economic status and low average incomes, making tobacco use a major contributor to health inequalities in morbidity and mortality [5,6].

Tackling the tobacco epidemic requires comprehensive and sustained efforts directed at various levels – the individual, the community and globally. Treatment and management approaches directed at an individual level stem from a recognition that tobacco use as a disease requires medical interventions. On the other hand, treatment and management approaches at community and global levels stem from a recognition of the contextual nature of smoking within society, and that smoking as a social and collective behaviour requires population-based interventions [7].

This chapter provides an overview of contemporary evidence on individual approaches and population-centred approaches to the treatment and management of tobacco use. Approaches at the individual level are discussed from a disease perspective giving consideration to a smoker's journey through treatment, including aspects such as identification,

Substance Abuse Disorders: Evidence and Experience, First Edition. Edited by Hamid Ghodse, Helen Herrman, Mario Maj and Norman Sartorius.
© 2011 John Wiley & Sons, Ltd. Published 2011 by John Wiley & Sons, Ltd.

assessment, motivation, treatment goals and access, as well as pharmacological and non-pharmacological interventions, bearing in mind individual-level determinants of tobacco use. Population-level approaches targeting social norms and attitudes are considered at community and global levels, bearing in mind the population-level determinants of tobacco use.

11.2   INDIVIDUAL-BASED TREATMENT AND MANAGEMENT APPROACHES

Individual-based treatment and management approaches aim to reduce tobacco use and its associated health and social hazards, through provision of treatment options targeting the individual tobacco user. Tobacco use, dependence and health consequences are recognized as a disease spectrum requiring medical attention [8]. In 1988 the US Surgeon General acknowledged the centrally rewarding properties of nicotine, isolated from tobacco leaves [9], and stated that:

> Cigarettes and other forms of tobacco are addicting; nicotine is the drug in tobacco that causes addiction; and that the pharmacological and behavioural processes that determine tobacco addiction are similar to those that determine addiction to drugs such as heroin and cocaine [10].

This statement recognizes the disease status of tobacco use and acknowledges the chronic relapsing nature of tobacco dependence.

As with any other disease accurate and comprehensive assessment, motivation, engagement of the individual and clear treatment goals are the cornerstones of successful treatment and management. A large majority of tobacco users express a wish to quit or reduce their smoking habit and a significant number do attempt quitting without seeking any help. Only a very small percentage (1–3%) of those attempting to quit without seeking help remain abstinent for 12 months [11]. This highlights the importance of attempting to provide a menu of evidence-based pharmacological and nonpharmacological treatment options and combinations of treatment modalities, tailored to the needs of the individual smoker, to facilitate successful treatment and management.

11.2.1   Identification, Assessment and Brief Interventions

The early identification and assessment of tobacco use is associated with early initiation of treatment and increased health benefits [12]. Brief interventions are opportunistic interventions especially designed to be provided within busy healthcare settings such as primary care settings, which on average take 5–10 minutes to deliver. Brief opportunistic interventions refer to the brief advice, discussion, negotiation and encouragement that can be delivered at opportune moments [13]. Despite variations in health-care systems in different countries a significant proportion (around 70%) of tobacco-users come into contact with their health-care providers [14] for a variety of reasons, putting health-care professionals in an ideal position to carry out effective identification and brief intervention.

Guidelines suggest that there are benefits in attempting to identify all tobacco users and providing brief interventions [13–16]. The *'Five As Framework'* [17] (*A*sk, *A*dvise, *A*ssess, *A*ssist and *A*rrange follow-up) provides an evidence-based approach for the identification of tobacco users and implementation of brief interventions within various settings.

All individuals coming into contact with the health-care system should be systematically *'asked'* about their use of tobacco. Recent clinical guidelines [16] suggest four main categories of patients – users willing to quit; users not willing to quit; once used tobacco but has since quit; and, never regularly used. Although, these categories are useful when determining appropriate interventions, they fail to categorize a proportion of tobacco users who do not use tobacco regularly but are still at low risk of exposure to tobacco toxins – that is the sporadic users. The following categories expand on those suggested in the guidelines, including the sporadic users, with some variations suggested for appropriate interventions:

- those who never used tobacco;
- those who are currently not using tobacco but have used tobacco sporadically in their lifetime;
- those who are currently abstinent but regularly used tobacco in the past;
- those currently using tobacco sporadically;
- those currently using tobacco regularly and are willing to quit;
- those currently using tobacco regularly and not willing to quit.

Recognition of which category an individual falls under provides the baseline for the second step – that is *'advising'* the tobacco user about the hazards associated with tobacco use and about the availability of suitable and efficacious treatment and management options. For example, those who never used tobacco can be encouraged to never be tempted to use tobacco and advised to avoid situations resulting in exposure to tobacco toxins. Current and past sporadic users can be advised to change this behaviour and on the addictive potential of nicotine. Regular users who are currently abstinent can be encouraged to maintain abstinence and advised to explore ways of preventing relapse and avoiding high-risk situations. Regular and current users, on the other hand, can be advised to quit or reduce the harm related to their tobacco use. The advice provided should be clear and match patient needs, expectations and goals, if it is to be effective and meaningful for the particular individual.

'Assessing' each individual's readiness to adhere to the advice offered is useful in determining and directing the next steps of the healthcare provider's intervention(s). Those willing to take on board the advice offered can be *'assisted'* to do so, whilst those not ready to take on the advice can be subjected to motivational techniques to *'assist'* them becoming ready for change. *'Arranging'* follow-up ensures consistency and continuity, provides opportunity for the individual to think about the advice provided, to analyse their relationship with tobacco and to come back with questions or feedback. It engages in relapse-prevention interventions and increases the chances of successful engagement in healthier lifestyles.

Identification and brief interventions are effective in promoting decreased exposure to tobacco toxins. Smoker's reports indicate that quit advice provided by clinicians tends to be perceived as a good motivator to stop smoking. Brief advice alone is likely to increase the quit rate by 1–3% [18], demonstrating the potential impact of adopting the *'Five A's Framework'* as a flexible and practical approach to addressing the health concerns related to tobacco exposure at an individual level.

11.2.2   Motivation

Assessing an individual's motivation to do something about their use of tobacco is a key element in determining the direction of treatment and management. Although motivation has generally been used to describe readiness at the individual level, the same concept can be used at the population level to describe the readiness of countries and organizations to engage in and implement tobacco-treatment interventions, initiatives, policies and control efforts.

A large proportion of tobacco users would like to give up their habit and makes several attempts at doing so. Globally, three out every four tobacco smokers, who report being aware of the adverse consequences of tobacco use, also report wanting to quit smoking [19], however, annual quit rates tend to be around 4% or less [20, 21]. Generally, tobacco users do not recognize or accept the hazardous potential of tobacco use until this becomes an integral part of their lifestyle, probably related to the fact that most tobacco-related hazards only manifest later on in life. Hence, generally those motivated or wishing to stop are those who are likely to find it more difficult to stop.

Motivation of individual tobacco users is usually measured by the keenness and willingness to seek and engage in treatment, and to achieve and maintain their identified treatment goals. On the flip-side of this, dropping out of treatment, not achieving treatment goals and not engaging or not seeking to engage in treatment is many times taken to indicate a lack of motivation. This view has been challenged by several authors, clinicians as well as tobacco users themselves, and although motivation can contribute to treatment failure, many other factors also play a role.

The degree of motivation at the point of initiation of treatment gives an indication of the degree of readiness for treatment at the point in time, but contrary to assumed belief, it was not found to predict treatment retention and tended to foster judgmental attitudes towards the individual tobacco user [22]. Motivation is dynamic and time specific, indicating the importance of a longitudinal approach to assessment of motivation, recognizing that it fluctuates over time [23]. Although a number of theories (for example, the 'stages of change' theory [24]; the 'social learning theory' [25]; and, the 'self-determination theory' [26] have been suggested as explanations of the underlying mechanisms of motivation, they all indicate that the degree of motivation is influenced by interpersonal interactions between the user and those involved in treatment. Such interactions have impact on the individual's perception of competence to achieve their treatment goals [26].

Vallerand and Thill [27] described motivation as a hypothetical construct explaining the external and internal forces influencing behaviour – that is, the forces that determine treatment seeking, initiation of treatment, engagement and retention in treatment. Internal forces include factors specific to the individual, for example, level of dependency, personality issues, relationship factors, various other life situations and treatment expectations. Amongst others, external forces include sociocultural attitudes, financial issues, service and therapist specifics.

It is therefore important to attempt to engage individuals assessed as having low levels of motivation to do something about their tobacco use, with the initial goals of treatment being to increase and/or maintain motivation levels and to increase the desirability of the treatment offered, increasing the chances of success of treatment.

11.2.3   Treatment and Management Goals

Identification, verification and ownership of the individual tobacco user's goals for treatment and management are key aspects of the treatment experience. Outcome and impact data [20, 21] indicate the importance of having a menu of intervention options suiting varying individual clinical needs, goals and motivation. Tobacco users willing to quit are generally encouraged to have *'cessation'* as their treatment goal; however, health-care practitioners frequently come across tobacco users who are less willing to abstain or have relapsed despite willingness to be abstinent or are willing to reduce their daily consumption as opposed to being abstinent perhaps through substituting with nicotine-replacement products.

Cessation of tobacco use refers to the achievement of abstinence. Evidence suggests that 'cessation' is the treatment goal associated with reduction in tobacco-related health risks resulting in improvement in the overall health of the smoker and that of the immediate and wider society. Several pharmacological and nonpharmacological treatment options are aimed at achieving abstinence, with annual quit rates of around 4% [20, 21]. The chronic relapsing nature of tobacco addiction is frequently translated into individuals engaging in smoking cessation interventions repeatedly with varying periods of abstinence. Even relatively short periods of abstinence can have beneficial effects.

A treatment goal of *sustained cessation and relapse prevention* protects the individual tobacco user and the public from the rapid reinstatement of tobacco use, increasing the chances of success of cessation interventions. Population-level approaches, such as smoke-free laws, banning smoking in closed public places, provide tobacco users with the choice of avoiding exposure to triggers for relapse – for example being exposed to other people smoking. In a recent review [28], behavioural interventions were not found to be effica-cious in preventing relapse, however, some pharmacological interventions, that is extended treatment with varenicline significantly reduced relapse.

Harm reduction refers to measures directed towards reducing tobacco-related harm. This goal recognizes the chronicity of addiction and the difficulty of achieving sustained cessa-tion and aims at achieving some control over tobacco use, reducing the harm consequent to the tobacco epidemic. A number of harm-reduction approaches have been identified [29]. Some of the more common individual-level approaches include, reducing the number of cigarettes smoked daily, using less-toxic tobacco products, partially substituting nico-tine with pharmacological agents and increasing the frequency and length of abstinence periods. Population-level approaches including health-promotion activities, such as public education on potential harms, increase the awareness of such harm and potentially increase the chances of early treatment seeking. Other measures, such as increasing the taxation on tobacco products also significantly reduce exposure to tobacco toxins – it is estimated that a 10% increase in tobacco prices, decreases tobacco consumption by 4–8% [3]. The long-term impact of harm-reduction approaches is unclear and there is insufficient evidence for long-term benefits; however, shorter-term benefits are more obvious and smokers can be encouraged to smoke less by using nicotine gum or inhalers [30].

11.2.4 The Stepped-Care Model for Treatment and Management

The stepped-care model for the treatment and management of tobacco-related problems is a useful cost-efficient approach to matching treatment goals, readiness for treatment and individual variation in treatment needs, with various treatment options. Goals of treatment and management may change with every treatment episode and within treatment episodes. A thorough and longitudinal assessment provides the basis for the setting of appropriate goals and treatment options.

In the stepped-care model, treatment interventions within a treatment system are set out schematically on a spectrum ranging from least intrusive, intensive and usually least expensive to increasing levels of intrusiveness, intensity and expense. Tobacco users are offered the least intrusive and least intensive treatment that meets their treatment goals – if this fails, treatment is stepped-up to a more intensive and intrusive treatment. The stepped-care model offers treatment options for all tobacco users, including those in their precontemplative stage of change [24].

A proposed scheme by Abrams *et al.* [31] provides a good example of how the stepped-care model can be implemented within the treatment system. Three treatment steps are proposed – with treatment intensity and cost ranging from minimal to moderate and maximum. Minimal treatment intensity options, mainly self-help interventions, are proposed as suitable for smokers with low dependence to nicotine, no history of treatment failure and no co-morbidity. Moderate treatment intensity options included brief intervention, pharmacological interventions such as nicotine replacement therapy and nonpharmacological interventions such as skills training and support are proposed as suitable for those with high levels of nicotine dependence but no co-morbidity. Maximum intensity treatment options, included specialist care and are proposed for smokers with high dependency levels and co-morbid disorders.

For the model to be effective the treatment scheme needs to be individualized and evidence based. Appropriate screening and assessment are key to identifying the nature of the problem, treatment needs and goals, for appropriate matching of intensity and intrusiveness of treatment options. Tobacco users with complex needs may need to be quickly stepped-up to more intensive treatment options or may need to enter the treatment system at the higher level of treatment intensity, guided by clinical judgement and individual choice. The model allows for a dynamic and flexible approach to treatment. The tobacco user remains the prime architect of a treatment package, matching their needs and goals, along with adequate clinical guidance [32,33].

The implementation of a stepped-care model can be applied both within individual-level interventions and population-level interventions. A vast literature demonstrates the effectiveness of interventions directed towards selected tobacco users, in particular those seeking treatment. Comparatively very little literature explores the effectiveness of a treatment system on the overall tobacco-related public-health concerns. An effective treatment system can be defined as one that captures all the population at risk of tobacco-related harm. Effective implementation of the stepped-care model to treatment systems can theoretically encompass all determinants of tobacco harm. A study [34] involving a large primary-care population explored the effectiveness of a stepped smoking cessation intervention based on the stages of change model. The results indicated that a stepped-care approach to treatment improved smoking-cessation rates irrespective of whether the smokers were ready to quit smoking. In another study on hospitalized smokers with coronary artery disease a stepped-care approach was associated with improved outcomes in the short term, but no improvement in the longer term [35]. The prevalence of smoking or tobacco use amongst individuals with mental illness is considerably higher than that of the general population. Another article recommended the implementation of the stepped-care model in individuals suffering from schizophrenia as an effective model that could be monitored through nicotine biomarkers [36].

Although further research is required to recommend a stepped-care approach, current literature indicates that the stepped-care model lends itself to a practical cost-effective treatment system for tobacco-related disorders.

11.2.5   Effective Treatment Access

Literature on healthcare systems for tobacco users suggests that the availability and access of treatment options is linked with success in reducing the tobacco use and the public's exposure to tobacco toxins [37–39]. Treatment access refers to the processes determining entry and utilization of a treatment system by an individual or population requiring such a system. Several processes have been identified as determining access, including the availability of the service/treatment option, the individual's expectations, attitudes and acceptability of the service, the physical/geographical accessibility of the service and many others [40–42]. Gulliford *et al.* [40] summarized the key processes determining access under four main headings (below) and consequently defined facilitation of treatment access as *'helping people to command appropriate health care resources in order to preserve or improve their health'*:

- *'Having access'*: This refers to tobacco users having adequate treatment and management options available, – that is the treatment exists within that population.
- *'Gaining access'*: Referring to the extent to which tobacco users gain access and the barriers that limit utilization of the available treatment. This is dependent on affordability of treatment options, physical accessibility and sociocultural acceptability.
- *'Gaining access to satisfactory health outcomes'*: Refers to the notion of treatment options being relevant and effective to achieve best possible outcomes.
- *'Access in the context of differing perspectives, health needs and cultural settings of diverse groups in society'*: Referring to the contextual relationship between availability and barriers and the varying personal and sociocultural needs, past experiences and expectations.

Access has also been described as a useful measure of quality of treatment provision [43]. This, together with other service characteristics such as service equity (i.e. being equally accessible to all those with equal needs), effectiveness and efficiency (i.e. being accessed by all those who are likely to achieve beneficial health outcomes and excluding all those who won't), service appropriateness (i.e. access meeting population need) and responsiveness (i.e. being efficient in responding to individual and population-identified need) reflect the quality of health care provision [40].

The majority of data on effective access of treatment systems for tobacco-related problems, has mainly demonstrated aspects of *'having access'* with very little reference to the other processes constituting access [37, 38]. For instance, a report on effective access to tobacco-dependence treatment in New Zealand [37] described the expansion of the treatment system to meet population demands and some initiatives implemented to make services accessible to more vulnerable groups such as the Maori population. Another report on tobacco-dependence treatment in England [38] described the treatment services, barriers to engaging the health care system in treatment for tobacco-related problems and epidemiological data on numbers accessing treatment. In both reports little was said on the impact of the treatment systems as dimensions of access. The majority of the literature also tends to explore the impact of one particular treatment option as opposed to looking at a whole treatment system. Further research on effective access is required to guide the development and improvement of the treatment and management of tobacco-related problems.

11.2.6 Pharmacological Interventions

Pharmacotherapy for the treatment and management of tobacco dependence is recommended for all individuals willing to engage in treatment, unless medically contraindicated or effectiveness is unclear (e.g. in pregnant women). Although pharmacotherapy on its own has proven efficacy – the combination of medication and nonpharmacological interventions is significantly more effective [15, 16].

11.2.6.1   Nicotine Replacement Therapy (NRT)

NRT is recommended as an appropriate first-line medication for treating tobacco dependence. It exerts its effects by delivering nicotine, replacing the nicotine absorbed from tobacco, alleviating nicotine-withdrawal symptoms and reducing the need for further tobacco use. It is available as a gum, sublingual tablet/lozenge, inhaler, nasal spray and transdermal patch.

There is little variation in effectiveness between the various formulations and the choice is usually determined by patient preference [44]. Nicotine gum is available in two doses – 2 and 4 mg. The gum should be chewed slowly and intermittently until a flavoured taste emerges and should then be held between the cheek and the gum for about 30 minutes, for absorption through the oral mucosa. The nicotine sublingual tablets are available in 1 mg, 2 mg and 4 mg doses. The tablets should be held in the mouth for absorption through the oral mucosa. The inhaler is also absorbed through the oral mucosa. In the nasal spray nicotine is absorbed nasally. One dose usually consists of 0.5 mg delivered to each nostril. It is generally recommended that to apply 1–2 doses per hour. Absorption through this route is rapid, suggesting that the nasal spray may be more suitable for those with high dependency to nicotine – but may still need to be combined with the transdermal patches [45]. The patches provide nicotine through transdermal absorption. They deliver nicotine over longer periods – usually 16 and 24 hours – and can deliver different doses ranging from 5 mg to 21 mg. The continuous release of nicotine suggests that patches could be useful in alleviating any fluctuations in withdrawal experiences, especially if used in combination with the nicotine gum.

NRT is generally well tolerated and the different formulations allow flexibility in appropriate treatment choice. A recent review [44] concluded that there was insufficient evidence to substantiate concern with use of NRT in patients with cardiovascular problems. One of the most common adverse events with use of nicotine patches is skin irritation – reported by more than half of those using the patch [46]. This tends to be mild and very rarely stops individuals from continuing their treatment. Other adverse effects include hiccups, gastrointestinal complaints and jaw and dental problems with the gum; buccal and nasal irritation, coughing and sore throat with the inhaler, nasal spray and tablets. Mouth ulcers and dryness of the mouth are also reported with the use of the tablets [44, 47, 48]. The use of NRT products by pregnant women is not contraindicated but should be avoided unless the benefits outweigh the risks [16, 49]. NRT use by breast-feeding patients should also be avoided or used intermittently, due to the presence of nicotine in breast milk [16, 49].

NRT increases the rate of long-term smoking cessation rate by 50–70% in smokers willing to quit, with high dependency levels. The 'number needed to treat' (NNT) – that is the number of individuals to be treated by NRT in order to get one successful quitter – is 23 [44]. There is little support for use of NRT products in individuals smoking less than 10–15 cigarettes per day [16, 49]. Similarly, there is little support for continuing to prescribe NRT products for individuals who have previously experienced treatment failure with NRT.

NRT is also useful when the treatment goal is harm reduction. The use of NRT gum or inhaler by smokers not willing to quit but seeking to reduce their tobacco problem is reported to increase the odds of reducing the number of cigarettes per day by at least 50%. The use of these NRT products can also increase the chances of achieving cessation following a short-period of reduction in cigarettes per day [30].

11.2.6.2 Bupropion

Bupropion is an anti-depressant with dopaminergic and adrenergic activities, and is recommended as first-line treatment in smoking cessation. It exerts its effects by blocking nicotine and reducing withdrawal symptoms and by relieving depressive mood associated with tobacco use and dependence [50–52]. Bupropion is as effective as NRT in achieving long-term cessation and the selection between NRT and bupropion depends upon individual preference. The NNT for bupropion is 18 [50]. Bupropion was not found to be effective in reducing daily intake of tobacco [30, 53].

The most common adverse events reported with use of bupropion are insomnia (in 30–40%), dry mouth (in 10%) and nausea. Other less common adverse events include allergic reactions and delayed hypersensitivity such as pruritus, angioedema, myalgia, and so on. An increased risk of seizures (reported to contribute to 7 seizures amongst 8000 individuals) following bupropion use has been reported especially when used by specific groups of individuals – those with a history of seizures, history of head trauma, eating disorder or history of alcohol withdrawal. Bupropion has also been reported as increasing the risk of neuropsychiatric symptoms such as agitation, hostility, low mood and suicidality, irrespective of previous history of mental illness [54]. It has been associated with 14 completed suicides and 17 suicidal attempts [54]. Bupropion has also been associated with deaths – however, the evidence is insufficient to infer causality [50].

The use of bupropion in pregnant women has not as yet been shown to be beneficial [16]. However, a study on its use in the first trimester showed that it was not associated with increased malformations, despite the association with spontaneous abortion [55]. The exposure of infants to bupropion through breast feeding is believed to be minimal [56].

11.2.6.3   Varenicline

Varenicline is a selective nicotine receptor partial agonist recommended as first-line treatment for nicotine dependence. It blocks the effects of nicotine by selectively activating the $\alpha_4\beta_2$ nicotine acetylcholine receptor, resulting in moderate but sustained dopamine release, which is believed to be the main mechanism counteracting nicotine-withdrawal symptoms [57].

Varenicline has proven efficacy in increasing the chances of cessation by two- to three-fold when compared to no medication. The 'number needed to treat' for varenicline is calculated at 10. Studies have also demonstrated moderately increased effectiveness with varenicline when compared to both bupropion and NRT [58,59]. Some benefit has also been demonstrated for using varenicline for relapse prevention [60], however, further research is required to substantiate this finding.

Concerns have been raised regarding the association between use of varenicline and the increased risk of psychiatric symptoms – mainly behaviour change, agitation, low mood and suicidal ideation. Varenicline has been temporally linked with a significant number of completed suicides [44] and suicidal attempts [54]. It is recommended that patients experiencing such symptoms should stop varenicline [54,61]. However, one study including individuals with concurrent mental illness reported no harm with use of varenicline within such a cohort [62].

Varenicline is contraindicated for use in pregnancy due to toxicity reported in animal studies. Animal studies also reported presence of varenicline in breast milk. It should be used with caution in individuals with kidney failure and a lower dose may need to be considered. It can also cause drowsiness, potentially impairing the ability to drive or operate heavy machinery. Other common side effects include nausea, which is reported to alleviate over time and can be prevented by dose titration [16, 49, 58].

11.2.6.4   Other Medications

Various other medications with different rationales for their effects on cessation of tobacco use have been proposed. Other anti-depressants such as *nortriptyline* have been used to assist smoking cessation. Nortriptyline has similar efficacy to bupropion and NRT in long-term smoking cessation. It is associated with a similar side-effect profile as tricyclic anti-depressants, however, when used at the low dose (75–150 mg) suitable for smoking cessation, side effects have less of an impact [50].

Selective serotonin uptake inhibitors have failed to show any beneficial effects on smoking cessation [50]. Similarly there is insufficient evidence to support the use of *anxiolytics* in smoking cessation [63]. *Clonidine* is a useful alternative to NRT or anti-depressants. Although further research is required, current research indicates it is effective in promoting smoking cessation and might be appropriate for use in individuals who could benefit from its sedative effects – for example smokers likely to experience anxiety related to smoking cessation [64].

A review [65] on *rimonabant*, a selective type 1 cannabinoid receptor antagonist, showed that 20 mg of rimonabant increased the chances of long-term smoking cessation by $1\frac{1}{2}$ times. Interestingly, rimonabant's effects of weight loss could be a beneficial effect for individuals not willing to quit due to the risk of weight gain. However, rimonabant was withdrawn from the European market as medication for weight loss due to its associations with mental disorders such as depression and suicidality. There was insufficient evidence for a role for rimonabant in maintaining cessation.

Nicotine antagonists (such as *mecamylamine*) are believed to exert their effects on smoking cessation through blocking the rewarding effects of nicotine. Studies show beneficial effects of mecamylamine on smoking cessation, especially, when used in combination with NRT. However, further evidence is required to substantiate this effect [66].

Silver acetate, when combined with cigarettes, produces an unpleasant metallic taste. It has been proposed as a medication to aid smoking cessation through pairing of the aversive stimulus (i.e. the unpleasant taste) with smoking. To date research suggests that the benefit of this treatment is minimal [67].

A more novel approach to pharmacotherapy is the nicotine vaccine. The rationale of the vaccine is to stimulate the production of anti-bodies, which bind to nicotine, preventing nicotine from crossing the blood/brain barrier and exerting its centrally rewarding effects. Interest for use of the vaccine amongst tobacco users is high and to date evidence suggests efficacy of the vaccine for sustained cessation especially at high anti-body levels [68,69].

11.2.7 Nonpharmacological Interventions

Non-pharmacological interventions can be offered individually or in groups and include a mixture of supportive approaches ranging from counselling to cognitive behavioural approaches such as problem-solving and coping-skills training to behavioural approaches and other approaches such as hypnotherapy and acupuncture. Below are some examples of nonpharmacological approaches.

11.2.7.1 Counselling

Individual and group counselling are effective in increasing treatment success rates. The length and number of counselling sessions have been linked to the success rate – in the way that chances of success are increased with the increase in intensity of counselling. Further research is required to support the appropriate matching of tobacco users with the most effective and cost-effective intensity and duration of counselling in line with the stepped-care model of treatment. However, current research points towards a dose–response relationship [16,70]. Further research is also required to explore what elements of 'counselling' have an impact on achieving treatment goals.

11.2.7.2 Problem-Solving and Social Support

Problem-solving, coping skills and stress management training and intratreatment social support are particularly reported to significantly increase abstinence rates. The strength of evidence for such components of therapy is not overwhelming, and it is likely that several confounding factors also play a significant role in treatment effectiveness [16].

11.2.7.3   Contingency Management

Contingency management has been implemented in a variety of settings to encourage engagement in treatment as well as to achieve cessation. In contingency management treatment goals and achieved targets are linked with incentives such as monetary rewards. Such approaches are effective in achieving early and medium-term quit rates, but are not so impressive in the long term, when the rewards are withdrawn [71].

11.2.7.4   Motivational Interviewing

Motivational interviewing techniques as applied to tobacco use aim to increase the likelihood that an individual engages in the process of achieving their identified treatment goals, whether these are cessation, prevention of relapse or harm reduction. It is *'directive'* and *'client centred'* and facilitates behaviour change through *'helping clients explore and resolve ambivalence'* to achieve their treatment goals [72]. Motivational interviewing is recommended for tobacco users, who are unwilling to quit [16]. Promoting motivation has been shown to increase the chances of future cessation attempts [16,73], but more research is required to support its effectiveness in decreasing relapse rates, achieving treatment goals and its implementation within programmes targeting special populations of tobacco users such as those with concomitant drug and/or alcohol use [74].

11.2.7.5   Aversive Techniques

In aversive techniques use of tobacco is paired with an unpleasant stimulus. It is based on the principles of 'classic conditioning' and aims to gradually condition tobacco use as an unpleasant experience. Several techniques have been suggested such as rapid smoking, rapid puffing, smoke holding, and so on. Rapid smoking is the one most commonly mentioned in the literature, and it involves taking puffs every 6–10 seconds, for 3 minutes or till they consume 3 cigarettes or till they feel they cannot smoke any more; resulting in unpleasant effects. Evidence supporting the effectiveness of such techniques is not robust [12,75].

11.2.7.6   Hypnotherapy and Acupuncture

Hypnotherapy and acupuncture are popular interventions despite their questionable efficacy. In hypnotherapy the desire to use tobacco is weakened through modification of the individual's perception of tobacco use. On the other hand, it is suggested that acupuncture reduces the symptoms of nicotine withdrawal. Reviews on both techniques demonstrate inconclusive results. In hypnotherapy, any beneficial effects could be consequent to non-specific factors such as the therapist–patient interaction. In acupuncture, short-term benefits may be evident, however, larger methodologically sound trials are required [76,77].

11.2.8   Combination Treatment

The effectiveness of the various recommended first-line medication in achieving long-term cessation is well documented in clinical guidelines [16]. Research on the effects of combined medication overall indicates a benefit in combining pharmacotherapies [78]. The combination of different formulations of NRT, such as the nicotine patch and inhaler and the long-term use of nicotine patch with the nicotine gum or nasal spray, is associated with improvement in cessation rates. Long-term benefit was reported with combining bupropion and the NRT patch [79]. No benefit was reported when combining nicotine patch with paroxetine [80]. Further evidence is required to support the use of combination therapies within various cohorts.

Similarly, the combination of medication and nonpharmacological treatment is associated with increased cessation rates [16]. Several studies reported that the combination of counselling or cognitive behavioural therapies and medication significantly improved the outcomes from counselling alone or medication alone [16, 78]. One interesting study reported enhanced outcomes with the combination of bupropion and counselling within the indigenous Maori population in New Zealand [81].

11.2.9   The Role of Family and Friends in Individual-Based Treatment

The use of tobacco by individuals has direct impact on their immediate environment, families, friends and other social networks and the dynamics of the relationships within the tobacco-user's world. Similarly, occurrences within the immediate environment, and behaviour and relationships of others impact on the initiation, nature and degree of tobacco use and tobacco treatment and management.

Children of smokers passively smoke at an early age. Early exposure to environmental tobacco and parental tobacco use are linked with tobacco use amongst young people. Smokers tend to seek relationships with other smokers and tend to marry smokers, consequently influencing each other's smoking behaviour – smoking the same number of cigarettes per day, maintaining each other's smoking behaviour and influencing the timing and outcome of treatment [82–84].

Involving family and friends within the treatment system determines the impact of individual-based treatment and management of tobacco use. Guidelines for the treatment of tobacco use recommend that family and social support interventions are made part of the treatment package [11]. Involving significant others can reduce the impact of tobacco use and increase the chances of favourable outcomes. As with treatment options for individuals with alcohol and drug problems, families and friends can be involved in a variety of interventions with varying degrees of intensity [85]. The stepped-care model for treatment could be applied to facilitate matching of individual needs and the needs of significant others with the various family-based interventions.

Further research is required in this area. Current literature has ranged from demonstrating no effect to minimal effect and to a more significant effect of the chances of quitting [11,86]. A large proportion of the literature focuses on cessation and relapse prevention as goals for treatment. The number of mechanisms involved in the interaction between the tobacco user and their immediate environment suggests that various alternative outcomes are at play and exploring harm reduction as a treatment goal may be more appropriate.

11.2.10   Treatment and Management within Specific Populations of Tobacco Users

Individual-based treatment approaches described above refer to specific treatment options without much reference to the effect of recommended treatment on individuals with particular needs.

The use of tobacco is highly prevalent amongst those with *mental illness*. Individuals with mental illness are twice as likely to smoke [87–89], when compared with the general population, highlighting the importance of identifying effective treatment options for this cohort of individuals. Generally, interventions for the general population have beneficial effects for individuals with mental illness [78]. In particular, the combination of bupropion (slow release) and NRT was reported as being effective in patients with schizophrenia, also having beneficial effects on the negative symptoms of schizophrenia and associated mood problems, mainly depression [90,91]. However, both bupropion and varenicline have been associated with psychiatric symptoms and their use within such a population would require adequate monitoring.

Tobacco dependence is also highly prevalent amongst individuals with *drug and/or alcohol dependency*. Pharmacological and nonpharmacological interventions and combinations of both are effective in individuals engaged in treatment for drug and/or alcohol problems [16]. However, further research around efficacy is required within this cohort. Some studies only report short-term benefits [92], while others suggested that treatment for tobacco dependence compromised outcomes for alcohol treatment [93].

The provision of treatment for individuals with *co-morbid physical conditions* is associated with enhanced outcomes. In individuals with co-morbid chronic obstructive airways disease intensive psychosocial interventions in combination with pharmacological agents is recommended [16]. The effectiveness of treatment in individuals with HIV remains unclear and further research on long-term outcomes is required [16]. In hospitalized patients intensive counselling during hospitalization together with post-hospitalization follow-up for at least 1 month was associated with increased rates of smoking cessation. Less-intensive counselling was not associated with any beneficial effects. Similarly, the addition of medication to intensive counselling, did not improve outcomes when compared to intensive counselling alone. Such findings indicate that hospitalization is an opportunistic period for tobacco users to engage in treatment [94].

Pharmacological and nonpharmacological interventions are effective in other specific groups such as *older tobacco users*, *ethnic minorities* and the *female population*. In women, advice to quit with a focus on hazards to children's health had significant benefits [16,95].

Water-pipe smoking, frequently seen in North Africa, some Mediterranean countries and some areas in Asia, is generally a social activity for families and friends, including women and young girls. It is erroneously perceived as being less hazardous and less addictive than other methods of tobacco use. Within such a group of smokers community-based approaches play a significant role in increasing the awareness of hazards related to water-pipe smoking. Further research on individual-based interventions is required [96]. Pharmacotherapies have not been shown to improve long-term outcomes in users of *smokeless tobacco*. On the other hand, studies demonstrated that behavioural interventions provided some benefit, particularly telephone counselling and oral examinations [97].

11.3 POPULATION-LEVEL TREATMENT AND MANAGEMENT OPTIONS

Population-level treatment and management options are wider reaching and are aimed at facilitating a supportive environment for a larger number of people, complimenting individual-based interventions. They play an important role within the treatment system – changing the community's perceptions around tobacco use, increasing awareness on tobacco-related hazards and promoting engagement in treatment goals and options. Community-based options recognize that tobacco use occurs within a broad social context and seeks to reduce population prevalence and tobacco-related harm by changing social norms [7, 98, 99]. Reducing the overall prevalence of smoking by 5% by 2020 is reported to result in significant reductions in tobacco-related health and social hazards [100, 101]. Population approaches have also been noted to widen the gap on social inequalities related to tobacco use. Population-level interventions have less impact on lower socio-economic groups in society, thus worsening health inequalities [5–7].

A large number of tobacco users attempt to stop using tobacco without seeking help or engaging in treatment. *Self-help materials* could be beneficial to those individuals not likely to seek help. The most widely used self-help materials are written materials such as patient leaflets; however, there are many other resources such as audio material, videos and computer games or programmes. Generic self-help materials provide a modest decrease in smoking-cessation rates. Individually tailored self-help materials provide better results than generic, although the overall benefit still remains very modest. Individually-tailored materials consist of interactive materials, often based on the stages of change model providing communities with information on treatment options matched to their change stages [102].

Mass-media campaigns have the benefit of reaching a large number of the population through various means – for example television, radio, newspapers, billboards, and so on. They increase awareness of associated hazards and treatment benefits, promote attitude change within society and enhance the public-health and political anti-tobacco initiatives [103]. It is unclear to what degree mass-media campaigns influence tobacco-use behaviour, however, overall, including mass-media campaigns in tobacco control programmes, they are effective in facilitating behaviour change [104].

Telephone quitlines are popular, accessible to various population groups, confidential and anonymous and cost effective. Within the UK, quitlines are estimated to reach 10% of the UK South Asian population of tobacco users [105]. Quitlines have the potential for being both 'reactive' (i.e. provide advice to individuals phoning in) and 'proactive' (i.e. provide ongoing advice through follow-up phone calls) [106]. It is difficult to measure the impact of telephone counselling, however, a recent review concluded that quitlines provide an effective route of access to support tobacco users, which is enhanced by proactive call-back. Calling back three to four times (as opposed to one or two times) increases the chances of cessation compared to other minimal interventions such as self-help materials [107]. Quitlines are generally believed to reach between 4 and 6% of the tobacco-using population [107, 108]. *Internet-based* online smoking cessation sites are also increasing in popularity. Online counselling provides the potential for an interactive mode of counselling likely to reach a large number of people including young tobacco users.

Population-level competitions and incentives, such as *quit and win* contests, are an effective way of encouraging tobacco users to engage in treatment goals through the offering of rewards for achievement of goals. Reports on the impact of contests are misleading, some studies reporting cessation rates of around 20% [103], while others report modest successes – that is around 1 in every 500 smokers stopping following 'quit and win' interventions [109]. Every 2 years the WHO coordinates an international 'quit and win' contest, including around 80 countries – this contest has an effective impact on tobacco users from developing countries [103, 109].

11.3.1   Tobacco-Control Legislation and Policy

Population-level measures of tobacco control, such as making it illegal to smoke in enclosed public places and having smoke-free workplaces, are effective measures aimed at achieving a supportive environment for smoking cessation, de-normalizing the use of tobacco, and protecting the population from the hazards of tobacco toxins. They are associated with significant reductions in prevalence and daily consumption and significant increases in willingness to quit and long-term quitting. High taxation on tobacco products is also associated with lower prevalence rates and higher quit rates. For instance, a 10% increase in the price of cigarettes is associated with a 4% reduction in demand in high-income countries and 8% reduction in low-income countries [110]. Other measures include regulation of contents of tobacco products; health warnings on tobacco packaging, regulation of tobacco advertising and sponsorship by the tobacco industry and regulation of tobacco supply. Bans on advertisements and promotion of tobacco products are associated with a 7% reduction in demand [110]. On the other hand, tobacco advertising and promotion were reported to be associated with increased prevalence of tobacco use by adolescents [111].

The commitment of the Government to ensure sustained decreased demand and increased environmental support and treatment, is reflected in the financial and human resource, allocated to both population-level and individual-level treatment and management.

11.3.2   International Treatment and Management Options

A global approach to the treatment and management of the tobacco epidemic is vital in addressing global demand and supply, protection of human lives and availability and access of treatment options. International organizations, such as the WHO Framework Convention on Tobacco Control (WHO FCTC), provide organizational structure and support for the sharing and distribution of information and guidelines and the promotion of funding, research and partnership bodies. Reports from champion countries implementing a comprehensive and coordinated approach to tackling the tobacco-use problem provide the opportunity for sharing and role modelling and overall encouragement for less-committed countries to engage in similar approaches.

The WHO FCTC came into force on the 27th February 2005 and is to date supported by 166 Parties. In 2008 the documentation *MPower* [3] was compiled describing six evidence-based tobacco control policies for global implementation:

- monitor tobacco use and prevention policies;
- protect people from tobacco smoke;

- offer help to quit tobacco use;
- warn about dangers of tobacco;
- enforce bans on tobacco advertising, promotion and sponsorship;
- raise taxes on tobacco.

Epidemiological data indicate that only 5% of the world's population are protected from environmental tobacco smoke, protected through bans on advertising, promotion and sponsorship and have available help to quit. Only 4–6% of the world's population receive appropriate warnings about the dangers of tobacco and only about half of the world countries have appropriate monitoring systems [3]. Such data highlights massive gaps in the global scene. The implementation of the *MPower* policies at a global level will significantly shrink the global tobacco epidemic.

11.4 CONCLUSION

The use of tobacco is everybody's problem. A comprehensive, coordinated, global approach to treatment and management of tobacco problems is vital for the success in controlling the tobacco epidemic. Availability and access to various individual-level and population-level treatment options with a treatment system have an impact on the willingness of individual tobacco users to determine their choice of treatment goals and their engagement in treatment options. The academic arena has provided us with robust evidence-based approaches for different population groups. The commitment of national governments to protecting the public from tobacco harm and providing a supportive environment is influential in altering social perception of tobacco use, denormalizing use and ensuring sustained public-health directives and tobacco-control initiatives. The coming together of various governments is instrumental to addressing both the demand and supply of tobacco use.

REFERENCES

1. Mathers, C.D. and Loncar, D. (2006) Projections of global mortality & burden of disease from 2002 to 2030. *PLoS Medicine*, **3** (11), e442, 2011–2030, from www.plosmedicine.org (accessed on 27 April 2009).
2. Peto, R., *et al.* (1996) Mortality from smoking worldwide. *British Medical Bulletin*, **52** (1), 12–21.
3. World Health Organization (2008) *WHO Report on the Global Tobacco Epidemic, 2008, The MPOWER Package*, World Health Organization, Geneva, Switzerland.
4. Mackay, J., Erikson, M. and Shafey, O. (2006) *The Tobacco Atlas*, 2nd edn, American Cancer Society, Atlanta.
5. Marmot, M. (2006) Smoking and inequalities. *Lancet*, **368**, 341–342.
6. Jha, P., Peto, R., Zatonski, W. *et al.* (2006) Social inequalities in male mortality, and in male mortality from smoking: indirect estimation from national death rates in England and Wales, Poland, and North America. *Lancet*, **368**, 367–370.
7. Frohlich, K. (2008) Is tobacco use a disease? *Canadian Medical Association Journal*, **179** (9), 880–882.

8. U.S. Surgeon General (2004) *The 2004 Surgeon General's Report – The Health Consequences of Smoking*, from http://www.cdc.gov/tobacco/data_statistics/sgr/sgr_2004/chapters.htm (accessed on 27 April 2009).

9. Henningfield, J.E. and Jasinski, D.R. (1988) Pharmacologic basis for nicotine replacement, in *Nicotine Replacement* (eds. O.F. Pomerleau and C.S. Pomerleau), Alan R. Liss, New York, pp. 35–61.

10. U.S. Department of Health & Human Services (1988) The Health Consequences of Smoking – Surgeon General's Report, Washington DC.

11. Fiore, M.C., Bailey, W.C., Cohen, S.J. *et al.* (2000) *Treating Tobacco Use and Dependence: Clinical Practice Guideline*, Department of Health & Human Services, Public Health Service. Rockville, MD, United States.

12. Ghodse, H. (in press) *Ghodse's Drugs 7 Addictive Behaviour: a Guide To Treatment*, 4th edn, Cambridge University Press, UK.

13. National Institute of Health & Clinical Excellence (2006) *Brief Interventions & Referral for Smoking Cessation in Primary Care & Other Settings*, Public Health Intervention Guidance No. 1, National Institute of Health & Clinical Excellence, UK.

14. Rigotti, N.A. (2002) Clinical Practice. Treatment of tobacco use and dependence. *New England Journal of Medicine*, **346**, 506–512.

15. Raw, M., McNeill, A. and West, R. (1998) Smoking cessation guidelines for health professionals. A guide to effective smoking cessation interventions for the health care system. *Thorax*, **53** (Suppl 5, Pt 1), S1–S19.

16. Fiore, M.C. *et al.* (2008) *Treating Tobacco Use and Dependence: 2008 Update*, United States Department of Health & Human Services, Public Health Service, USA.

17. American Psychiatric Association (1996) Practice guideline for the treatment of patients with nicotine dependence. *American Journal of Psychiatry*, **153** (10 Suppl), S1–S31.

18. Stead, L.F., Bergson, G. and Lancaster, T. (2008) Physician advice for smoking cessation. *Cochrane Database of Systematic Reviews* **2**. DOI: 10.1002/14651858.CD000165.pub3.

19. Jones, J.M. (2006) *Smoking habits stable; most would like to quit*, from http://www.gallup.com/poll/23791/Smoking-Habits-Stable-Most-Would-Like-Quit.aspx (accessed on 24 April 2009).

20. Messer, K., Pierce, J.P., Zhu, S.H. *et al.* (2007) The California Tobacco Control Program's effect on adult smokers: (1) Smoking cessation. *Tobacco Control*, **16** (2), 85–90.

21. West, R. (2006) *Background smoking cessation rates in England*. From www.smokinginengland. info/Ref/paper2.pdf (accessed on 3 June 2009).

22. Miller, W.R. (1985) Motivation for treatment: a review with special emphasis on alcoholism. *Psychological Bulletin*, **98**, 84–107.

23. Reeve, J. (1992) *Understanding Motivation and Emotion*, HBJ Publishers, Montreal.

24. Prochaska, J.O. and DiClemente, C.C. (1986) Toward a comprehensive model of change, in *Treating Addictive Behaviours* (eds. W.R. Miller and N. Heather), Plenum, New York, pp. 3–27.

25. Bandura, A. (1977) Self-efficacy: toward a unifying theory of behavioral change. *Psychological Review*, **84** (2), 191–215.

26. Deci, E.L. and Ryan, R.M. (1985) *Intrinsic Motivation and Self-Determination in Human Behavior*, Plenum, New York. From Simoneau, H. and Bergeron, J. (2003) Factors affecting motivation during the first six weeks of treatment. *Addictive Behaviours*, **28**, 1219–1241.

27. Vallerand, R.J. and Thill, E. (1993) *Introduction à la psychologie de la motivation*, Montréal: Étude Vivante. From Simoneau, H. and Bergeron, J. (2003) Factors affecting motivation during the first six weeks of treatment. *Addictive Behaviours*, **28**, 1219–1241.

28. Hajek, P., Stead, L.F., West, R. *et al.* (2009) Relapse prevention interventions for smoking cessation, *Cochrane Database of Systematic Reviews* **1** (Art. No.: CD003999). DOI: 10.1002/14651858.CD003999.pub3.

29. Shiffman, S., Gitchell, J.G., Warner, K.E. *et al.* (2002) Tobacco harm reduction: Conceptual structure and nomenclature for analysis and research. *Nicotine & Tobacco Research* **4** (Suppl 2), S113–S129.

30. Stead, L.F. and Lancaster, T. (2007) Interventions to reduce harm from continued tobacco use. *Cochrane Database of Systematic Reviews* 3 (Art. No.: CD005231). DOI: 10.1002/14651858.CD005231.pub2.

31. Abrams, D.B., Orleans, C.T., Niaura, R. *et al.* (1996) Integrating individual and public health perspectives for treatment of tobacco dependence under managed health care: A combined stepped care and matching model. *Annals of Behavioral Medicine*, **18**, 290–304.

32. Piasecki, T.M. and Baker, T.B. (2001) Any further progress in smoking cessation treatment? *Nicotine & Tobacco Research*, **3**, 311–323.

33. Smith, S.S., Jorenby, D.E., Fiore, M.C. *et al.* (2001) Strike while the iron is hot: can stepped-care treatments resurrect relapsing smokers? *Journal of Consulting and Clinical Psychology*, **69**, 429–439.

34. Cabezas, C., Martin, C., Granollers, S. *et al.* (2009) Effectiveness of a stepped primary care smoking cessation intervention (ISTAPS study): design of a cluster randomised trial. *BMC Public Health*, **9**, 48.

35. Reid, R., Pipe, A., Higginson, L. *et al.* (2003) Stepped care approach to smoking cessation in patients hospitalized for coronary artery disease. *Journal of Cardiopulmonary Rehabilitation* **23** (3) (May–Jun), 176–182.

36. McChargue, D.E., Gulliver, S.B. and Hitsman, B. (2003) Applying a stepped-care reduction approach to smokers with Schizophrenia. *Psychiatric Times*, September, 78.

37. Price, L. and Allen, M. (2003) *New Zealand: Effective Access to Tobacco Dependence Treatment*, World Health Organization. From http://www.who.int/tobacco/research/cessation/en/best_practices_new_zealand.pdf (accessed on 31 July 2009).

38. Raw, M. and McNeill, A. (2003) *Tobacco Dependence Treatment in England*, World Health Organization. From http://www.who.int/tobacco/research/cessation/en/best_practices_england.pdf (accessed on 31 July 2009).

39. Curry, S.J. (2001) Bridging the clinical and public health perspectives in tobacco treatment research: Scenes from a tobacco treatment research career. *Cancer Epidemiology, Biomarkers & Prevention* **10** (April), 281–285.

40. Gulliford, M., Morgan, M., Hughes, D. *et al.* (2001) *Access to Health Care: Report of a scoping exercise for the National Co-ordinating Centre for NHS Service Delivery and Organisation R & D (NCCSDO)*, NCCSDO, London.

41. Aday, L.A. and Anderson, R.M. (1981) Equity of access to medical care: a conceptual and empirical overview. *Medical Care*, **19** (Supplement), 4–27.

42. Pechansky, R. and Thomas, W. (1981) The concept of access. *Medical Care*, **19**, 127–140.

43. Maxwell, R.J. (1984) Quality assessment in health. *British Medical Journal*, **288**, 1470–1472.

44. Stead, L.F., Perera, R., Bullen, C. *et al.* (2008) Nicotine replacement therapy for smoking cessation. *Cochrane Database of Systematic Reviews* **1** (Art. No.: CD000146). DOI: 10.1002/14651858.CD000146.pub3.

45. Sutherland, G., Stapleton, J., Russell, M.A.H., Jarvis, M. *et al.* (1992) Randomized controlled trial of nasal nicotine spray in smoking cessation. *Lancet*, **340**, 324–329.

46. Fiore, M.C., Jorenby, D.E., Baker, T.B. and Kenford, S.L. (1992) Tobacco dependence and the nicotine patch. Clinical guidelines for effective use. *JAMA*, **268**, 2687–2694.

47. Wallstrom, M., Sand, L., Nilsson, F. and Hirsch, J.M. (1999) The long-term effect of nicotine on the oral mucosa. *Addiction*, **94**, 417–423.

48. Schneider, N.G., Olmstead, R.E., Nides, M. *et al.* (2004) Comparative testing of 5 nicotine systems: initial use and preferences. *American Journal of Health Behavior*, **28**, 72–86.

49. BMJ (2008) *British National Formulary: 56*, September, 2008. BMJ Group, London.

50. Hughes, J.R., Stead, L.F. and Lancaster, T. (2007) Antidepressants for smoking cessation. *Cochrane Database of Systematic Reviews* 1 (Art. No.: CD000031). DOI: 10.1002/14651858.CD000031.pub3.

51. Cryan, J.F., Bruijnzeel, A.W., Skjei, K.L. and Markou, A. (2003) Bupropion enhances brain reward function and reverses the affective and somatic aspects of nicotine withdrawal in the rat. *Psychopharmacology (Berl)*, **168**, 347–358.

52. Lerman, C., Roth, D., Kaufmann, V. *et al.* (2002) Mediating mechanisms for the impact of bupropion in smoking cessation treatment. *Drug and Alcohol Dependence*, **67**, 219–223.

53. Hatsukami, D.K., Rennard, S., Patel, M.K. *et al.* (2004) Effects of sustained-release bupropion among persons interested in reducing but not quitting smoking. *American Journal of Medicine* **116** (3), 151–157.

54. Osterweil, N. (2009) *Chantix and Zyban to Receive Boxed Warnings for Serious Neuropsychiatric Symptoms*, Medscape, LLC (07/01/2009) Medscape Medical News © 2009.

55. Chun-Fai-Chan, B., Koren, G., Fayez, I. *et al.* (2005) Pregnancy outcome of women exposed to bupropion during pregnancy: a prospective comparative study. *American Journal of Obstetrics & Gynecology*, **192** (3), 932–936.

56. Haas, J.S., Kaplan, C.P., Barenboim, D. *et al.* (2004) Bupropion in breast milk: an exposure assessment for potential treatment to prevent post-partum tobacco use. *Tobacco Control*, **13**, 52–56.

57. Sands, S.B., Brooks, P.R., Chambers, L.K. *et al.* (2005) *A new therapy for smoking cessation: varenicline, a selective nicotinic receptor partial agonist [SYM10C]*. Society for Research on Nicotine and Tobacco 11th Annual Meeting. 20–23 March 2005; Prague, Czech Republic. 2005, p. 14.

58. Cahill, K., Stead, L.F. and Lancaster, T. (2008) Nicotine receptor partial agonists for smoking cessation. *Cochrane Database of Systematic Reviews* 3 (Art. No.: CD006103). DOI: 10.1002/14651858.CD006103.pub3.

59. National Institute for Health and Clinical Excellence (2007) Varenicline for smoking cessation. From http://www.nice.org.uk/nicemedia/pdf/TA123Guidance.pdf (accessed 14th April 2008). National Institute for Health & Clinical Excellence, London.

60. Tonstad, S., Tonnesen, P., Hajek, P. *et al.* (2006) Effect of maintenance therapy with varenicline on smoking cessation: a randomized controlled trial. *JAMA*, **296** (1), 64–71. [clinicaltrials.gov ID: NCT00143286].

61. Food & Drug Administration (2008) FDA issues Public Health Advisory on Chantix. From http://www.fda.gov/NewsEvents/Newsroom/PressAnnouncements/2008/ucm116849.htm (accessed 24th June 2009).

62. Stapleton, J.A., Watson, L., Spirling, L.I. *et al.* (2008) Varenicline in the routine treatment of tobacco dependence: a pre-post comparison with nicotine replacement therapy and an evaluation in those with mental illness. *Addiction*, **103** (1), 146–154.

63. Hughes, J.R., Stead, L.F. and Lancaster, T. (2000) Anxiolytics for smoking cessation. *Cochrane Database of Systematic Reviews* 4 (Art. No.: CD002849). DOI: 10.1002/14651858.CD002849.

64. Gourlay, S.G., Stead, L.F. and Benowitz, N. (2004) Clonidine for smoking cessation. *Cochrane Database of Systematic Reviews* **3** (Art. No.: CD000058). DOI: 10.1002/14651858. CD000058.pub2.

65. Cahill, K. and Ussher, M.H. (2007) Cannabinoid type 1 receptor antagonists (rimonabant) for smoking cessation. *Cochrane Database of Systematic Reviews* **4** (Art. No.: CD005353). DOI: 10.1002/14651858.CD005353.pub3.

66. Lancaster, T. and Stead, L.F. (1998) Mecamylamine (a nicotine antagonist) for smoking cessation. *Cochrane Database of Systematic Reviews* **2** (Art. No.: CD001009). DOI: 10.1002/14651858.CD001009.

67. Lancaster, T. and Stead, L.F. (1997) Silver acetate for smoking cessation. *Cochrane Database of Systematic Reviews* **3** (Art. No.: CD000191). DOI: 10.1002/14651858.CD000191.

68. Leader, A.E., Lerman, C. and Cappella, J.N. (2010) Nicotine vaccines: Will smokers take a shot at quitting? *Nicotine & Tobacco Research* **12** (4), 390–397.

69. Cornuz, J., Zwahlen, S., Jungi, W.F., *et al.* (2008) A vaccine against nicotine for smoking cessation: a randomized controlled trial. *PLoS One* **3** (6), e2547.

70. Lancaster, T. and Stead, L.F. (2005) Individual behavioural counselling for smoking cessation. *Cochrane Database of Systematic Reviews* **2** (Art. No.: CD001292). DOI: 10.1002/14651858.CD001292.pub2.

71. Cahill, K. and Perera, R. (2008) Competitions and incentives for smoking cessation. *Cochrane Database of Systematic Reviews* **3** (Art. No.: CD004307). DOI: 10.1002/14651858. CD004307.pub3.

72. Miller, W.R. (1983) Motivational interviewing with problem drinkers. *Behavioural Psychotherapy*, **11**, 147–172.

73. Butler, C.C., Rollnick, S., Cohen, D. *et al.* (1999) Motivational consulting versus brief advice for smokers in general practice: A randomized trial. *British Journal of General Practice*, **49**, 611–616.

74. Lai DTC., Qin, Y. and Tang, J.L. (2008) Motivational interviewing for smoking cessation. *Cochrane Database of Systematic Reviews* **1** (Art. No.: CD006936). DOI: 10.1002/14651858. CD006936.

75. Hajek, P. and Stead, L.F. (2001) Aversive smoking for smoking cessation. *Cochrane Database of Systematic Reviews* **3** (Art. No.: CD000546). DOI: 10.1002/14651858.CD000546.pub2.

76. Abbot, N.C., Stead, L.F., White, A.R. and Barnes, J. (1998) Hypnotherapy for smoking cessation. *Cochrane Database of Systematic Reviews* **2** (Art. No.: CD001008). DOI: 10.1002/14651858.CD001008.

77. White, A.R., Rampes, H. and Campbell, J. (2006) Acupuncture & related interventions for smoking cessation. *Cochrane Database of Systematic Reviews* **1** (Art. No.: CD000009). DOI: 10.1002/14651858.CD000009.pub2.

78. Ranney, L., Melvin, C., Lux, L. *et al.* (2006) Systematic review: Smoking cessation intervention strategies for adults and adults in special populations. *Annals of Internal Medicine*, **145**, 845–856.

79. Jorenby, D.E., Leischow, S.J., Nides, M.A. *et al.* (1999) A controlled trial of sustained-release bupropion, a nicotine patch, or both for smoking cessation. *New England Journal of Medicine*, **340**, 685–691. [PMID: 10053177].

80. Killen, J.D., Fortmann, S.P., Schatzberg, A.F. *et al.* (2000) Nicotine patch and paroxetine for smoking cessation. *Journal of Consulting & Clinical Psychology*, **68**, 883–889 [PMID: 11068974].

81. Holt, S., Timu-Parata, C., Ryder-Lewis, S. *et al.* (2005) Efficacy of bupropion in the indigenous Maori population in New Zealand. *Thorax*, **60**, 120–123 [PMID: 15681499].

82. Venters, M.H., Jacobs, D.R., Luepker, R.V., Maiman, L.A., Gillum, R.F. (1984) Spouse concordance of smoking patterns: The Minnesota heart survey. *American Journal of Epidemiology*, **120** (4), 608–616.

83. Gulliver, S.B., Hughes, J.R., Solomon, L.J. and Dey, A.N. (1995) An investigation of self-efficacy, partner support and daily stresses as predictors of relapse to smoking in self-quitters. *Society for the Study of Addiction to Alcohol & other Drugs*, **90**, 767–772.

84. Roski, J., Schmid, L.A. and Lando, H.A. (1996) Long-term associations of helpful and harmful spousal behaviours with smoking cessation. *Addictive Behaviors*, **21** (2), 173–185.

85. Ghodse, A.H. and Galea, S. (2005) Families of people with drug abuse, in *Families & Mental Disorders: From Burden To Empowerment* (eds. N. Sartorius, J. Leff, J.J. Lopez-Ibor *et al.*), World Psychiatric Association, John Wiley & Sons, England, pp. 161–193.

86. Park, E.W., Schultz, J.K., Tudiver, F.G. *et al.* (2004) Enhancing partner support to improve smoking cessation. *Cochrane Database of Systematic Reviews* **3** (Art. No.: CD002928). DOI: 10.1002/14651858.CD002928.pub2.

87. Hughes, J.R. *et al.* (1986) Prevalence of smoking among psychiatric outpatients. *American Journal of Psychiatry*, **143**, 993–997.

88. Lasser, K. *et al.* (2000) Smoking and mental illness: a population-based prevalence study. *Journal of the American Medical Association*, **284**, 2606–2610.

89. McNeill, A. (2001) *Smoking and Mental Health – a Review of the Literature*, SmokeFree London Programme, London.

90. Evins, A.E., Cather, C., Rigotti, N.A. *et al.* (2004) Two-year follow-up of a smoking cessation trial in patients with schizophrenia: increased rates of smoking cessation and reduction. *Journal of Clinical Psychiatry*, **65**, 307–311.

91. George, T.P., Vessicchio, J.C., Termine, A. *et al.* (2002) A placebo controlled trial of bupropion for smoking cessation in schizophrenia. *Biological Psychiatry*, **52**, 53–61.

92. Prochaska, J.J., Delucchi, K. and Hall, S.M. (2004) A meta-analysis of smoking cessation interventions with individuals in substance abuse treatment or recovery. *Journal of Consulting & Clinical Psychology*, **72**, 1144–1156 [PMID: 15612860].

93. Joseph, A.M., Willenbring, M.L., Nugent, S.M. and Nelson, D.B. (2004) A randomized trial of concurrent versus delayed smoking intervention for patients in alcohol dependence treatment. *Journal of Studies on Alcohol*, **65**, 681–691 [PMID: 15700504].

94. Rigotti, N., Munafo', M.R. and Stead, L.F. (2007) Interventions for smoking cessation in hospitalised patients. *Cochrane Database of Systematic Reviews* **3** (Art. No.: CD001837). DOI: 10.1002/14651858.CD001837.pub2.

95. Yilmaz, G., Karacan, C., Yoney, A. *et al.* (2006) Brief intervention on maternal smoking: a randomized controlled trial. *Child Care Health Dev*, **32**, 73–79.

96. Maziak, W., Ward, K.D. and Eissenberg, T. (2007) Interventions for waterpipe smoking cessation. *Cochrane Database of Systematic Reviews* **4** (Art. No.: CD005549). DOI: 10.1002/14651858.CD005549.pub2.

97. Ebbert, J., Montori, V.M., Vickers-Douglas, K.S. *et al.* (2007) Interventions for smokeless tobacco use cessation. *Cochrane Database of Systematic Reviews* **4** (Art. No.: CD004306). DOI: 10.1002/14651858.CD004306.pub3.

98. Secker-Walker, R., Gnich, W., Platt, S. and Lancaster, T. (2002) Community interventions for reducing smoking among adults. *Cochrane Database of Systematic Reviews* **2** (Art. No.: CD001745). DOI: 10.1002/14651858.CD001745.

99. Ockene, J.K. (1992) Are we pushing the limits of public health interventions for smoking cessation? *Health Psychology*, **11**, 277–279.

100. Peto, R. and Lopez, A.D. (2001) Future worldwide health effects of current smoking patterns, in *Critical Issues in Global Health* (eds. C.D. Koop, C. Pearson and M.R. Schwarz), Jossey-Bass, New York, pp. 154–61.

101. Frieden, T.R. and Bloomberg, M.R. (2007) How to prevent 100 million deaths from tobacco. *Lancet*, **369**, 1758–1761.

102. Lancaster, T. and Stead, L.F. (2005) Self-help interventions for smoking cessation. *Cochrane Database of Systematic Reviews* **3** (Art. No.: CD001118). DOI: 10.1002/14651858. CD001118.pub2.

103. Costa e Silva, V.L. (2003) *Policy Recommendations on Smoking Cessation & Treatment of Tobacco Dependence*, World Health Organization, Geneva, Switzerland.

104. Bala, M., Strzeszynski, L. and Cahill, K. (2008) Mass media interventions for smoking cessation in adults. *Cochrane Database of Systematic Reviews* **1** (Art. No.: CD004704). DOI: 10.1002/14651858.CD004704.pub2.

105. South Asian Social Researcher's Forum (2001) *An Evaluation of the Services of Asian Quitline*, UK.

106. Lichtenstein, E., Glasgow, R.E., Lando, H.A. *et al.* (1996) Telephone counselling for smoking cessation – rationales and metaanalytic review of evidence. *Health Education Research*, **11**, 243–257.

107. Stead, L.F., Perera, R. and Lancaster, T. (2006) Telephone counselling for smoking cessation. *Cochrane Database of Systematic Reviews* **3** (Art. No.: CD002850). DOI: 10.1002/14651858. CD002850.pub2.

108. Owen, L. (2000) Impact of a Telephone Helpline for Smokers who called During a Mass Media Campaign. *Tobacco control*, **9**, 148–154.

109. Cahill, K. and Perera, R. (2008) Quit and Win contests for smoking cessation. *Cochrane Database of Systematic Reviews* **4** (Art. No.: CD004986). DOI: 10.1002/14651858.CD004986. pub3.

110. World Bank (1999) *Curbing the Epidemic: Governments and the Economics of Tobacco Control*, The International Bank for Reconstruction and Development, World Bank, Washington, DC.

111. Lovato, C., Linn, G., Stead, L.F. and Best, A. (2003) Impact of tobacco advertising and promotion on increasing adolescent smoking behaviours. *Cochrane Database of Systematic Reviews* **3** (Art. No.: CD003439). DOI: 10.1002/14651858.CD003439.

12.1 Challenges in Reducing the Disease Burden of Tobacco Smoking

Coral Gartner, Ph.D and Wayne Hall, Ph.D

School of Population Health, University of Queensland, Brisbane, Queensland, Australia

Cigarette smoking became the dominant form of tobacco use in most of the developed world by the mid-twentieth century. This followed development of the flue-curing method that produced more acidic smoke that was easier to inhale into the lungs, and the invention of the Bonsack cigarette-making machine that reduced the cost of manufactured cigarettes. By the middle of the twentieth century the increase in cigarette smoking had produced an epidemic of lung cancer, a hitherto rare disease. Smoking was established as an important cause of premature mortality through pioneering epidemiological studies, such as Doll and Hill's cohort study of British male doctors [1], and the landmark US Surgeon General's *Report on Smoking and Health* in 1964 [2].

By the beginning of the twenty-first century in high-income countries, the cigarette-smoking epidemic has reached a stage in which smoking prevalence in both men and women is declining and lung-cancer incidence has passed its peak in men and women [3]. Nonetheless, around 1 in 5 adults continue to smoke in these countries and new smokers continue to be recruited. Furthermore, as described in Chapter 9, special populations within these countries, such as indigenous peoples and those with co-morbid mental illnesses, continue to have a very high smoking prevalence [4, 5]. Tobacco use is strongly correlated with and can be a substantial contributor to social disadvantage. As smoking becomes more concentrated in socially disadvantaged groups, more research will be needed into what policies are most effective in reducing smoking in these populations [6].

The smoking epidemic has yet to peak in low- and middle-income countries, where the majority of the world's smokers now live. The large multinational tobacco companies have responded to greater restrictions on tobacco marketing and decreasing smoking prevalence in their traditional markets by targeting low- and middle-income countries with aggressive tobacco marketing campaigns [7]. As a consequence, even though smoking has declined in high-income countries, the total number of tobacco-attributable deaths is

Substance Abuse Disorders: Evidence and Experience, First Edition. Edited by Hamid Ghodse, Helen Herrman, Mario Maj and Norman Sartorius.
© 2011 John Wiley & Sons, Ltd. Published 2011 by John Wiley & Sons, Ltd.

projected to rise globally from 5.4 million in 2005 to 6.4 million in 2015 and 8.3 million in 2030 [8]. Tobacco smoking will remain a substantial international public health issue for decades to come without concerted international efforts to reduce its prevalence.

Policies to reduce tobacco smoking in developed countries have been dominated by demand-reduction strategies such as taxation, advertising bans, pack warnings and mass-media campaigns. Supply-reduction strategies have been limited to minimum purchase age laws and strategies to combat tobacco smuggling and an illicit tobacco market. These population-level strategies have been favoured because they produce much greater declines in smoking prevalence by discouraging the uptake of smoking amongst young people and encouraging cessation amongst current smokers.

It is difficult to measure the effect of these individual tobacco control policies on population smoking prevalence because most populations have been exposed to multiple policies that probably work together to create a culture in which smoking has been 'denormalized' [9]. There is, nevertheless, good evidence to support the effectiveness of many tobacco control policies [10,11]. As discussed in Chapter 10, increased taxation is one of the most effective public health policies to reduce tobacco consumption. A meta-analysis of 86 published studies found the mean price elasticity for tobacco products was −0.48, meaning that for every 10% increase in price, tobacco consumption fell by 4.8% [12]. Mass-media campaigns of anti-smoking advertising are also highly effective at encouraging smoking cessation and discouraging smoking initiation. Wakefield *et al.* found that presenting anti-smoking advertisements on television at a frequency that exposed each person to around 4 ads per month decreased smoking prevalence by 0.3 percentage points [13]. A similar decrease was obtained by increasing the costliness of a pack of cigarettes by 0.03% of gross average weekly earnings. Complete tobacco advertising bans including sports sponsorship, and prominent graphic health warnings on cigarette packs are also effective strategies [11,14].

The WHO Framework Convention on Tobacco Control (FCTC) has been a major achievement in international tobacco control (see Chapter 10 for background of the FCTC). The FCTC stipulates a minimum set of tobacco control strategies that signatory countries must commit to implementing. These include many of the most effective population level strategies, such as advertising bans, tobacco taxation and pack health warnings.

THE FUTURE OF TOBACCO CONTROL IN DEVELOPED COUNTRIES

Smoking remains the largest preventable cause of premature mortality even in countries that have implemented the majority of the FCTC provisions. If smoking prevalence continues to decline at current rates, smoking will still be an important public-health issue for decades to come in countries with the most rigorous tobacco-control policies, such as Australia [15] and the USA [16]. Modelling of projected smoking prevalence if current trends continue indicate that if nothing changes adult smoking prevalence will be around 14% in Australia and 17% in the USA in 2020. Smoking prevalence would plateau just under 10% in Australia and just under 16% in the USA around the year 2050 [15, 16].

It is clear that strategies beyond the FCTC provisions are needed to produce major reductions in smoking prevalence in developed countries with strong tobacco-control policies [17,18]. In Australia, for example, current cessation rates would need to double to achieve an adult smoking prevalence below 10% by 2020.

Improving Smoking-Cessation Rates

The currently available pharmacological cessation aids are discussed in Commentary 12.3. These consist of nicotine-replacement therapy in the form of gum, patches, inhalators, lozenges, sublingual tablets and nasal sprays; the anti-depressants bupropion and nortripty-line; and varenicline, a selective nicotine receptor partial agonist. New approaches, such as a nicotine vaccine, are also under development. Nonpharmacological approaches include opportunistic brief interventions during contact with health services and individual or group counselling. When considered as clinical interventions, the high risk of premature mortality and serious morbidity from continued smoking means that even the modest efficacy of available smoking cessation aids make them cost-effective interventions [19].

Despite the widespread availability of pharmacological aids that double the chances of successfully quitting smoking, the majority of quitters continue to quit unassisted or 'cold turkey' [20]. The low impact of cessation aids on overall population smoking prevalence has led some tobacco-control advocates to argue for abandonment of publicly funded cessation clinics in favour of greater investment in public-health campaigns to encourage smokers to quit. Concerns that promotion of cessation aids could overmedicalize quitting and erode smokers' confidence in their ability to quit have also been expressed [21]. However, others point to the low success rate of unassisted quit attempts and argue that a greater impact could be achieved by encouraging more smokers to use effective cessation aids and services that should be judged as clinical interventions rather than a public-health measure [22].

Harm-Reduction Strategies

The only harm-reduction strategies that have been widely supported in the tobacco-control community have been those that reduce the harms to nonsmokers through public smoking bans. These primarily aim to protect nonsmokers from exposure to second-hand smoke but have the secondary benefit of reducing the number of cigarettes smoked by smokers and promoting quitting by reducing the opportunity to smoke [23].

Other forms of tobacco-harm reduction (THR) – such as promoting safer methods of using tobacco – remain deeply controversial. This is in large part due to the failure of attempts to develop safer, low-tar or light cigarettes and so on. Opponents of THR cite the tobacco industry's misleading promotion of so-called 'light' or 'low-tar' cigarettes as less-harmful cigarettes. These offered little or no health benefit and discouraged many smokers from quitting [24].

These concerns have less force when applied to nonsmoked forms of tobacco. Most of the harms arising from tobacco use are byproducts of inhaling tobacco smoke rather than the effects of nicotine. The possibility therefore exists that the harm from smoking could be reduced by encouraging smokers who are unable or unwilling to quit to switch to much less harmful methods of obtaining nicotine such as low-nitrosamine smokeless tobacco (LNSLT) or pharmaceutical nicotine (PN). This strategy has not been officially adopted in any country and proposals to trial it have been the subject of strong debate [25].

Advocates of this form of THR point to the experience in Sweden where the increased use of a form of LNSLT known as 'snus' amongst men has been associated with a decline in smoking and tobacco-related disease. Concerns have also been raised about how the tobacco industry may use less-harmful tobacco products to dilute the effect of other tobacco-control strategies, such as public smoking bans [26]. Opponents of THR have argued for more concerted efforts to get smokers to quit using behavioural and pharmacological aids.

New Approaches to Demand Reduction

A number of strategies have been proposed to reduce the demand for cigarettes by reducing their everyday availability and the marketing appeal of branded packaging.

Tobacco retail display bans are either being implemented or discussed in a number of developed countries (e.g. Australia, Canada). These point-of-sale cigarette pack displays, known as 'powerwalls', are typically positioned prominently at eye level behind the sales counter of convenience stores, supermarkets and so on. They arguably promote tobacco use by familiarizing children with tobacco products and tempting recent quitters to relapse [27, 28]. Hence, removing these displays is advocated as a way to further denormalize tobacco use and assist quitters to remain abstinent.

Mandatory plain packaging for all tobacco products is a policy that aims to eliminate the promotional messages associated with pack designs [29]. In countries with extensive advertising bans, the cigarette pack is an important marketing tool that conveys brand imagery. Like retail display bans, mandatory plain packaging for tobacco products can be seen as an extension of tobacco advertising bans.

Other recently adopted or discussed strategies include bans on smoking in cars when children are present [30] and including smoking scenes as a factor that is considered in film classifications [31]. All these policies represent incremental additions to existing strategies and are unlikely to have large impacts on smoking prevalence even on their advocates' most optimistic assumptions.

Producing a steeper decline in smoking prevalence will be a major policy challenge. It may require more radical approaches to tobacco control such as: reducing the addictiveness of cigarettes by mandating an incremental decrease in the maximum nicotine content to zero [32]; cap and trade systems whereby the amount of smoked tobacco that can be sold is gradually reduced to zero [20]; reducing the number of retailers who are permitted to sell smoked tobacco [33]; implementing a regulated market model where tobacco products are only sold by a government-run authority with a mandate to reduce smoking prevalence [34]; and smoker licensing that would require smokers to obtain a licence before being permitted to purchase cigarettes [35].

These strategies could potentially produce a faster decline in smoking prevalence. The challenge in implementing them is twofold. First, they represent major departures from existing tobacco control strategies and so will require major efforts to build public and political support for them. Secondly, there is also no evidence on their likely effectiveness because no countries have introduced them [18]. Their effectiveness can therefore only be judged if and when they are implemented.

REFERENCES

1. Doll, R., Peto, R., Boreham, J. *et al.* (2004) Mortality in relation to smoking: 50 years' observations on male British doctors. *British Medical Journal*, **328**, 1519.

2. US Surgeon General's Advisory Committee on Smoking and Health (1964) *Smoking and Health*, US Public Health Service, Office of the Surgeon General, Washington, DC.

3. Lopez, A.D., Collishaw, N.E. and Piha T. (1994) A descriptive model of the cigarette epidemic in developed countries. *Tobacco Control*, **3**, 242–247.

4. Lasser, K., Boyd, L., Woolhandler, S. *et al.* (2000) Smoking and mental illness: a population-based prevalence study. *Journal of the American Medical Association*, **284**, 2606–2610.

5. Baker, A., Ivers, R.G., Bowman, J. *et al.* (2006) Where there's smoke, there's fire: high prevalence of smoking among some sub-populations and recommendations for intervention. *Drug and Alcohol Review*, **25**, 85–96.

6. Ogilvie, D. and Petticrew, M. (2004) Reducing social inequalities in smoking: can evidence inform policy? A pilot study. *Tobacco Control*, **13**, 129–131.

7. Dağli, E. (1999) Are low income countries targets of the tobacco industry? *International Journal of Tuberculosis and Lung Disease*, **3**, 113–118.

8. Mathers, C.D. and Loncar, D. (2006) Projections of global mortality and burden of disease from 2002 to 2030. *PLoS Medicine*, **3**, 2011–2030.

9. Chapman, S. (1993) Unravelling gossamer with boxing gloves: problems in explaining the decline in smoking. *British Medical Journal*, **307**, 429–432.

10. World Bank (1999) *Curbing the Epidemic: Governments and the Economics of Tobacco Control*, World Bank, Washington, DC.

11. Levy, D.T., Chaloupka, F. and Gitchell, J. (2004) The effects of tobacco control policies on smoking rates: a tobacco control scorecard. *Journal of Public Health Management and Practice*, **10**, 338–353.

12. Gallet, C.A. and List, J.A. (2003) Cigarette demand: a meta-analysis of elasticities. *Health Economics*, **12**, 821–835.

13. Wakefield, M.A., Durkin, S., Spittal, M.J. *et al.* (2008) Impact of tobacco control policies and mass media campaigns on monthly adult smoking prevalence. *American Journal of Public Health*, **98**, 1443–1450.

14. Hammond, D., Fong, G.T., McDonald, P.W. *et al.* (2003) Impact of the graphic Canadian warning labels on adult smoking behaviour. *Tobacco Control*, **12**, 391–395.

15. Gartner, C.E., Barendregt, J. and Hall, W.D. (2009) Predicting the future prevalence of cigarette smoking in Australia: how low can we go and by when? *Tobacco Control*, **18**, 183–189.

16. Mendez, D., Warner KE. (2004) Adult cigarette smoking prevalence: declining as expected (not as desired). *American Journal of Public Health*, **94**, 251–252.

17. Chapman, S. (2008) Global perspective on tobacco control. Part II. The future of tobacco control: making smoking history? *International Journal of Tuberculosis and Lung Disease*, **12**, 8–12.

18. Gartner, C.E. and McNeill, A. (2010) Options for global tobacco control beyond the Framework Convention on Tobacco Control. *Addiction*, **105**, 1–3.

19. Song, F., Raftery, J., Aveyard, P. *et al.* (2002) Cost-effectiveness of pharmacological interventions for smoking cessation: a literature review and a decision analytic analysis. *Medical Decision Making*, **22**, s26–s37.

20. Hall, W.D. and West R. (2008) Thinking about the unthinkable: a de facto prohibition on smoked tobacco products. *Addiction*, **103**, 873–874.

21. Chapman, S. (1985) Stop-smoking clinics: a case for their abandonment. *The Lancet*, **325**, 918–920.

22. Britton, J. (2009) In defence of helping people stop smoking. *The Lancet*, **373**, 703–705.

23. Chapman, S., Borland, R., Scollo, M. *et al.* (1999) The impact of smoke-free workplaces on declining cigarette consumption in Australia and the United States. *American Journal of Public Health*, **89**, 1018.

24. Hughes, J.R. (2001) Do "light" cigarettes undermine cessation? *Tobacco Control*, **10**, 41i–42i.

25. Gartner, C.E., Hall, W.D., Chapman, S. *et al.* (2007) Should the health community promote smokeless tobacco (snus) as a harm reduction measure? *PLoS Medicine*, **4**, 1703–1704.

26. Carpenter, C.M., Connolly, G., Ayo-Yusuf, O.A. *et al.* (2009) Developing smokeless tobacco products for smokers: an examination of tobacco industry documents. *Tobacco Control*, **18**, 54–59.

27. Wakefield, M.A., Germain, D., Durkin, S. *et al.* (2006) An experimental study of effects on schoolchildren of exposure to point-of-sale cigarette advertising and pack displays. *Health Education Research*, **21**, 338–347.

28. Wakefield, M.A., Germain, D. and Henriksen, L. (2008) The effect of retail cigarette pack displays on impulse purchase. *Addiction*, **103**, 322–328.

29. Freeman, B., Chapman, S. and Rimmer M. (2008) The case for the plain packaging of tobacco products. *Addiction*, **103**, 580–590.

30. Freeman, B., Chapman, S. and Storey P. (2008) Banning smoking in cars carrying children: an analytical history of a public health advocacy campaign. *Australian and New Zealand Journal of Public Health*, **32**, 60–65.

31. Charlesworth, A. and Glantz, S.A. (2005) Smoking in the movies increases adolescent smoking: a review. *Pediatrics*, **116**, 1516–1528.

32. Bonnie, R.J., Stratton, K. and Wallace, A.L. (eds.) (2007) *Ending the Tobacco Problem: A Blue-print for the Nation*, National Academies Press, Washington, DC.

33. Cohen, J.E. and Anglin, L. (2009) Outlet density: a new frontier for tobacco control. *Addiction*, **104**, 2–3.

34. Borland, R. (2004) Taming the tigers: the case for controlling the tobacco market. *Addiction*, **99**, 529–531.

35. Chapman, S. and Liberman, J. (2005) Ensuring smokers are adequately informed: reflections on consumer rights, manufacturer responsibilities, and policy implications. *Tobacco Control*, **14**, ii8–ii13.

12.2 Public Health and Tobacco Use

Pim Cuijpers, Ph.D.

*Department of Clinical Psychology, Vrije Universiteit, Amsterdam,
The Netherlands*

The three chapters on the epidemiology, prevention, treatment and management of tobacco use and dependence clearly show the enormous impact this problem has on modern societies. With an expected 1000 million premature deaths during this century (see Chapter 7), tobacco use is definitely one of the most important public health problems at this time. If tobacco were discovered now for the first time, no health administration would allow it to be introduced in national economies as a new drug. So, in fact, public health is constantly fighting the relics of the past.

From another perspective one could state that public-health and clinical professionals are trapped in a struggle with commercial companies who try to make a profit on a lethal drug. Public-health and clinical professionals have to solve the remaining problems that are left over after commercial companies have had their profits. The public-health sector is constantly repairing the damage resulting from lack of control of tobacco industries. The chapter on prevention clearly shows that tobacco industries are actively involved in trying to get young people to use tobacco because they '*would be out of business in 25 to 30 years because they will not have enough customers to stay in business*' (see Chapter 8).

Because the budgets that the commercial companies have for their marketing strategies are much larger than those assigned to public health, the struggle does not seem fair. As described in the chapter on epidemiology, the tobacco industries have developed very sophisticated methods of marketing and had the budgets to do so (see Chapter 7). The public-health sector with limited resources, a completely different set of methods, has not been very much of a match for these industries.

And although there are some successes of the public-health sector, the tobacco industries also have their successes. With strong political support, the past decades have seen a successful and considerable reduction of tobacco use in Western countries. As indicated in the chapter on epidemiology, however, tobacco production and consumption has more than doubled in developing countries over the same period. And while the prevalence of smoking amongst men has peaked in many countries, it continues to climb amongst women. These

Substance Abuse Disorders: Evidence and Experience, First Edition. Edited by Hamid Ghodse, Helen Herrman, Mario Maj and Norman Sartorius.
© 2011 John Wiley & Sons, Ltd. Published 2011 by John Wiley & Sons, Ltd.

trends make it clear that although the tobacco use can be successfully reduced, the efforts to realize this are huge and the outcome of this fight is still not clear.

On the other hand, the chapter on treatment and management of tobacco use shows that the methods to reduce tobacco use have been well developed in the past decades. All three chapters stress the need for a comprehensive, coordinated and global approach to treatment and management of tobacco problems. It has also become clear that single strategies may be effective on an individual level, but not enough to realize a substantial reduction of tobacco use and the associated disease burden. Apart from strong policy measures and international coordination, including a nonsmoking policy in public places and tax increases, it needs aggressive countermarketing campaigns, interventions on the level of the community, and individual interventions to support smoking cessation. There should be little doubt that such a comprehensive approach is the most successful strategy to reduce tobacco use.

This is an important message for public-health and clinical professionals anywhere in health care. Although many doctors and other health professionals only work with tobacco users on an individual level, they have to realize that their efforts to stimulate and help patients to quit smoking are only one small part of a comprehensive strategy stimulating the smoker to quit. From this perspective, it is very harmful when individual doctors who smoke themselves do not stimulate their patients to quit as well. The same is true the ideas supported by many professionals in mental-health care that the smoking of chronic psychiatric patients should be seen as self-medication or as 'even the last pleasures of life' left to these patients. To quit smoking is a message that should be supported by all people working in health care. It may be necessary to organize specific campaigns aimed at health professionals stimulating them to support the overall comprehensive approach of the tobacco epidemic.

There is no lifestyle with a larger impact on public health than tobacco use. Tobacco is a major threat to public health. Public-health and clinical professionals are learning better and better how to deal with this threat. A comprehensive, coordinated, global approach to treatment and management of tobacco problems is vital for the success in controlling the tobacco epidemic. Each individual professional should play his or her role in reducing this threat. The three chapters on epidemiology, prevention, treatment and management of tobacco use and dependence provide an excellent resource for public health and clinical professionals who want to get an overview of the current knowledge on this topic.

12.3 Decreasing the Health Hazards of Tobacco: Necessary and Possible, But not Easy

Ahmad Mohit M.D.

Department of Psychiatry, Iran University of Medical Science, Tehran, Iran

Commenting on chapters about Tobacco is not easy. On the one hand, consumption of tobacco is still the most common amongst all dependence producing substances; and on the other hand, it is probably the substance with both the least inhibition and social stigma and greatest known health hazard. The other side of the reality is that, in many places, particularly the industrially developed countries of Europe, Western Pacific and North America, some effective measures have been taken and the results in decreasing tobacco consumption and its health hazards can be shown statistically. But when we look globally and particularly at poorer, developing countries; we observe two opposite facts. The first is that almost in every country there are some regulations regarding taxation, pricing, the age limit for buying tobacco products and smoke-free areas. At the same time, the reality in the same countries is that, getting your hand on a pack of cigarette is practically as easy as buying a bottle of milk; and tobacco products, particularly cigarettes, are used with minimum concern for the existing regulations and/or the health of nonsmokers. The tobacco companies may have lost some markets in the developed world, but no doubt they have gained more, through regular trade or smuggling, in other parts of the world.

Looking at the global condition of tobacco use through the World Health Organization's Atlas [1], there is a global trend of decreasing consumption (or deceasing in the rate of increase of consumption) of tobacco. However, this trend is very slow and is much more evident in industrially developed and richer countries. For instance, in China alone an astronomical number of 300 million men smoke. Smoking amongst women is much less and this is particularly true for the less-developed countries. However, the trend of women's smoking is on the rise. Children and adolescents are also in danger. . . .

The chapter on prevention addresses the issues of prevention with emphasis on the youth. The comprehensive, holistic approach to the problem of tobacco use is what is suggested

Substance Abuse Disorders: Evidence and Experience, First Edition. Edited by Hamid Ghodse, Helen Herrman, Mario Maj and Norman Sartorius.
© 2011 John Wiley & Sons, Ltd. Published 2011 by John Wiley & Sons, Ltd.

by this chapter for prevention. The writers emphasize that adopting a strategy that focuses only on one age group, one gender or one causal factor cannot have lasting effects. Instead, they suggest broad strategies aiming *'to denormalize tobacco use; reduce accessibility and affordability; provide information and regulate tobacco products'*. Even when the issue of smoking amongst children and youth is concerned, they suggest that the *'strategies should be embedded in a more comprehensive, broader strategy including the environment where children and youth live'*. And, this seems to be the greatest strength of this chapter.

The four strategic approaches to prevention of tobacco use should be used as headlines of detailed programmes. Here are some thoughts regarding each of these approaches:

Denormalization is changing the social attitude towards a behaviour that is considered normal. Changing a social and even an individual attitude is a very complex undertaking. Individual attitudes are formed through the whole process of development and are affected by deep-rooted cultural beliefs and emotions associated with them. Denormalization has perhaps been the greatest cause of most success stories regarding decreasing demand for tobacco consumption. Until the end of the decade of 1970, consumption of tobacco, particularly in the form of smoking was accepted as a norm. Cigarettes were as much a part of an everyday family basket as bread was; it was accepted and consumed without any concern. Only children and adolescents, and in some cultures women felt a sense of shame, fear or awkwardness attached to using tobacco.

Denormalization does not only mean taking away the normality of the behaviour of tobacco consumption. It also means denormalization of the business and industry that is associated with the consumption of tobacco. It means working towards considering and presenting the work of tobacco companies an abnormal, unhealthy business of 'The intentional sale of a defective product that is both addictive and lethal' [2].

As a practical step to write this commentary, the author organized informal meetings with 3 groups of people in Tehran, the capital city of Iran. 1 : 7 University students 20–23 years old of mixed gender. 2 : 7 well-known men and women intellectuals including one novelist and poet, a sociologist, a painter, a movie director, a professor of philosophy, an architect and a psychiatrist 3 : 7 ordinary working people with occupations ranging from teacher to shop keeper to taxi driver and housewife. All three groups were asked to discuss and answer the following question:

> Considering the fact that there is no doubt regarding the harmful effects of tobacco consumption, particularly smoking cigarettes; what comes to your mind as a means to decrease this habit?

Although there were different and very diverse suggestions in all the areas of availability, affordability, accessibility and health promotion and education; what all three groups agreed without using any technical term was methods based on 'denormalization'. And one common conclusion amongst them was that smoking has decreased only in those sections of the population where denormalization has worked. Here are a few interesting examples taken from their discussions:

- 20 years ago, when we gathered for an evening party, everybody smoked inside the room with no inhibition. Now, visibly more people feel awkward and self-conscious of smoking indoors. They either don't smoke at all or go out to an open space like a balcony for smoking.

- Years ago, taxi and bus drivers and even some passengers smoked inside public means of transportation without feeling that it is something inappropriate and harmful. It is no longer so.
- Although there are still some offices where smoking is not forbidden; people think twice before smoking in an office space. It is as if a kind of moral police is stopping them from lighting a cigarette.
- There was also another point of agreement: no matter what methods we take, total elimination of tobacco use is only 'Wishful Thinking'. Therefore, we need to have programmes of *Harm Reduction* for those who continue smoking and also passive smokers.

Although this nonformal experiment does not fulfil the necessary criteria for a research trial; it is nevertheless an indication of the feeling of a cross-section of the people in a large city in a country that is being rapidly urbanized and in some aspects industrialized. A country that is neither very poor and underdeveloped, nor an industrially developed one.

In the area of reducing *accessibility* and *affordability,* in many countries attempts to increase taxes and adopting age limits to purchase tobacco products started as early as the decade of 1970s and even earlier. But what made these a global commitment was the *World Health Organization's Framework Convention on Tobacco Control (FCTC)* [3]. Chapter 6 of this convention specifically deals with pricing, taxation and age limits and requires the member states to enact and reinforce legislation in these areas in order to make tobacco products less accessible and available for all, particularly the youth. This and other articles like article 16 that deals with sales to and by minors, article 12 regarding education are of particular importance in this area. These measures were in different ways being practiced in many different European and American countries for decades before this convention was established; and as a result, according to Ilana Crome in the chapter on epidemiology of the present book: '*While tobacco production and consumption has declined dramatically in developed countries over the last thirty years, it has more than doubled in developing countries over the same period (Davis et al., 2007)*'. Now, with an internationally agreed upon document at hand, an instrument for action is also available. But, are the same methods and regulations going to be as effective in the developing world?

There are a number of reasons for optimism and no doubt, some equally strong reasons for pessimism. One reason for optimism is that according to the World Health Organization [4], *Several countries have already shown that smoking rates can be reduced. These successes can be reproduced by any responsible nation, but only through immediate, determined, and sustained governmental and community action.* There are also examples of successful programmes in developing countries; which indicate that success in these countries is possible. But, in reality we deal with a major problem that is on the rise. Looking at the last page of the WHO Tobacco Atlas shows this bleak future side by side with some hope, but reminds us that the best we can say about the future is uncertain. According to Dr. Sue Galea the author of the chapter on treatment of this book: *Tobacco use is a risk factor for 6 out of the 8 leading causes of death worldwide. In 2005, the worldwide total tobacco-attributable deaths were estimated to be 5.4 million/year. In 2015 this is projected to rise to 6.4 million/year and by 2030 to 8.3 million/year. This increase is projected to be mainly attributable to a significant increase in mortality in low-income and middle-income countries.* This is a very gloomy prediction, which amongst other things shows that efforts to decrease tobacco consumption have little chance of success in low- and middle-income developing countries. Why is it so?

Reasons are many and range from lack of facilities for proper schooling, sport and pastime to high stress level in daily life, low level of health education, uncertainty about the future, direct and indirect pressure by the tobacco industry that includes corruption, as well as other reasons. Research in each of these areas and many more are absolutely necessary.

CONCLUSION

As mentioned at the beginning of this article, discussing an issue like tobacco is not easy. In almost the entire world, in spite of all health hazards that are proven and to a large extent known by the public; tobacco is still a legal and easily attainable substance. Many of the drugs that are abused do not have as many dangerous health consequences as tobacco. But, tobacco products particularly cigarettes are available to the majority of the people, even in those countries with the most scientific, legal, civil and human restricting regulations. Almost all other drugs of abuse they are recognized as such, but, – to be honest – cigarettes are still a part of daily life. This has started to be broken in a number of countries, but not for most of the world. The mosquito of tobacco – as Dr. Gro Harlem Brundtland a previous Director General of World Health Organization had said – is strongly at work and most of the world are not ready or informed to face it. Why? Because, dealing with this mosquito is not as easy as other agents of epidemics. We have more questions in dealing with this mosquito than solutions. That is why at this final stage, I would like to put the finishing point to this comment, not by answers, but by a few questions:

- Considering all sides of a complex issue; what other actions are realistically possible to take, particularly in developing countries?
- Can we find ways to know why what has worked in some countries cannot work in others?
- What would be the tobacco-industry's reaction? And, how to deal with it?
- Is it possible to redirect the industry towards other lines of productivity and profiting? Can the experiences for crop replacement in other areas help? How?
- How can we correctly study the cultural, social, economic and other aspects of the '**Whole**' picture of tobacco use and address them in the areas of supply, demand and harm for each country and even community?

REFERENCES

1. World Health Organization (Jay Mackay & Michael Erikson authors) (2002) *Tobacco Atlas*, pp. 24–28.
2. *Garfield Mahood, Executive Director, Non-Smokers' Rights Association* From Tobacco Industry Denormalization (TID) www.nsra-adnf.ca.
3. World Health Organization (2003) Framework Convention on Tobacco Control (FCTC), ISBN 92 4 159101 3.
4. WHO (2002) Tobacco Atlas, p. 32.

12.4 Overcoming State Addiction to Tobacco Industry

Robert West, BSc, PhD

Department of Epidemiology and Public Health, University College London, London, UK

Tobacco use, and particularly cigarette smoking is responsible for more deaths than all other forms of substance misuse put together, with an estimated annual toll of 4.9 million currently [1]. Progress has been made towards reductions in prevalence in many countries, most notably in North America, Western Europe, Australia and New Zealand: in many of these countries it has fallen to under 25% [2]. However, this is being offset by increases in other countries, particularly in Asia where smoking prevalence amongst women is set to rise from currently low levels of under 10% to more than 20% as a product of westernization and tobacco-company marketing.

The three chapters in this volume reveal a very important truth: we know what to do to dramatically reduce tobacco use and save many millions of human lives each year. Tobacco use is a field of study that is rich in high-quality data on epidemiology, pharmacology, psychology and sociology. We know that if countries such as China and India were to establish a 10-year tobacco control strategy of the kind already enacted by countries such as Canada, including bans in promotion, large price increases, strongly enforced smoking restrictions, mass-media campaigns, and programmes to help addicted smokers to stop, the lives of millions of their citizens would be spared [1].

So, what are the prospects that this kind of action will be taken, and that countries that have already made progress will do more to reduce the death toll further? The answer at present has to be 'not good'. The barriers to mounting effective campaigns to reduce tobacco use are numerous and challenging but they all boil down to a simple equation: for individuals and institutions making decisions about what to do, there is a greater incentive to do nothing or engage in modest and largely ineffective policies than to take action that will make a substantial difference. The measures that the tobacco industry fears most are those that put up the financial cost to the consumer, and these should lie at the heart of any strategy. This needs to involve large tax increases and strong internationally coordinated measures to

Substance Abuse Disorders: Evidence and Experience, First Edition. Edited by Hamid Ghodse, Helen Herrman, Mario Maj and Norman Sartorius.
© 2011 John Wiley & Sons, Ltd. Published 2011 by John Wiley & Sons, Ltd.

combat smuggling. The problem of course is that such measures may be unpopular and there may be a negative impact of the economy of countries that are involved in growing tobacco or manufacturing tobacco products. In addition, many countries have state-owned tobacco industries on which they rely for a major proportion of their income.

So, in a real sense many states around the world are addicted to the tobacco industry. Like individual tobacco users they recognize that it is harming the health of their populations and they have expressed a clear desire, through subscribing to the Framework Convention on Tobacco Control, to become 'tobacco-free' [3]; but they find that they need it. So, they take marginal and largely ineffective actions and shy away from doing what is necessary to address it seriously.

So what can be done to change things? For the individual addict to change, he or she has to come to a deep realization that change is better than the status quo. There has to be a change of heart as well as mind. This can be a matter of timing. An event occurs that shakes the individual out of complacency or there is a build up of dissatisfaction until a small trigger is enough to tip him or her into a new way of thinking. But that is just the start. For many individuals, what is needed then is a plan of campaign. To avoid recidivism, actions need to be taken to establish a strong footing for the new life. The barriers need to be anticipated and plans developed concerning how they are going to be overcome.

For states to overcome addiction to the tobacco industry they need to arrive at a deep realization that they would be better off without their dependence on tobacco. Unfortunately, for many of the individuals in positions of power, this is not the case. They benefit from tobacco use either directly through financial contributions from tobacco companies or indirectly from the economic activity relating to the tobacco industry. In that case, other individuals or organs of the state must bring pressure to bear to incentivise those decision makers to act in the best interests of the state. This can perhaps be achieved through social pressure but it needs orchestration, coordination and mobilization of public opinion. Nongovernmental organizations can play a role here. In the UK, ASH (Action on Smoking and Health) was established by British doctors concerned about government inaction once the dangers of smoking became evident. At first, this was an effective pressure group but now it is considered an important ally of government in developing and implementing policy.

There can be no doubt that attempts to force the issue will be met with hostility and concerted resistance from the tobacco industry and its apologists. These people have huge resources at their disposal and with billions of dollars at stake we can assume that they will continue to behave as they have done in the past – to obfuscate, muddy the waters, provide excuses and deny facts – to prevent effective tobacco-control measures being adopted.

Every country will have different challenges and opportunities with regard to tobacco-control interventions. Financial resources are a major problem but so are human resources. A first step in developing a tobacco-control strategy will be to build capacity in that country – a cadre of professionals with a detailed understanding of tobacco control and how it can be put into effect. There would be merit, therefore, in going much further than has been done to date to establish capacity-building programmes in countries that currently lack expertise. This is potentially something that could be undertaken under the auspices of the FCTC, but it would require resources. The task would be to identify a non-governmental organization in every country that could play the kind of role that ASH played in the UK in the 1960s and 1970s and to provide training, mentoring and support to build them into effective campaigning and advisory bodies. Funding for such an initiative could come from such bodies as the Gates Foundation or the Bloomberg fund.

Of paramount importance in all of this is that tobacco-control advocates work in a united fashion and avoid denigrating policy options that do not fit with their particular set of values. For example, some tobacco-control advocates have argued against provision of assistance for smokers wanting to stop [4]. The argument put forward is that most smokers manage to stop without such assistance and resources are better spent establishing conditions that make smoking less attractive. The fact that most smokers stop without assistance simply reflects the fact that very few smokers *use* assistance. Thus, if 1000 smokers try to stop without help and their chances of success are 5% [5], this will yield 50 ex-smokers. If 100 try to stop with help and their chances of success are four times those of the unaided quitters at 20% [6], this will yield 20 ex-smokers, less than half those who quit unaided. The solution is obviously not to abandon assistance as an option but to try to get more people to use it.

In summary, as is evident from the chapters in this volume, we are fortunate in the case of tobacco in having good evidence for what can be done to avert the massive death toll. The most important issue facing the world is how to get governments to put effective tobacco-control policies into place when as nation states many of them are addicted to tobacco as an industry. As with individuals, the first step is achieving a deep realization of the need for change and then planning an effective campaign to achieve that change. For many countries this will require nongovernmental organizations to take a lead. There is a huge task ahead in identifying and building capacity in those organizations. This will be costly and will require support from countries with more developed tobacco-control programmes. This can be achieved under the auspices of the FCTC and there are potential sources of funding that could be used to achieve this. No doubt there will be concerted resistance from the tobacco industry and its apologists and any tobacco-control initiative will need to put considerable resources into fighting this resistance.

REFERENCES

1. World Health Organisation (2008) *WHO Report on the Global Tobacco Epidemic: the MPOWER Report*, WHO, Geneva.
2. Mackay, J., and Eriksen, M.P. (2006) *The Tobacco Atlas*, World Health Organisation, Geneva.
3. WHO (2003) *Framework Convention on Tobacco Control*, World Health Organisation, Geneva.
4. Chapman, S. (2009) The inverse impact law of smoking cessation. *Lancet*, **373** (9665), 701–703.
5. Hughes, J.R., Keely, J. and Naud, S. (2004) Shape of the relapse curve and long-term abstinence among untreated smokers. *Addiction*, **99** (1), 29–38.
6. West, R., McNeill, A. and Raw, M. (2000) Smoking cessation guidelines for health professionals: an update. Health Education Authority. *Thorax*, **55** (12), 987–999.

12.5 The Framework Convention on Tobacco Control: The Importance of Article 14

Robyn Richmond, PhD, MA, MHEd

School of Public Health and Community Medicine, University of New South Wales, Kensington, Australia

The World Health Organization's Framework Convention on Tobacco Control (FCTC) has a number of core measures to reduce tobacco use globally. The FCTC recommends public-health measures including: taxes on tobacco products, price increases, legislation, restriction on the sale and advertising of cigarettes and on smoking in public places, large warning labels positioned on cigarette packs, and the involvement of health professionals in providing advice to smokers to quit [22, 23]. The FCTC is described in the chapter on Tobacco Prevention by Blanco, Silva and Monteiro. This commentary focuses on the role of health professionals in smoking cessation and concerns about populations at risk from tobacco use.

IMPORTANCE OF HEALTH PROFESSIONALS IN THE TREATMENT OF SMOKERS

Article 14 of the FCTC identifies the importance of health professionals in the treatment of smokers and recommends that countries develop evidence-based treatment guidelines. It states that 'each Party shall develop and disseminate appropriate, comprehensive and integrated guidelines based on scientific evidence and best practices, taking into account national circumstances and priorities, and shall take effective measures to promote cessation of tobacco use and adequate treatment for tobacco dependence' [1]. The chapter by Crome and Mumafo on Tobacco Epidemiology identifies the important role that health professionals have in smoking cessation.

Substance Abuse Disorders: Evidence and Experience, First Edition. Edited by Hamid Ghodse, Helen Herrman, Mario Maj and Norman Sartorius.
© 2011 John Wiley & Sons, Ltd. Published 2011 by John Wiley & Sons, Ltd.

Health professionals are effective in encouraging smoking cessation and include doctors, nurses, dentists, pharmacists, social workers and psychologists [2–7, 20]. The Cochrane Database has reviewed evidence from 41 trials involving 31 000 smokers and reported that there was a significant increase in cessation when smoking-cessation advice is provided by health professionals [8]. Indeed, spending more time has a more positive outcome according to the US Clinical Practice Guideline [7]. Providing smoking-cessation advice provides a good return on investment. It is cost effective compared to a number of medical interventions such as mammography, Pap smears, high cholesterol and high blood pressure [9, 10]. In a review conducted in New Zealand, Shearer and Shanahan found that quitline services in combination with pharmacotherapy were the most cost effective of smoking-cessation interventions.

The chapter by Crome and Mumafo identifies education as the important first step, and they comment that it is not being comprehensively carried out in medical schools. As medical practitioners of the future, medical students should be taught about tobacco-control strategies and smoking-cessation methods during their education [6]. A decade ago we conducted a world-wide survey on the teaching about tobacco in medical schools. We recently repeated this survey and received responses from 665 medical schools from 109 countries. We found that only 11% taught a specific module on tobacco in the first survey, but this had increased to 27%; 40% integrated teaching about tobacco with other topics ten years ago but this had increased to 77% [6]. We found an encouraging increase in the extent of teaching on tobacco in medical schools over ten years. Similar initiatives are undertaken with other student health professionals.

CLINICAL PRACTICE GUIDELINES

Over the past few years we have seen many countries develop clinical practice guidelines for smoking cessation. Guidelines are generally based on evidence from clinical trials and promote interventions of proven benefit. The survey of guidelines located on the treatobacco.net web site, found that 31 countries have guidelines and most are based on guidelines developed in the US and UK and use the Cochrane database as their source. They have broad support from medical and professional societies, two thirds recommend access to quitline services, and they recommend available medications for smoking cessation that are predominantly the nicotine gum and patch, bupropion and varenicline [1].

HIGH-RISK POPULATIONS WHO USE TOBACCO

There are a number of subpopulations who have a high burden from their tobacco use. The chapter by Crome and Mumafo on Tobacco Epidemiology identifies many of these groups. They include women, including pregnant smokers, adolescents, those with a psychiatric illness such as depression and schizophrenia, those with medical co-morbidities such as coronary heart disease, respiratory diseases and cancer, those who misuse alcohol and illicit drugs, and those from low socioeconomic backgrounds such as prisoners [11]. Guidelines for smoking cessation identify these subpopulations at risk and have made evidence-based recommendations for smoking cessation including treatment flowcharts or algorithms for brief interventions based on the 5As (ask about smoking status, advise to stop, assess willingness to quit, assist by prescribing and referring for support, and arrange follow up for further support) and motivational interviewing [2, 7, 12, 24]. The chapter by Galea on Treatment and Managements describes the 5As approach and important components of smoking-cessation treatment in some detail.

The burden of tobacco use on one of these high-risk groups is described. Smoking in people with mental-health problems is common with estimates ranging from 50 to 80% [13]. In Australia, 73% of men and 56% of women with psychosis were smokers [14] compared to the general populations where there are 21% of smokers [15]. Mortality rates due to cardiovascular disease amongst people with severe mental disorders are twice those in the general population [21]. Cardiovascular disease occurs more frequently and accounts for more premature death than suicide amongst people with schizophrenia [16]. People with schizophrenia and bipolar disorder have much higher rates of cardiovascular risk factors such as smoking, obesity, dyslipidaemia, hypertension and diabetes, and less access to medical care than people without schizophrenia [16, 17]. This unhealthy lifestyle and lower knowledge of cardiovascular risk factors provides a focus for more comprehensive interventions amongst people with severe mental disorders [18]. In our randomized controlled trial of 298 heavy smokers with a psychotic disorder, we found that a significantly higher proportion of smokers who completed all treatment sessions had stopped smoking compared to controls [19]. As smoking rates in the general population decrease, the presence of tobacco use amongst those with a mental-health problem become more apparent in general or family practice [12]. These subpopulations at risk, like the other vulnerable and disadvantaged groups should be offered smoking-cessation interventions that are efficacious.

The main conclusions of this commentary are that focus needs to be increased on the important role that health professionals play in providing evidenced-based brief smoking-cessation advice to smokers. There is also an imperative to focus on those at high risk from the burdens of smoking, as these groups continue to have high smoking rates.

REFERENCES

1. Raw, M. and Slevin, C. (2007) A survey of tobacco dependence treatment guidelines and systems in 45 countries. Available at http://www.treatobacco.net/en/uploads/documents/Publications/HC3%20RAW%20Treatment%20survey.pdf (accessed on 1st March, 2010).

2. Zwar, N.A., Richmond, R.L., Davidson, D. and Hasan, I. (2009) Postgraduate education for doctors in smoking cessation. *Drug and Alcohol Review*, **28** (5), 466–473.

3. Gordon, J., Albert, D.A., Crews, K.M., and Fried, J. (2009) Tobacco education in dentistry and dental hygiene. *Drug and Alcohol Review*, **28** (5), 517–532.

4. Sarna, L., Bialous, S.A., Rice, V.H. and Wewers, M.E. (2009) Promoting tobacco dependence treatment in nursing education. *Drug and Alcohol Review*, **28** (5), 507–516.

5. Williams, D.M. (2009) Preparing pharmacy students and pharmacists to provide tobacco cessation counselling. *Drug and Alcohol Review*, **28** (5), 533–540.

6. Richmond, R., Zwar, N., Taylor, R. *et al.* (2009) Teaching about tobacco in medical schools: a worldwide study. *Drug and Alcohol Review*, **28** (5), 484–497.

7. Fiore, M.C., Bailey, W.C., Cohen, S.J. *et al.* (2000) *Treating Tobacco Use and Dependence. Clinical Practice Guideline*, US Department of Health and Human Services. Public Health Service, Rockville, MD.

8. Stead, L.F., Bergson, G. and Lancaster, T. (2008) Physician advice for smoking cessation. *Cochrane Database of Systematic Reviews* **2** (Art. No.: CD000165). DOI: 10.1002/14651858. CD000165.pub3.

9. Shearer, J. and Shanahan, M. (2006) Cost effectiveness analysis of smoking cessation interventions. *Australian and New Zealand Journal of Public Health*, **30**, 428–434.

10. Cornuz, J., Gilbert, A., Pinget, C. *et al.* (2006) Cost-effectiveness of pharmacotherapies for nicotine dependence in primary care settings: a multinational comparison. *Tobacco Control*, **15**, 152–159.

11. Richmond, R.L. and Zwar, N. (2010) Treatment of tobacco dependence. Chapter 39, in *Tobacco – Science, Policy and Public Health*, 2e (ed. N. Gray), Glyph International, Bangalore, India.

12. Zwar, N., Richmond, R., Borland, R. *et al.* (2004) *Smoking Cessation Guidelines for Australian General Practice: Practice Handbook*, Department of Health and Ageing, Australia.

13. Hughes, J.R. (1993) Pharmacotherapy for smoking cessation: unvalidated assumptions, anomalies, and suggestions for future research. *Journal of Consulting and Clinical Psychology*, **61** (5), 751–60.

14. Jablensky, A., *et al.* (2002) People living with psychotic illness: An Australian study 1997–98 an overview. p. iii–22.

15. Australian Institute of Health and Welfare (2005) *2004 National Drug Strategy Household Survey*. Australian Institute of Health and Welfare, Canberra.

16. Hennekens, C. (2007) Increasing global burden of cardiovascular disease in general populations and patients with schizophrenia. *Journal of Clinical Psychiatry*, **68** (Supp 4), 4–7.

17. Kilbourne, A.M., *et al.* (2008) Improving medical and psychiatric outcomes among individuals with bipolar disorder: a randomized controlled trial. *Psychiatric Services*, **59** (7), 760–768.

18. Osborn, D., *et al.* (2007) Physical activity, dietary habits and Coronary Heart Disease risk factor knowledge amongst people with severe mental illness. *Social Psychiatry and Psychiatric Epidemiology*, **42** (10), 787–793.

19. Baker, A., Richmond, R., Haile, M., *et al.* (2006) A randomized controlled trial of a smoking cessation intervention among people with a psychotic disorder. *American Journal of Psychiatry*, **163**, 1934–1942.

20. Richmond, R. (2009) Editorial: Education and training for health professionals and students in tobacco, alcohol and other drugs. *Drug and Alcohol Review*, **28** (5), 463–465.

21. Weiss, A.P. *et al.* (2006) Treatment of cardiac risk factors among patients with schizophrenia and diabetes. *Psychiatric Services*, **57** (8), 1145–1152.

22. WHO Framework Convention on Tobacco Control (2003) World Health Organization. Geneva, Switzerland.

23. MPOWER 2009 (2009) *WHO Report on the Global Tobacco Epidemic, 2009: Implementing Smoke-Free Environments*, World Health Organization, Geneva, Switzerland.

24. Zwar, N., Richmond, R., Borland, R. *et al.* (2007) Smoking cessation pharmacotherapy: an update for health professionals. Melbourne: Royal Australian College of General Practitioners, Reviewed and updated April 2009.

12.6 Comments Regarding Epidemiology of Tobacco Use, Tobacco Use: Prevention and Tobacco Abuse: Treatment and Management

Yu Xin, M.D.

Institute of Mental Health, Peking University, Beijing, China

In the war against tobacco, health professionals and the public were in the weaker position from the very beginning. The World Health Organization's International Classification of Diseases didn't include tobacco use until the version of ICD-9 released in 1977, in which tobacco was listed as 'nondependent tobacco use disorder', code 305.1 [1]. Although it was categorized as 'nondependent', this item included several conditions such as tobacco used to the detriment of a person's health or social functioning, tobacco dependence and excessive use of tobacco products. It was the first time that the international scientific world formally recognized that tobacco was an addiction problem, even in an ambiguous expression. In contrast, however, the tobacco industry made a lot of effort both with marketing strategies and augmenting the addictive properties of nicotine. When more and more confidential files from tobacco companies were exposed to the public, we were astonished to find out that those companies had done much more than scientists to understand the pharmacology of nicotine let alone the commercial aspects of cigarettes selling. There are many explanations for this unequal situation, but obviously, while the scientific world hadn't regarded tobacco as a psychoactive substance that might be its main attribute. When tobacco companies tried to increase the nicotine concentration in each cigarette, or improved the filter technique to make nicotine inhalation more rapid, scientists were still arguing whether tobacco was only psychologically addictive or whether it produced physical dependence [2]. The slow response of academia is also reflected in the scarcity of high-quality research papers on tobacco use as well as some key issues: the operational diagnostic criteria of tobacco-use disorder, the objective biomarkers of nicotine addiction, global epidemiological data

Substance Abuse Disorders: Evidence and Experience, First Edition. Edited by Hamid Ghodse, Helen Herrman, Mario Maj and Norman Sartorius.
© 2011 John Wiley & Sons, Ltd. Published 2011 by John Wiley & Sons, Ltd.

on tobacco use particularly in developing countries, risk factors in special populations and the cost-effectiveness assessment of comprehensive intervention programs on tobacco cessation.

In the first half of the twentieth century, communicable disease seemed more prevalent in developing countries and noncommunicable disease in developed countries. But this situation changed during the late phase of the last century. While communicable diseases such as malaria and tuberculosis are still prevalent, noncommunicable disease such as diabetes, stroke, cancer, and heart disease are becoming more prevalent particularly in fast-growing developing countries like India and China [3]. It is clearly demonstrated that in developed countries such as the US, in the adult population the incidence rate of smoking along with heart disease and stroke is declining, while it rises sharply in developing countries. In these developing countries, where impairment of social and economical development is always serious, certain populations are more vulnerable than others to tobacco and tobacco-related health problems. For example, in China, there are more than 300 million people suffering from hypertension, most of whom live in the rural areas and haven't received treatment in their lifetime [4, 5]. Moreover, for other lifestyle-related disease such as heart disease, stroke, cancer and diabetes, the fastest growing population of tobacco users comes from socioeconomically disadvantaged groups like rural residents, migrant workers and low-income/unemployed city dwellers [6]. Smoking is certainly not the only contributor but is certainly one of them. The epidemiological data showed that the smoking rate was much higher in rural residents and migrant workers. However, explicit and informative studies are seldom conducted in those so-called fast-growing developing countries and even scarcer in those vulnerable populations.

The treatment and management of tobacco-related health problems absolutely need the involvements of many parts of the society besides the health sector, particularly the input from government. Considering the huge current smoking population and the increasing potential smoking population in teenagers, 'treatment and prevention' strategy needs to be carefully weighed. To prevent people becoming new smokers via various measures such as reduction of the supply of tobacco products, limiting access to cigarettes and treating tobacco dependence either in clinical settings or communities, totally relies on a comprehensive policy that covers tobacco plantation, production, sales, and management of health-related problems. Being a party to the WHO Framework Convention on Tobacco Control doesn't necessarily mean that actions are taken automatically. Although smoking-related death rates are going up quickly globally and particularly in developing countries, the death toll is sometimes not as eye-catching as the increase in economic returns from the tobacco industry. Of course, health economists can calculate in detail the cost of smoking-related health loss even in international dollars [7]. However, the disease-related health cost and premature-death-induced productivity loss are not as direct as the income from cigarettes taxation. Moreover, health economics is still a 'developing science' in most of the developing countries. Due to the lack of expertise and necessary information, health economic data yielded for economic burden of a specific disease is often full of shortcomings and obvious questions. Health economics is not a 'better than nothing' study. A paradoxical and corrupt health economic report will not only mislead the decision makers but at worst mean that they never take further actions. Unfortunately, in fact these 'health economic' studies keep coming out with discrepant results.

Medicine should be the hero in the prevention and treatment of tobacco use. But which speciality should take the responsibility of looking after smoking patients who seek medical help? Chest physicians? Because smoking can induce respiratory disease. Heart doctor? Because smoking can increase the risk of coronary heart disease and hypertension. Neurologist? Because smoking can make memory decline in mid-life [8]. Or psychiatrist since smoking itself is an addiction behaviour and increases the risk of depression and other mental diseases [9]. In modern hospitals medicine is highly specialized. The demarcation of these specialties is somehow a '*de facto*' condition . It varies by countries, sometimes by hospitals. Since smoking was defined as a disease only three decades ago, it is still looking for its 'right location' in hospitals. 'Accept' or 'decline' treatment programs for tobacco use as one of the professional coverage sometimes depends on the availability of extra resources. The pragmatic attitude prevalent in medical professionals toward treatment of smoking makes it difficult to disseminate knowledge of tobacco-use disorders and establish specialist team focusing on this issue. Worse than that, the basic information that should be known by physicians of every discipline is not well known. A survey showed that only 6% of physicians had heard of the tobacco-dependence treatment guidelines and 1% knew about the symptoms of nicotine withdrawal [10]. The medical world seems far from well prepared to meet the health challenges of tobacco use. Although we understand the need could be tremendous in terms of treatment and management of tobacco use, we haven't done much to understand how to provide effective services.

Unlike the wars against other illegal drugs such as heroin or cocaine, tobacco control is more difficult to reach a unanimous agreement amongst and within the societies. Medical professionals, however, need to be politically sensitive, publicly smart, and scientifically rigorous to lead the allies in fighting against the enemy of the biggest epidemic in human history.

REFERENCES

1. (1975) *International Statistical Classification of Diseases*, World Health Organization, Geneva.

2. Carmo, J.T., Andres-Pueyo, A. and Lopez, E.A. (2005) The evolution in the concept of smoking. *Cad Saude Publica*, **21** (4), 999–1005.

3. Daar, A.S., Singer, P.A. and Persad, D.L. *et al.* (2007) Grand challenges in chronic non-communicable diseases. *Nature*, **450** (7169), 494–496.

4. Pang, W., Li, Z. and Sun, Z. *et al.* (2010) Prevalence of hypertension and associated factors among older rural adults: results from Liaoning Province, China. *Med Princ Pract*, **19** (1), 22–27.

5. Xiaohui, H. (2008) Urban-rural disparity of overweight, hypertension, undiagnosed hypertension, and untreated hypertension in China. *Asia Pac J Public Health*, **20** (2), 159–169.

6. Siahpush, M., Brown, A. and Aanonsen, N.O. (2002) *Social Inequalities in Smoking*, VicHealth Centre for Tobacco Control, Victoria.

7. Welte, R., König, H. and Leidl, R. (2000) The costs of health damage and productivity losses attributable to cigarette smoking in Germany. *Euro J Public Health*, **10**, 31–38.

8. Nooyens, A.C., van Gelder, B.M. and Verschuren, W.M. (2008) Smoking and cognitive decline among middle-aged men and women: the Doetinchem Cohort Study. *Am J Public Health*, **98** (12), 2244–2250.

9. Grabowska, P., Targowski, T., Rozynska, R. *et al.* (2005) Alexithymia and depression: relationship to cigarette smoking, nicotine dependence and motivation to quit smoking. *Przegl Lek*, **62** (10), 1004–1006.

10. Kerr, M. (2008) Few Physicians Fully Aware of Tobacco Dependence Treatment Guidelines. *Reuters Health Information*. [Online] available: http://nodope.co.za/index.php?option=com_content&view=article&id=29:few-physicians-fully-aware-of-tobacco-dependence-treatment-guidelines&catid=4:international-media&Itemid=25(2010/3/5).

Index

Note: page numbers in *italics* refer to figures, those in **bold** refer to tables

Substance Abuse Disorders: Evidence and Experience, First Edition. Edited by Hamid Ghodse, Helen Herrman, Mario Maj and Norman Sartorius.
© 2011 John Wiley & Sons, Ltd. Published 2011 by John Wiley & Sons, Ltd.

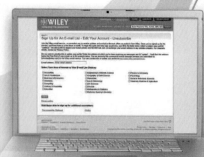